Praise for *Teaching Power Yoga for Sports*

"I feel that I get the most benefits from Gwen Lawrence's yoga as part of my recovery routine, with her restorative postgame yoga. I find my soreness reduced, and I gain flexibility and feel ready for the week ahead!"

Kerry Wynn, Defensive End for the New York Giants

"I have been doing yoga with Gwen Lawrence for the past six years, and I find it to be a necessary part of my training routine. Gwen takes her time to guide each of us through every one of the positions, thoroughly explaining the importance of each stretch. Gwen is personable and knowledgeable, and she brings a gentle spirit to each class."

Mark Herzlich, Linebacker for the New York Giants

"Since coming to the New York Giants, working with Gwen Lawrence has been a great addition for me in my training and recovery routines. Her yoga sessions allow me to set aside time to focus solely on improving flexibility, strength, and power-through movements designed perfectly for football players."

Ryan Nassib, Former Quarterback for the New York Giants

"The fact that Gwen knows the sports—she takes the time to get to know the different positions and the different needs of the specific athlete she's working with. And I think that's what sets Power Yoga for Sports apart. . . . It's just one of those things that I gotta incorporate into my life every day."

Amani Toomer, Former Wide Receiver for the New York Giants

"I have worked with Gwen for only a couple of months and I have recognized tremendous gains in my flexibility, core strength, and balance, which are essential to staying healthy and explosive. I consider myself lucky to have learned as much from Gwen as I have in such a short time."

Kevin Boothe, Former Offensive Guard for the New York Giants

"She conducts class with tremendous professionalism and makes it challenging to the athletes. She relates very well to our players and commands their respect. I believe that Gwen is an outstanding yoga coach who provides a valuable experience for those athletes who consistently participate in her class."

Jerry Palmieri, Former Strength and Conditioning Coach for the New York Giants

"I'm a triathlete. The swimming part was the hardest for me because my technique wasn't very good. Then I met Gwen Lawrence and her innovative method, Power Yoga for Sports. Since then, I've gotten more flexibility and I improved my swimming technique, becoming faster and breaking my personal records! Thank you very much, Gwen."

Gabriel Ruivo, Personal Trainer and Triathlete

TEACHING
POWER YOGA
FOR SPORTS

GWEN LAWRENCE

Library of Congress Cataloging-in-Publication Data

Names: Lawrence, Gwen, author.
Title: Teaching power yoga for sports / Gwen Lawrence.
Description: Champaign, IL : Human Kinetics, [2019] | Includes
   bibliographical references.
Identifiers: LCCN 2018028445 (print) | LCCN 2018036357 (ebook) | ISBN
   9781492572749 (ebook) | ISBN 9781492563068 (print)
Subjects: LCSH: Hatha yoga. | Athletes--Training of.
Classification: LCC RA781.7 (ebook) | LCC RA781.7 .L38 2019 (print) | DDC
   613.7/046--dc23
LC record available at https://lccn.loc.gov/2018028445

ISBN: 978-1-4925-6306-8 (print)

Permission notices for material reprinted in this book from other sources can be found on pages xvii-xviii.

The web addresses cited in this text were current as of August 2018, unless otherwise noted.

Senior Acquisitions Editor: Michelle Maloney; **Developmental Editor:** Laura Pulliam; **Senior Managing Editor:** Amy Stahl; **Copyeditor:** Kevin Campbell; **Proofreader:** Laura Stoffel; **Graphic Designer:** Sean Roosevelt; **Cover Designer:** Keri Evans; **Cover Design Associate:** Susan Rothermel Allen; **Photograph (cover):** Kevin Ferguson/© Human Kinetics (left) and MIGUEL RIOPA/AFP/Getty Images (right); **Photographs (interior):** Kevin Ferguson/© Human Kinetics, unless otherwise noted; **Visual Production Assistant:** Joyce Brumfield; **Photo Production Manager:** Jason Allen; **Photo Asset Manager:** Laura Fitch; **Senior Art Manager:** Kelly Hendren; **Illustrations:** © Human Kinetics; **Printer:** Premier Print Group

We thank the The Duncans at The Centre in Purchase, New York, for assistance in providing the location for the photo shoot for this book.

Printed in the United States of America   10 9 8 7 6 5 4 3 2 1

Human Kinetics
P.O. Box 5076
Champaign, IL 61825-5076
Website: www.HumanKinetics.com

In the United States, email info@hkusa.com or call 800-747-4457.
In Canada, email info@hkcanada.com.
In the United Kingdom/Europe, email hk@hkeurope.com.

For information about Human Kinetics' coverage in other areas of the world,
please visit our website: **www.HumanKinetics.com**

E7267

I have had many great people influence, support, and inspire me along my career journey, from Tom Coughlin to Frank Gifford, but the single biggest motivator for my creativity and inventiveness is hands-down my soulmate and best friend, my husband Teddy.

It is through his journey through college sports and professional athletics that I was privileged to be his ride-or-die—to share in the successes, listen to complaints, and confront injuries, ups, downs, and diagnoses—an experience that helped me to develop my company, which now serves people in 18 countries and 28 states. It is my goal to reach as many athletes and coaches as I can to help them to be proactive to health, not reactive to injury. My husband was pivotal in creating my love of sports and helping me to understand that I can serve best by saving athletes the pain of injury, the loss of playing time, and potentially the loss of their positions. I thank him for his sacrifices to make me happy, whole, and the best woman I can be. He blessed me with three great, athletic sons who are completely on board in this journey that has become a family philosophy.

To my sons, Brooks, Tyrus, and Cal, who have always told me they love and support me, and how proud they are of me; they will never know how much I appreciate those words. As a modern mom you can often be conflicted about working and not staying home, but their clear, authentic, pure love makes it clear to me that I have made the best decisions for our family and have been a role model they can be honored to call Mom. It is through their love that I never doubted I could do anything I set out to do.

CONTENTS

POSE FINDER

(continued)

Pose Finder *(continued)*

FOREWORD

I cannot claim to be a great student of the principles of yoga or Power Yoga for Sports. However, I have seen the benefits of yoga and athletic fitness experienced by my athletes. Gwen Lawrence led my players in yoga exercises for 12 years. She is a highly motivated individual who is able to apply the principles of Power Yoga for Sports to meet the specific needs of athletes. Yoga provides exercises that work around each person's physical limitations, which is beneficial because many professional athletes have a history of injuries that limit them from moving their bodies in a full range. Whether it's an arthritic knee or an ailing back, it is important to be able to manipulate an exercise so that the individual can benefit from the movement and to see imbalances and help correct the imbalances before they inevitably lead to injury.

I have seen Gwen's routines benefit my athletes in a number of ways. My players' flexibility and joint range of motion were increased; because of these gains, they were able to demonstrate better positional skills on the football field and improved strength training techniques in the weight room. For anyone who is familiar with yoga or Power Yoga for Sports, this would not be much of a surprise since increased flexibility is a primary foundation of the exercises. These exercise routines assisted my athletes in recovering from games as well as multiple practices. The exercises and controlled breathing promoted a revitalization of the body and mind that helped them get ready for the next game in a shorter amount of time.

In 2015 I gave Gwen the task of teaching our coaches and players about mindfulness. After the third session, I asked her to give us examples of how mindfulness could be applied to everyday life. For the next hour and a half, we heard story after story of our troops returning to the United States in extremely stressed and unproductive states of mind as well as stories of law enforcement officers, firefighters, and other emergency first responders all transformed to stress-free and productive states of mind through months of mindfulness and yoga. Hearing those stories only increased my understanding of how these techniques would help my athletes succeed. I am very glad to have learned the techniques and secrets of Power Yoga for Sports.

As both a player and a coach, I have always believed, and still do, that a hard-working, disciplined, and focused approach has led to the successes I've experienced on the football field and in life. What I've also been able to do is to continue to grow as a coach. When I arrived in New York, Gwen was already a part of the Giants training staff. Yoga was very new to me, so I decided to have a meeting and find out what it was all about. From that first meeting until the time I left the Giants, I knew this training could help my players, my coaches, and me. Each year we would discuss how to best implement the training, and each year we added more and more to our training schedule. Seeing how my players and coaches responded to the teaching and training made me realize the unique opportunity we had that very few, if any, of the other teams had. There was clearly a direct correlation between players' training on a regular basis and remaining healthy during the season. The 2007 offensive line was a key factor in our Super Bowl run that year, and the majority of them trained during the team sessions and additionally on their own time that season. In all, I realized then and now how important Gwen was as a part of our training staff. I look back now and realize I was thinking outside the box to continue to have this as a part of our training because yoga was perceived so differently when I first started. I came to believe in this program, and that is why she remained with the New York Giants. She brought to us a unique way of helping ourselves; we were able to keep our best players on the field and playing at their best for an entire season. I owe a tremendous amount of gratitude to Gwen for her years of helping our players perform at their best. It is her dream to create curriculum changes and add Power Yoga for Sports as a major in the academics areas of study; this book is the first step.

This book is for everyone, including our athletes; businesspeople; active duty military personnel; and tactical professionals such as our police officers, firefighters, and emergency responders who have experienced both physical and mental stress and want an edge to go to the next level of health and fitness. I believe that the routines in this book will assist these men and women in their quest to return to a healthy lifestyle. Finally, with this book, everybody will have access to the techniques previously learned only by the trainees Gwen has taught in 18 countries and 28 states to date.

Tom Coughlin, Former Head Coach of the New York Giants

PREFACE

I want you to be excited about this learning journey. But I also want you to understand the depth and layers of my path that make me uniquely qualified to bring you this trademarked, time-tested system of training, Power Yoga for Sports.

My journey has been long, and it seems that it developed over the course of a well-defined series of events that I followed. I have been a dancer since the age of three and a working fitness professional since the age of 18. From the age of 15, I spent countless hours watching my now-husband play baseball and be actively pursued by the professional scouts of Major League Baseball. Through that experience, I learned how to interact with coaches, trainers, and, most importantly, the scouts. I sat with them for two doubleheaders every weekend; I asked questions, and we shared arm speed times on our stopwatches. I learned firsthand what a prospect needed to do in order to make it to the next level. Looking back, this was valuable both to my education and to the development of my unique system.

After majoring in art and dance in college, I immediately went back to school to become a licensed massage therapist. I worked with physical therapists, doctors, and chiropractors, picking their brains and learning as much as I could. Eventually I became a massage therapist to the stars. This experience gave me a deep knowledge of how the body works and recovers from injury, how to train to maximize performance, and how to work successfully with elite, high-profile athletes and celebrities.

On the first day of labs in massage school, the professor asked each of us why we wanted to learn these skills and what our dreams were. As we went around the room, students shared stories of noble goals: to work with the sick, to rehabilitate the disabled, and so on. When it was my turn, I proudly stated, "I want to work with professional athletes!" The room erupted with laughter, and I suppose that was a blessing because it ignited a fire in me to accomplish that dream. I mention this because whether you picked up this book to help your own Little Leaguer or whether you aspire to follow in my path, know that you can do it, no matter what anybody else says.

Over the years, I've learned the skills to make it in my business today: to effectively connect with the coaches and trainers on the professional, college, high school, and Little League teams I train. I constantly consult with them on the needs of their athletes, which may include dealing with past or present injuries, and I work with them on how to effectively improve their already grueling training regimens. Power Yoga for Sports practitioners exist to enhance the effectiveness of an athlete's arduous training routines, not to reinvent the wheel.

As a yoga teacher, you should be inspired to study and understand anatomy for the rest of your life. Once when I was teaching a professional football team, I talked about stretching the hamstrings and, believe it or not, a player asked me, "Where is my hamstring?" I cannot stress enough that it is your job to be great and to continue to study and learn for the rest of your life so you can share your vast knowledge and gain the trust of the best in their field. It is not unusual for me to see Coach Tom Coughlin, previously of the New York Giants, and to have him shake my hand and ask me how "my team" (the Giants) is doing! Professional coaches even email me for advice about their own training needs. This is how valuable and trusted you can become.

It is my passion to know how the games are played, the duties of each position, and the qualities the coaches look for from power players at each position. This helps me to create Power Yoga for Sports programs to maximize results while minimizing time, honing in on specific needs and leaving out the fluff! Athletes are already burdened with crammed schedules. We need to be concise and efficient in how we use the available time to help them achieve the best results. Players tell me every day how Power Yoga for Sports is the hardest workout they have ever done and how they wish they had started it as youth athletes. They immediately understand how this system is relevant to their game and position and how it can help to reduce injuries and ultimately lengthen their careers.

Finally, I have a unique ability to read bodies; I can analyze my athletes for imbalances and asymmetry that inevitably (if unaddressed) will lead to injury. I consider it a curse and a gift. It is a curse because I can never seem to turn it off, and it is a gift because what I see has great potential to prevent injuries before they happen. In this book, you too will learn to see those imbalances.

The first time I saw Alex Rodriguez, I instantly noticed that his torso was torqued to the right. I tested his eye dominance and found that he was right-eye dominant, so I knew he was at a great disadvantage in properly tracking the pitches he faced. I had to bring him back to center and open his neck rotation as much as possible to give him the best view of his pitcher with the least amount of effort. People around the world send photos to me to analyze their posture, and I'm able to help relieve some of their nagging, mysterious pains. Alignment issues lead to musculoskeletal disorders and injuries, resulting in lost playing time and ending an athlete's career. Athletes' efforts to enhance performance will be wasted if they don't start by first preventing injuries. Let's become proactive to health rather than reactive to injury.

I am excited to present this book to all yoga teachers, coaches, athletes, and trainers who want to be the best they can be and who understand the importance of my life's work and are interested in saving athletes the pain of injury, the loss of playing time, the possible loss of position, and even the loss of their ability to earn money for a longer period of time. This book eliminates your need to reinvent the wheel. I am sharing my trade secrets to live the amazing life and career I do, to understand the needs of athletes, and to become indispensable in their lives. Power Yoga for Sports trainees understand that good is the enemy of great. Now is the time to commit to great.

Power Yoga for Sports Code of Ethics

I demand that any practitioner of my system proudly adhere to a code of ethics to protect yourself, the integrity of Power Yoga for Sports, and the athletes you work with. This code of conduct is a summary of acceptable ethical and professional behavior by which all Power Yoga for Sports-certified teachers and practitioners willingly agree to conduct the teaching and business of yoga and to protect the athletes they work with. One of the most important aspects of Power Yoga for Sports is protecting the practice's reputation in professional athletics because this helps in developing long-term relationships based on trust.

The Power Yoga for Sports Code of Ethics is as follows:

1. You must leave being a fan at home. Being a professional means treating clients at the elite level as you would any other clients.

2. Never ask for autographs from your athlete clients.

3. Never ask an athlete or coach for favors.

4. Never ask for tickets; only accept them when they are offered.

5. Respect the rights, dignity, and privacy of all students, players, and coaches.

6. Avoid words and actions that constitute sexual harassment or could be deemed offensive.

7. Never express your personal problems to your athletes; they should feel you are there to enhance their lives.

8. Adhere to all local government and national laws that pertain to yoga teaching, hands-on adjusting, and business.

9. Uphold the integrity of the vocation by conducting yourself in a professional and conscientious manner.

10. Acknowledge the limitations of your skills and scope of practice and, where appropriate, refer students to alternative instruction, advice, treatment, or direction.

11. Create and maintain a safe, clean, and comfortable environment for the practice of yoga.

12. Actively encourage diversity by respecting all students regardless of age, physical limitations, race, creed, gender, ethnicity, religious affiliations, or sexual orientation.

13. Never take pictures during a session without permission, except pictures that will be seen only by the client (for demonstration use or to improve the client's understanding of his issues). Never post pictures of your athletes, take selfies when teaching, or take any other photo that could compromise your job (and violate NCAA standards, when applicable).

14. Maintain the privacy of all athletes' injuries, limitations, and problems at all times.

ACKNOWLEDGMENTS

Aside from my family, I would love to thank the New York Giants for the privilege of being their yoga coach for 18 seasons, the New York Knicks for their years of support, and the New York Red Bulls, the New York City Football Club, the New York Rangers, the New York Mets, and the New York Yankees for trusting me with the well-being of their players. My thanks also go to all the professional trainers who unendingly let me pick their brains.

I would love to thank all my pros who looked to me to help them through thick and thin, every day encouraging me by their words and inspiring me to forge on in a male-driven world because I was making a change.

Thank you to the people in my community who have never wavered in their support for me, including Tom Coughlin, Bob Fletcher, Bill Swerfager, Rod Mergardt, Rhonda Clements, Bryce Kuhlman, Michael Watkins, Nevine Michaan, and Nick Benas.

Thanks to my outstandingly supportive publishing group at Human Kinetics, especially Michelle Maloney, Laura Pulliam, and Amy Stahl.

Finally, I would like to thank my top Power Yoga for Sports team and trainees, including Jim Berti, Ali Caulfield, Kim Polivko, and Judy Dimon who understand and trust the dream and the process I have created.

CREDITS

The following credit lines are for sport position photos that appear alongside each corresponding yoga pose photo on the following pages:

Football

Page 203, squat: Michael Chang/Getty Images
Page 204, goddess: John Rivera/Icon Sportswire via Getty Images
Page 204, extended side angle: Scott W. Grau/Icon Sportswire via Getty Images
Page 204, straddle forward bend twist: Zach Bolinger/Icon Sportswire via Getty Images
Page 205, face-down shoulder stretch: David Rosenblum/Icon Sportswire via Getty Images
Page 205, lunge twist: Todd Kirkland/Icon Sportswire via Getty Images
Page 205, crescent lunge: David Rosenblum/Icon Sportswire via Getty Images
Page 206, half hero's: Carlos Herrera/Icon Sportswire via Getty Images
Page 206, warrior 2: Scott W. Grau/Icon Sportswire via Getty Images
Page 206, revolving triangle: Harry How/Getty Images
Page 207, tree pose: Patrick Gorski/Icon Sportswire via Getty Images
Page 207, low push-up: Peter G. Aiken/Getty Images
Page 207, chair: Elsa/Getty Images
Page 208, warrior 3: Jonathan Daniel/Getty Images
Page 208, opposite-arm opposite leg: David Allio/Icon Sportswire via Getty Images

Soccer

Page 214, lunge twist: Tony Quinn/Getty Images
Page 215, wheel of life: Tony Quinn/Icon Sportswire via Getty Images
Page 215, reclining big toe pose: Brian A. Westerholt/Getty Images
Page 215, warrior 3: Jamie Schwaberow/NCAA Photos via Getty Images
Page 216, revolving triangle: Rich Graessle/Icon Sportswire via Getty Images
Page 216, hero's pose: Joel Auerbach/Getty Images
Page 216, low push-up: Doug Stroud/NCAA Photos/NCAA Photos via Getty Images
Page 217, face-down shoulder stretch: Francesco Pecoraro/Getty Images
Page 217, wrist openers: Harry How/Getty Images

Basketball

Page 220, locust: Jonathan Daniel/Getty Images
Page 220, crescent lunge: Justin Tafoya/NCAA Photos via Getty Images
Page 221, straddle forward bend: Robert Johnson/Icon Sportswire via Getty Images
Page 221, extended side angle: Bob Levey/Getty Images
Page 221, standing crescent: Christian Petersen/Getty Images
Page 222, wheel of life: Tom Pennington/Getty Images
Page 222, revolving triangle: Tony Quinn/Icon Sportswire via Getty Images

Baseball and Softball

Page 225, three-legged dog: David Ellis/Getty Images
Page 226, warrior 1: Paul Bereswill/Getty Images
Page 226, warrior 2: Jonathan Daniel/Getty Images
Page 226, warrior 3: Merle Laswell/Icon Sportswire via Getty Images
Page 229, squat: Mark Cunningham/MLB Photos via Getty Images
Page 230, camel: Victor Decolongon/Getty Images
Page 230, warrior 2: Paul Bereswill/Getty Images
Page 233, extended-leg side plank: Mike McGinnis/Getty Images
Page 233, split: Ron Vesely/MLB Photos via Getty Images
Page 234, crescent lunge: Brian D. Kersey/Getty Images
Page 234, wheel of life: Sarah Sachs/Arizona Diamondbacks/Getty Images
Page 234, locust: Mark Cunningham/MLB Photos via Getty Images
Page 235, squat: Christian Peterson/Staff/Getty Images
Page 235, warrior 2: Joe Robbins/Getty Images
Page 235, chair: John McCoy/Getty Images
Page 236, lunge twist: Bob Levey/Getty Images

Hockey

Page 239, frog: Marc Sanchez/Icon Sportswire via Getty Images
Page 239, lunge twist: Dean Mouhtaropoulos/Getty Images
Page 239, eagle pose: Mike Ehrmann/Getty Images
Page 240, boat pose: Brett Holmes/Icon Sportswire via Getty Images
Page 240, half side squat: Michael Martin/NHLI via Getty Images

Why Athletes Need Power Yoga for Sports

Teaching yoga to athletes is a great responsibility. The needs of an athlete differ from those of a yogi. Athletes typically do not have the flexibility a typical yoga practitioner has; their sport sets them up for imbalanced work on the field of play, which sets them up for imbalances that can lead to injury. A typical yogi has unlimited time to devote to the practice of yoga, and the goals of a typical yoga class are inner peace, increased sensitivity to stress, and improved flexibility through discipline. While these are all important to athletes, you must be sensitive to the specific training demands of competitive sports. Athletes must invest time in activities that will produce peak performance, and their goals may also include longevity in their sport and injury prevention.

Teachers of Power Yoga for Sports must address their athletes' training demands, the most probable potential injuries, tasks on the field of play, body type, and common movements when they develop classes geared toward their athletes' goals. Teachers must often develop routines on the fly that align with daily injury assessments and complaints. Typical yoga teachers teach classes in line with what they are feeling, but those who teach Power Yoga for Sports (PYFS) have to feel the needs of others. Therefore, as you teach PYFS, you need to stay up to date on all of your athletes' injuries and with the latest research on sport sciences.

In this book, we focus on balance within the athlete's body and its importance in injury prevention. You will learn functional strength moves that will humble the most muscular athletes and moves that will help them to improve their flexibility and range of motion. You will also learn to cultivate mental toughness, which involves training the athlete to stay in difficult poses using mindfulness and breathing techniques to go the distance. And, finally, you will learn to teach athletes to focus so that, instead of just robotically performing yoga moves, they focus their minds and detach from distractions both on and off the field. Power Yoga for Sports can take athletes to the next level.

Why should I try yoga?

You should be open to trying whatever it takes to make the best health decisions for your life, and you should create a schedule of working out and training your body. When exploring yoga for the first time, commit to doing 5 to 10 sessions before you decide whether you like it or not. This will give your body a chance to experience change. Try different styles of yoga and teachers because they all bring their own emphasis to the practice.

SIX FACETS OF THE POWER YOGA FOR SPORTS SYSTEM

Over the course of creating Power Yoga for Sports, I boiled its effectiveness down to six components: balance, strength, flexibility, mental toughness, focus, and breathing. Each component has been carefully thought out and is pivotal to athletes' ability to reach their potential. In baseball, a great player is called a five-tool athlete; in Power Yoga for Sports, I teach the six tools. No single tool can create excellence on its own; they build on each other, and at different times athletes must focus on different areas to improve. Yoga is not just all about stretching.

Balance

Balance can be understood in two ways: in terms of dynamic equilibrium and in terms of the body's symmetry and alignment. Following the Power Yoga for Sports program and following routines laid out in this book, an athlete will develop better proprioceptive, physical balance. You can simply think of this form of balance as your ability to maintain your base of support. In physics and in art, a line of gravity is used to define balance. Improving your balance involves improving your ability to keep your line of gravity over your base of support by shifting an imaginary plumb line from your chin (if standing) directly over the base of support.

Balance in relation to Power Yoga for Sports is the ability to move your body accurately and efficiently while playing your sport. It also involves being agile enough to change position on a dime without falling or losing your bearings.

Balance and Your Body's Sensory Systems

Maintaining balance requires the coordination of three different sensory systems in your body: the vestibular system, the somatosensory system, and the visual system.

Vestibular System

The vestibular system consists of the sense organs in your head, specifically your ears, which regulate your equilibrium and give your brain directional information about head position and change of position and about your movement in relation to what is moving around you. The best thing you can do to improve this system is go barefoot as much as possible, as is done in yoga. A common practice in yoga to improve balance is to use *drishti*, or a point of focus, in which you rest your gaze on a chosen point during yoga practice and movement. Focusing on a fixed point improves your concentration in a game situation because it's easy to become distracted when your eyes are moving around to take in your surroundings or to monitor the actions of your opponent. Drishtis also help in establishing proper alignment.

Learn the Game

Learning the game is a mainstay of making a difference as a PYFS teacher. Most athletes do not have a lot of downtime; in the time they do have, it may be hard for them to commit to a basic yoga class.

PYFS offers much more than flexibility training, and it offers it in usable lengths of time that are easy for an athlete to commit to. We boil down the 5,000-year-old art of yoga not only to exactly what athletes need but, more importantly, to what each person needs for a particular position in a particular sport. This is part of our commitment to making the best use of an athlete's time. PYFS teachers are not trying to make athletes into yogis—in fact, just the opposite. We are learning about the athlete's world, the ins and outs, the good and the bad. Then we can create classes that have a substantial impact and require the least amount of time. There is no reason to train an athlete to go through a vinyasa with the ultimate goal of being able to do a split if that is not relevant to her sport or position, and it likely won't be unless she happens to play first base in baseball or softball. We train for the purpose of improving the game play and the player, and that purpose must be imprinted on the mind of the PYFS teacher.

So how do you know what your players' needs are? Learn the game. First, watch games live or on TV. Make a conscious effort to watch not as a fan but as someone looking for

- common movements on the field,
- how athletes move,
- the duties of each position,
- how the movements of each position differ,
- the big movements the body makes,
- the subtle movements,
- the difference between offensive and defensive play, and
- the most common injuries of this sport and how you could teach movements that better prepare the athlete and help to prevent such injuries.

Second, work closely with coaches, trainers, and doctors to learn about the athletes, their training, and their performance. Ask questions such as these:

- What is going on with the team?
- What injuries currently plague the players?
- What common complaints do they hear from players?
- Why do they think these injuries are happening?
- Where are they in the training cycle?
- How can you serve the team more effectively?
- Are they fatigued from travel?
- What are their plans and expectations of you for a session?
- Would recovery yoga poses be beneficial?

A PYFS teacher enhances the athletes' already grueling training regimen; you are there to check in with the coaches and trainers daily, weekly, or monthly. When they know they can trust you, you will be more effective, and they will understand your intentions and your value to their team.

Somatosensory System

The somatosensory system comprises nerves called proprioceptors in your muscles and joints along with the pressure and vibration sensors in your skin and joints. These receptors are sensitive to stretch or pressure in the surrounding tissues. With any movement of the legs, arms, hands, or other body parts, sensory receptors react by carrying impulses to the brain to maintain balance and prevent a fall. You can observe this in yoga. Have you ever tried a warrior 3 pose and felt the constant and subtle actions of all the small muscles in the foot and ankle as you held your position? Try right now to simply stand in a quiet room in mountain pose with your arms down by your sides and your eyes closed. Notice the vacillations in your feet; that is the somatosensory system at work. To improve it, regularly practice your yoga, giving special attention to balance poses on one foot. (See standing poses in chapter 5.)

Visual System

The visual system relies on your eyes to figure out where your head and body are in space and your location in space relative to other objects or players on the field. To help improve your vision, you should limit the time you are exposed to blue light interference from sources such as a TV or computer. Avoid eyestrain as much as possible; for example, read in proper lighting, and allow your eyes to rest for six to eight hours a night. You need to have good eyes, good ears, and healthy muscles and joints to be properly balanced. One practice for improving the visual system is to vigorously rub your hands together until they become hot, then lean your elbows on a table and cup your hands over your eyes. In my experience, this practice allows the healing heat to penetrate the eyes, then the optic nerve, and eventually the brain to relax and release tension.

When you take care of your vestibular, somatosensory, and visual systems and follow the Power Yoga for Sports routines, your movements become smoother and easier. This will help you to become more effective at your sport. Working on balance will certainly help you on the field. Your body must be able to support compromising positions that your sport puts you in. If you have better balance, acrobatic plays will be commonplace for you; your performance will improve, and you will have less risk of injury.

Balance and Symmetry of Your Body

The second part of balance, and the one that is more important to the Power Yoga for Sports system, is symmetry of the muscles and the alignment of the body, taking into consideration all external bumps and torques. Most sports are one-side dominant: You throw from one side, your kick strength is stronger on one side than the other, your serve is one-side dominant, and so on. The sport that may be the most innately symmetrical is swimming. Each of us has a dominant side, so you can never be perfectly symmetrical. However, with careful mindfulness and body awareness, you can become immediately aware when you are too far off balance. Power Yoga for Sports can teach you to understand asymmetries and address them before they become imbalances. Be proactive in preventing injury, rather than reactive in recovering from injury.

Think of it this way: Symmetry problems are like caring for a car. If you never rotate the tires on your car, you may end up driving on a misaligned car with a balding tire that eventually ruptures. Or think of a monster truck—those absurdly large trucks with extremely large tires to match! Now imagine replacing the passenger-side tires of that monster truck with tires meant for a small two-door sedan. Sounds ridiculous, right? It is the same with your body. Unfortunately, we are often more careful with our cars than we are with our own bodies. Imagine the damage the monster truck would sustain to the undercarriage and how terribly it would drive. I see people walking around every day with absurd misalignments in their bodies, and it pains me.

To help athletes to address their imbalances, you must understand the planes of the body and their relation to movements. Figure 1.1 shows the three planes the body moves in—sagittal, frontal, and transverse. If you take into consideration imbalances, tight spots, knots, and excess scar tissue in conjunction with these planes of motion, I believe it will be easier for you to understand why asymmetries can cause the body to move awkwardly and, even worse, to incur tears and strains.

Take a look at the sagittal plane, which slices the body in half down the middle to create a perfect right side and left side. This is the plane in which the body performs flexion and extension, such as bending forward or extending into a backbend, and the even more detailed flexion of the knees and front of the shoulders. When you look at the body and visualize the sagittal plane, you can better identify left- and right-side imbalances that are out of the ordinary. You can also visualize all the movements done on the sagittal plane that must not cross the cut wall—for example, kicking the leg straight out in front, not across the body because that movement would break through the wall.

Next, recognize the frontal plane. The frontal plane divides the body into a front and a back. This is not symmetrical like the sagittal plane (the front of your body looks different than the back of your body), but you can spot asymmetry here when you see people who are too far forward on their feet and overload the front or too far back and overload the back. You can also identify

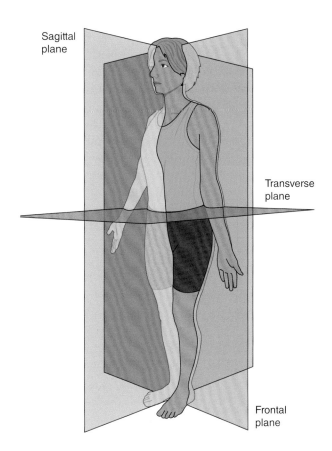

Figure 1.1 Three planes of motion: sagittal, transverse, and frontal.

imbalance here if you see someone with poor posture and a hunched back. The frontal plane is where the movement of abduction (moving away from the midline) happens—for example, performing a side kick or raising your arm straight out to the side. The body also adducts (moves back toward the midline of the body) in this plane; squeezing your inner thighs together or bringing your arms toward the body are examples of adduction.

Finally, we analyze the transverse plane. This plane separates the body at the waist to form a top body from the waist up and a bottom body from the waist down. This plane is an important one for athletes because the transverse plane is where rotation of the spine occurs. Every sport requires athletes to twist their bodies to generate torque or to create a large field of vision. If you do simple seated twists, you can immediately notice which side you twist toward more easily and which side presents more resistance.

Movement in the transverse plane can seriously affect your level of play. For example, imagine you are running toward the goal in a soccer game while dribbling the ball in front of you. You move effortlessly to the left, but you are more limited in your ability to rotate to the right. In this case, you might lose some field of vision on the tight side, and opponents might sneak up on you more easily from this side and steal the ball. Opposing coaches can pick this out on films of your performance, and they can target your weak right-side skills as vulnerability. Power Yoga for Sports can help you to address these asymmetries and make corrections so you can excel. This idea comes back into play when we discuss the importance of eye dominance and symmetry of the eyes in chapter 2.

Strength

In Power Yoga for Sports, we address how to build functional strength by practicing well-designed strength-building poses. A common misconception of yoga is that it does not build strength. Nothing could be further from the truth when you practice forms of yoga such as PYFS. Try holding a forearm plank for two minutes and let me know if your shoulders are not screaming and your core is not challenged to the fullest while the sweat drips down your face. Enough said!

Functional strength training should be thought of in terms of a movement range. As athletes and lay people, we perform a wide range of movements like jogging, running, jumping, lifting, pushing, pulling, bending, twisting, turning, standing, starting, and stopping, all related to our body planes and axis of movement. To improve functional strength, we must train to improve the relationship between the nervous and muscular systems. The goal of functional training is to make improvements in one movement enhance the performance of another movement.

Many athletes train on machines that do not accommodate movement beyond the movements typical of a sport. A movement that isolates a joint and muscle—such as a leg extension's impact on the quadriceps—is simply training that muscle. In fact, machines often force movements onto people who may not be able to do them well because of compression on the joints or because of a machine's one-size-fits-all design. Athletes can still use machines and free weights, as long as they stay mindful of how they feel, thinking about their position in their sport and the common movements they are called on to perform. Power Yoga for Sports concepts will help you to get to the next level, but you should remain loyal to your strength and conditioning coaches. You should perform strength training appropriate to the training cycle and cardiovascular training appropriate to the sport, in addition to PYFS.

Flexibility

One of the cornerstones of Power Yoga for Sports is our treasured equation:

$$Strength + Flexibility = Power$$

Over the years, I've heard excuses from professional athletes to the tune of, "I cannot get too flexible; I will lose strength," or "If I get too flexible, I will pull a muscle."

Remember we are talking about equalizing strength with flexibility and trusting in the knowledge of strength and conditioning specialists and yoga coaches to do that. Yes, if athletes lack muscle tone and are very flexible, they may not achieve significant power gains, but serious athletes don't need to worry about that. On the other side of the coin, athletes who are strong but not flexible could be increasing their risk of injury. Consistent with our emphasis on symmetry, I believe that an athlete should try to be equally strong and flexible.

Let's look at this in terms that are easy to understand, with a bow and arrow analogy. Imagine a bow that is so strong that it will not break, and the bowstring is so tight you cannot pull it all the way back. You release the arrow, and what happens? It probably hits the ground short of the target or reaches the target without much impact. Now let's think of a bow that is so strong it will not break, and the bowstring is so supple you can pull the arrow all the way back to your ear. When you release the arrow, what happens? Power, power, power and, with practice, a bull's-eye! Another very clear demonstration of the balance between strength and flexibility is in the nearly poetic performance of elite gymnasts. One would never say flexibility has inhibited them; on the contrary, their perfect balance propels them into flips and twists second to none.

Flexibility is the missing piece. My athletes spend countless hours on strength and lifting because it looks so good, and the first thing to be nixed from their training is flexibility work. They ignore it because it can be painful and can take a long time to see results and also because their egos take a hit when they are not good at something. The routines in this book help athletes to learn long, deep holds to increase flexibility and to actually love them.

Yoga is famous for improving flexibility. With PYFS, we do flexibility training with long, deep holds to better increase flexibility and to create outstanding regenerating, restorative classes.

The Best Rehabilitation Technique Is Prevention

Make the best use of an athlete's time. Whether you are teaching professionals or Little Leaguers, the training you provide might be set aside if training time is limited. Athletes may resort to the lame group stretches we have seen them warming up with for decades. These typically do not enhance flexibility. They may simply reveal to athletes where they are tight; if they then skip hurriedly through the stretches or even cheat at them, what is the point?

Yoga can and should be an important part of every athlete's training. Some athletes find that yoga works best for them when done pregame or prepractice, while others prefer it after a game or practice. We are all different, from skeletal structure to muscle to life experiences; encourage athletes to find what works best for them so they can reap the best and quickest rewards.

The idea is to slow down and open the body through passive stretching, breathing, and time. Athletes perform a limited number of poses in a typical 30- to 60-minute session, holding poses for anywhere from 3 to 15 minutes as they sink deeper into each pose. During these long holds, the muscles relax much more than they do during the typical two-second stretches on the field that we all learned in middle school. Athletes feel more confident than they might with other types of yoga because we use props such as bolsters, blankets, and blocks to support the body. Our slower-paced classes are usually a welcome respite in their training, and they are often performed on recovery or rest days. The sessions can result in decreased muscle soreness, decreased risk of injury, greater range of motion in the joints, and improved performance.

A common misconception when stretching is that you should go hard until it hurts. This causes the body to resist and the mind to start negotiating an out, resulting in no improvements. That type of hard-core flexibility training may be appropriate for very advanced athletes like gymnasts or dancers, but even they do not make that the majority of their flexibility training. The key to increasing flexibility is for an athlete to

- identify the spots that are the tightest and that impede sport performance,
- perform flexibility work consistently to preserve gains and continue to improve,
- listen to the body while holding poses and adjust if needed, and
- breathe.

Athletes who follow these guidelines are more apt to stick to the plan and see greater improvements. The idea is to get deeper into the poses than the last time you performed them. Factors that may impede progress include inappropriate poses performed after games, intense soreness, anxiety and stress, or adverse temperatures. Encourage athletes to keep the following in mind in order to optimize results:

- Perform poses in a warm, not hot, room. I prefer to warm up the body to stretch from the inside out, not the outside in. Athletes who feel great in a hot room may push too far too quickly and risk negating their gains with an injury.
- Include a recovery or rest day in the training cycle.
- Perform poses after the body is warmed by activity such as aerobic training or a warm-up plan. (We'll talk more about warming up in chapter 4; simple plans for flexibility, along with full regeneration routines, are provided in chapter 10.)
- Breathe in and out of the nose and deep into the abdomen while stretching.

No lesson on flexibility would be complete without mentioning compression and tension and the difference between the two. In simple terms, tension is the sensation of tissues being pulled;

this is what we typically feel when we ease into our stretches. This could be described as itchy, deep, warm, or hurting so good. When you feel tension in a muscle, you know that eventually it will improve and flexibility will increase. Compression is the sensation of tissues being pinched or pressed and is painful in a different way. If we feel compression, we have to recognize that this is the ultimate limit to our range of motion, and there is no pushing through it. It is truly the inability to go deeper due to the shape of the bones and joints, and it is unchangeable.

Downward dog is a great way to demonstrate the difference between compression and tension. While you tune into your shoulder joint, notice that it is shallow and vulnerable and susceptible to injury. If you raise your arm above your head, as is done in downward dog, and tune into the sensation in your chest and even your armpit, you will probably feel muscle tension, especially if you have very developed musculature. If, however, you feel a pinch on the top of the shoulder, and the feeling is almost a stuck feeling like you cannot go any farther, that is compression of the bony structure, and you should stop.

We cannot eliminate all risks in a yoga practice or stretching regimen, but we should do our best. As a teacher of Power Yoga for Sports, you must pay special attention if you do any hands-on adjustments. You must learn to distinguish feelings of compression from those of tension, and you should never push a client past compression. Each state and country has its own regulations for hands-on adjustments while teaching, and it is your responsibility to know your local regulations and to always ask your clients for permission to adjust their posture. Understanding the difference between tension and compression does not eradicate all danger; even seasoned yogis and gymnasts who are not overly aggressive can strain themselves. Even in restorative yoga, injury is possible if a person is not mindful of their movements and their body's signals.

What are yin yoga and yang yoga?

Yin yoga is slowly paced; poses are typically held for relatively long periods of time. For beginners, poses range from one to three minutes in duration. More advanced practitioners hold poses for up to 10 minutes each. Yin yoga is a practice of surrender in order to affect the body deeply into the connective tissues. Yang yoga is a more dynamic form of yoga. It is a flowing, moving style that builds strength and endurance and aims to generate heat in the body.

Focus

Focus is critical to being a superior athlete, and there are two types of focus worthy of our discussion. Externally, athletes can focus their eyes and their gaze for better physical balance; internally, they can focus on finding calm in uncomfortable situations by not allowing distractions to draw their attention away from a game or goal. Physical balance is perfected when an athlete finds that visual focal point. For example, when performing challenging tree poses, a person who is not focused and is looking around at others will certainly fall.

Finding calm in an uncomfortable situation is the essence of sports and an important part of finding that internal focus. There will be times when an athlete wants to rest, walk off the field, or argue a play, taking his mind off the task at hand and ultimately hurting performance (we discuss this in detail in chapter 3 on mindfulness practices). I want my athletes so focused on their purpose that they do not look for the exit door, the easy way out, or any other way than the winning way. One of the phrases we use in the Power Yoga for Sports Manifesto is, "Trying is an excuse for future failure." After all, Nike doesn't say, "Just try it!" A successful athlete needs to know that games are won and lost in the last quarter, period, hole, or set, so staying in the game and knowing you cannot stop means you need to find a way to dig deep. Long, deep holds in yoga teach you that like nothing else.

Mental Toughness

Mental toughness comes into training when we are challenged to hold poses using strength, flexibility, and breath. This type of training trains the physical body, and it also prepares the athlete for difficult game situations. "Don't run for the exit door" is another quote we use to convey the importance of mental toughness. Beyond focus, mental toughness is the second most not-talked-about quality of the great athlete. It's the desire to want it, to win, and to be better than the next person no matter what it takes. Sticking to the most challenging yoga poses—complicated, twisty, breathing, and balancing—teaches athletes to find their zone and succeed, translating those same lessons and feelings into their game.

Mental toughness is being that person who rises from defeat, disadvantage, and loss with confidence, unfazed and ready to get back out there and turn the page, living in the present moment. Having stellar mental toughness gives an athlete the ability to perform at a high level no matter how high the stakes are, how intense the pressure is, or how extreme the stress level is. It doesn't matter how the athlete performed in the past under the same circumstances. Mental toughness can be understood as the bridge to the best performance. A great way to illustrate mental toughness is to think about boot camp and the Marines. The green hopefuls may come in strong, ready, and wanting to be Marines, but it is the trainee who can get past the almost abusive training who will ultimately save lives in combat situations. That Marine has learned mental toughness. It is built simply through commitment, consistency, and preparedness. Toughness is often described as being a muscle to train and build; the more you challenge it and stick to your goals, the better and more developed it becomes.

If you were to ask your athletes what percentage of their game depends on being mentally strong, they would probably say 50 percent or higher. If this is true, what are they doing to train for the mental game? Even if you think only 20 percent of the game is mental, I would ask again, what are they doing to train for the mental game? If the answer is nothing, then they are automatically at a 20 percent disadvantage. Against athletes of the same size and ability who train for the mental game, athletes who do not mentally train are at an even greater disadvantage. PYFS trains the mental game by teaching goal setting and visualization techniques; these are described in chapter 3.

Breathing

Breathing is the cornerstone of life. Proper breathing in athletics and sport performance can make or break the outcome. Rib and lung openers and yogic breath work can increase lung capacity and even help relieve exercise-induced asthma symptoms, while nasal or belly breathing can increase calm while decreasing stress and anxiety.

Some athletes experience pregame anxiety. Anxiety is a natural reaction to pressures in the environment and part of the preparation for the fight-or-flight response. This is our body's primitive and automatic response that prepares it to act in a way that saves us from harm. It is an innate reaction that ensures our survival or even avoidance of injury. Sports and competition promote similar reactions because they often pose a threat to the ego or to the success of an athlete's play. Whenever the rigors of training or competition appear to surpass an athlete's ability, anxiety is likely to result if she is untrained in techniques to sideline it. Sports place a number of stressors on athletes. The game can be physically exhausting; athletes can face superior opponents; hostile fans yell, judge, and may verbally abuse them; and athletes can be faced with less-than-stellar weather conditions that challenge the body. However many of these elements they face, well-trained athletes can refocus their stress, breathe, and reveal a calmer attitude to succeed.

Breathing techniques taught in this book will enable you to teach your athletes longevity on the field, ease of play, and a look of effortlessness. Breathing seems to be something we think we already know how to do. Teaching your athletes how to breathe is essential to their success.

Common Breathing Issues

Some athletes have exercise-induced asthma. Power Yoga for Sports can help with this condition by teaching your athlete rib-expanding stretches to increase lung capacity. Particularly helpful would be poses like standing crescent pose, wheel of life, and triangle pose. It is important to teach athletes to breathe in and out through the nose and deep into the belly. This technique calms the body to lessen the severity of asthmatic episodes. Breathing through the nose for athletes who play outside is especially important because the nose cools or warms the incoming air for the body to accept more easily. When the weather outside is cold and you breathe through your mouth, your throat is more likely to constrict and activate asthmatic symptoms. The habit of coming off the field and maintaining nasal belly breathing shuts down the fight-or-flight response. Breathing through the mouth is a default method if you are stuffy or if you are in a stressful situation and need your body to respond appropriately.

TRAINING CYCLE BASICS

Since ancient times, there have been many forms of developing or training physical abilities. When you teach athletes Power Yoga for Sports, it is important to consider where they are in their training cycle. Conditioning programs are developed according to where an athlete is in his competitive season. Break training into preseason, in-season, and off-season periods. You should know where your athletes are in this cycle, and you should prepare programs so the athletes peak at the perfect time and are in regeneration phases when necessary.

Preseason is the longest period and is the time when you teach your athletes more aggressively. This is when you incorporate strength-building yoga routines and when you go harder on specific flexibility training. Always make your plans in cooperation with the team's lead strength and conditioning coaches.

In season, your athletes will taper off their aggressive training and focus more on their sport-specific moves. This is the perfect time to design restorative programs that will regenerate each athlete for the next competition. Game day also involves more mental training, visualization, and the use of mindfulness skills. The chief concern is knowing they did all they could to train and to perform their best.

Off-season is the best time for athletes to explore different types of yoga and how their bodies best respond to different techniques. They can alternate vinyasa and aggressive classes with regeneration and long holds. It is important for athletes to use this time to excel at their visualization skills so that they become rote for them during the season.

What does *vinyasa* mean?

Vinyasa means breath-synchronized yoga poses, which are often associated with a continual flowing series of poses.

It should be clear by now that if you want to train athletes and include yoga, Power Yoga for Sports is the technique to use. We've learned what Power Yoga for Sports is and how your athletes will benefit from your teaching. Now, let's explore the alignment of the body and its importance to the success and longevity of an athlete's career. Detecting problems in alignment is another cornerstone of the Power Yoga for Sports teachings.

2

Anatomy, Alignment, and Assessment

To be the best Power Yoga for Sports teacher you can be, you must commit to understanding bones, muscles, and basic anatomy. Too often yoga teachers graduate from training without proper attention to anatomy. I believe that if you want to be the best at manipulating athletes' bodies so they become more efficient, less prone to injury, and in better balance, anatomical study is critical to your success. A brief review is provided here, but I suggest you commit to lifelong, self-motivated human structure studies to make yourself better than the rest. It will only add to your success.

ANATOMY

The human body is the tool for play in sports. Part of your job is to understand its structure, movements, and performance capabilities. As a Power Yoga for Sports teacher, you should know all the muscles and bones by heart. It adds to your credibility, and your athletes will trust in you, knowing they are getting the best attention and care. Many athletes do not know basic anatomy and structure, which makes it more important for PYFS teachers to offer sound instruction and informed reasoning for their teachings.

Bones

Bones provide our support structure, and our movements are enabled through joints. You must study this support structure so you can understand how the configuration of bones and joints affects each athlete. Everyone has the same bones, but each athlete's bones are shaped somewhat differently, creating resistance and inabilities that vary from one person to another. The same is true for joints. Each athlete has the same joints, but, considering variations in bone shape, they can all move somewhat differently from one person to the next. Some athletes can move smoothly with grace and no restrictions, while others appear to get stuck in their range of motion. Whatever your athlete's needs or restrictions are, there is a resolution in training to address them. Take a look at figure 2.1 for the names and locations of the bones of the human skeletal system.

Muscles

Muscles are critical to understanding how the movement of the bones occurs. Continuous review of a muscle's origin (where the muscle starts), insertion (where the muscle attaches to bone or

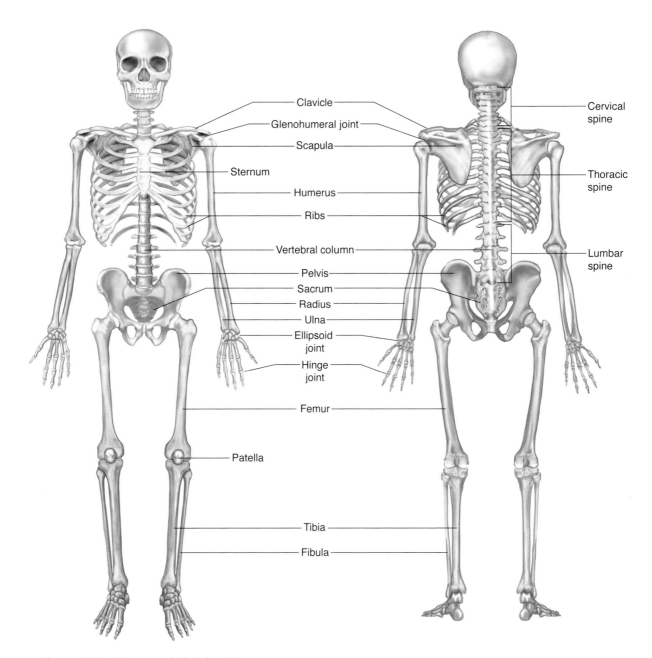

Figure 2.1   Human skeletal system.

soft tissue), and location is recommended for any professional who works with athletes. Athletes need to know the game they play and the plays they are required to make; you need to know the muscles they use and the shape they must be in to achieve their goals.

There are 640 muscles in the human body. They come in three types:

- Skeletal muscles, which perform voluntary movements and are attached to bones or tendons
- Smooth muscles, which perform involuntary movements of internal systems such as the digestive system and respiratory system
- Cardiac muscle, which performs the involuntary action of regulating the heart

For the sake of general yoga, we focus on skeletal muscles since it is these muscles that are directly impacted by playing sports and these muscles that we must learn to stretch and align. See figure 2.2 to review the human muscular system.

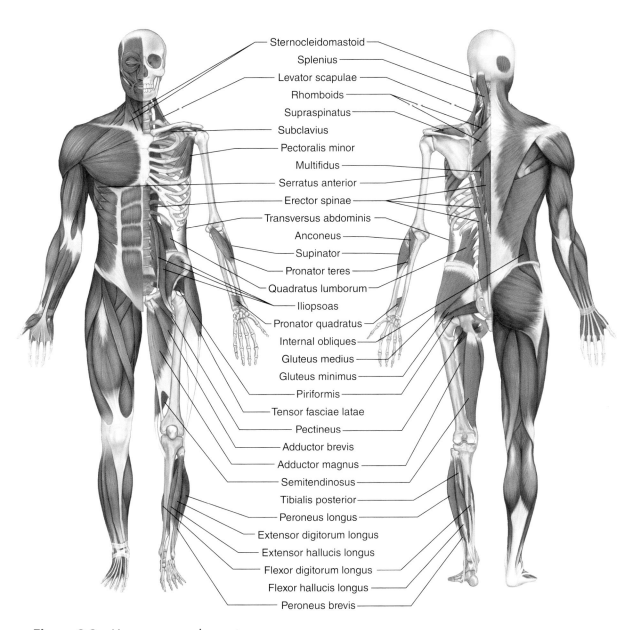

Sternocleidomastoid
Splenius
Levator scapulae
Rhomboids
Supraspinatus
Subclavius
Pectoralis minor
Multifidus
Serratus anterior
Erector spinae
Transversus abdominis
Anconeus
Supinator
Pronator teres
Quadratus lumborum
Iliopsoas
Pronator quadratus
Internal obliques
Gluteus medius
Gluteus minimus
Piriformis
Tensor fasciae latae
Pectineus
Adductor brevis
Adductor magnus
Semitendinosus
Tibialis posterior
Peroneus longus
Extensor digitorum longus
Extensor hallucis longus
Flexor digitorum longus
Flexor hallucis longus
Peroneus brevis

Figure 2.2   Human muscular system.

ALIGNMENT

Before you determine the yoga poses that best fit an athlete's body and sport, you need to understand the movement skills required of that sport and how those movements affect alignment. Study the sport as much as you can, either in person or by watching videos or television. Consult with coaches and trainers, and consider these questions:

- Does the sport involve or require endurance, such as being able to run several miles during competition?
- Does the sport involve or require quick agility moves, such as those of receivers and defensive backs in football who change direction on a dime?
- Does the sport involve or require diving, such as when a soccer goalkeeper makes a save?
- Does the sport involve or require twisting motions, as in basketball, football, or baseball?
- Does the sport involve or require jumping, like a basketball or volleyball player must do?
- Does the sport involve or require static movement that is powered from the core, as in skiing?

- Does the sport involve or require mental strength, like that of a quarterback or pitcher?
- Does the sport involve or require upper-body-driven movement, as in golf or swimming?
- Does the sport involve or require lower-body-driven movement, like running or playing as a football receiver?

These questions will help you to understand what the sport requires and what types of movement skills an athlete must develop or maintain to excel in that sport. Yoga can enhance or improve those skills with regular practice of the poses and techniques you will learn in later chapters. When you feel you have a comprehensive grasp of a sport's demands, you can begin to visualize poses that

How the Body Moves

The bones and joints work together as the body moves. Most movements have an opposite movement, referred to as an antagonistic movement. The comparisons here describe these pairs of movements.

Flexion and Extension

Flexion and extension are performed in the sagittal plane. Flexion refers to a movement that decreases the angle between two body parts. For example, when the knee flexes, the ankle moves closer to the glutes. Extension refers to a movement that increases the angle between two body parts. Extension of the knee straightens the lower limb and increases the angle back to 180 degrees.

Abduction and Adduction

Abduction is a movement away from the midline of your body, just as abducting someone is to take them away. For example, abduction of the shoulder raises the arms to the sides of the body. Adduction is a movement toward the midline. Adduction of the hip squeezes the legs together.

Medial and Lateral Rotation

Medial and lateral rotation describes the movement of the limbs around their long axis. Medial rotation is a rotational movement toward the midline. It is sometimes referred to as internal rotation. Imagine if you were to rotate your straight legs to point the toes inward toward each other; this is medial or internal rotation of the hip. Lateral rotation is a rotating movement away from the midline. In this example, this would mean rotating your legs so the toes point out and away from each other.

Elevation and Depression

Elevation refers to movement up; for example, lifting the shoulder in a shrug. Depression refers to movement in an inferior or down direction, such as moving from a shrug through neutral and pressing the shoulders lower than normal.

Pronation and Supination

Pronation and supination can sometimes seem confusing. If you are lying in a supine position, you are on your back; prone is lying on your belly.

Dorsiflexion and Plantarflexion

Dorsiflexion and plantarflexion are terms used to describe movements at the ankle. They refer to the surfaces of the foot; the dorsum is the top of the foot, and the plantar surface is the bottom of the foot. Dorsiflexion refers to flexion at the ankle so that the foot points up, stretching the Achilles tendon and calf. Plantar flexion refers to movement at the ankle so that the foot points down.

complement the athlete's current training and add challenge. Remember the six facets of PYFS that we learned about in chapter 1. Then you can start to consider additional relevant information to help you formulate the most effective routines for your athletes.

Observe and Question

When you watch games or competitions, drill down to the specifics. Think of the different positions within the sport. For example, baseball pitchers, catchers, and outfielders all move differently throughout a game, and they each benefit from yoga techniques that are specific to their positions. It's incredibly important for you to consider the duties of each athlete on the field of play and how that person's body moves. This type of thinking is what separates PYFS from a "regular" yoga class. Also keep in mind that not only do you want to strengthen the body for repetitive sport positions, you also want to include poses that unwind the body and relieve the constant stress from those repetitive positions. A good example would be a catcher's squat, where the stress is on the back and hips. In this case, an inverted table is a good pose to use to open the hip flexors.

What game-related improvements will athletes see once they start yoga?

After one to three months of consistent sport-specific practice (two to four times a week), your athletes will experience freely moving joints, better functional strength, improved body symmetry, and better breath control. These improvements support ease of movement on the field, increased power of movement, accuracy of execution, and better recovery after games.

Also, look for repetitive movements. Is there a natural movement that is regularly made in the position and sport you are observing? Of course there is, so stretch and strengthen the commonly used muscles and joints. Sports tend to be one-side dominant; therefore, they create imbalances. Be aware of misalignments that are born of repetitive moves. Learn about the injuries that are most common to each position in a sport. These can often be traced back to imbalances that come from overuse. The challenge is how to correct for these imbalances. We can never make the body perfect because there is always a dominant side (righty or lefty), but we can lessen the asymmetry and make it more manageable.

Also, listen to your players. They will offer clues and straight-up complaints about their nagging aches and pains. At the beginning of each class, ask if there are any new injuries, aches, or pains, and be ready to adjust your routine on the fly to accommodate these ailments. PYFS coaches should remember their players' injuries and complaints and use that information to prepare routines and classes. This makes for successful PYFS teachers who can think on their feet and prove their value. A good way to observe imbalances with your athletes is to begin class with simple assessment poses to help you direct the class for the best results; we cover assessments in the next section of this chapter.

Teach Self-Awareness

It is critical when teaching athletes that you give them tools that not only make sense to them but also allow them to learn and assess on their own. Do not worry; they will always come back to you for classes! But giving them tools to succeed outside class is invaluable. Suggest ways that they can change how they see their bodies. I often take pictures (without showing the face or other identifiable clues so there is no threat to their privacy) so they can see with their own eyes what I am telling them is going on with their symmetry and their bodies. It has been my experience that when an athlete can see her issues, they become more real to her, and she becomes more motivated to fix the problems.

Practice this yourself as a teacher: take notice of asymmetry, misalignments, and other physical clues that can be addressed. As you teach a Power Yoga for Sports class, give the athletes helpful cues to feel their feet in their shoes, the clothes on their bodies, and the symmetry in their form. Too often they are so focused on the workout, game, or opponent that they tune out of their bodies, to their detriment. They need to learn to feel their clothing, the ground beneath them, the impact of the weather on their skin, and their rate of respiration. Being in tune with their bodies and their surroundings can help them to better regulate their bodies to maximize performance, not to mention reduce injuries if something feels or looks off.

This idea of both feeling and seeing the body is critical for athletes. They should look for asymmetries, bumps, bulges, or misalignments, which tend to be precursors to injuries created by imbalances. Encourage them to look in the mirror and truly see, not just look. They should follow the outline of their form and compare both sides daily. They must be advocates for their own bodies to reap long-term rewards and longevity. It is your job as their Power Yoga for Sports coach to teach them to understand and notice body alignment so that they do not ignore and therefore train misalignments.

Why is body symmetry so important?

Just as an aligned car is important to performance, safety, and efficiency, the body must be in balance to work at its best. The more in balance the body is, the more effortless the movements and the lower the risk of injury.

Address Injuries

When misalignments, overuse, or accidents cause injury, athletes must take precautions to allow the affected area to heal and rehabilitate. As you work with trainers, medical staff, and athletes who are managing acute or chronic injuries, it's important to understand more about how these might affect other areas of the body and how your work with the athletes can encourage healing.

In the yoga world, we look at the body in a holistic way, which is different from how other health professions may view it. If you have a shoulder injury and go to a doctor, the doctor will likely treat the shoulder only. Yoga teachers look at the entire body and the impact the shoulder injury might have on the rest of the body.

If you have an injury, the effect it has on your body is fascinating. For example, what starts as a hip injury can manifest in many different ways. The crisscross effect explains that when you compensate for an injury by altering your posture and alignment, you may create an imbalance on the opposite side of the body. For example, an athlete who injures the right hip may develop problems in the left knee or left calf as it takes on the extra load while the athlete favors the injured right side. Also, gait and posture may change whether the athlete is aware of it or not. He may begin to limp, setting the stage for compensations that can produce muscular imbalances and asymmetry in both the upper and lower body. Tightness from an injury impedes how the body moves in all three planes and can therefore affect the fluidity of play. You must watch your athletes from all angles and pay attention to how they move.

When an athlete has an injury or tight spot, observe the area around that spot, and watch how the athlete moves it. Consider the athlete with a hip injury that could lead to knee issues. In this example, if the hips can remain supple in all directions, the hip socket can absorb the shock and the potential energy from powerful and perhaps sudden movements, sparing the susceptible knee from possible damaging impacts. If a football defensive back has hips that are too tight while he is cutting and changing direction, the energy of his motion has to go somewhere—if not into the hips, then into the knee area, where it can create problems. This is a common injury in nearly every sport that requires the use of legs against the ground.

Keeping the hips strong and flexible can have mental and emotional benefits as well. Emotions like stress, trauma, fear, and anxiety are held in the hips. The next time you have a difficult day or are suffering from a serious trauma that life dealt you, you may find that you have a hard time working on your hips. This means you need to focus on them more. You also need to make sure that as you relax in the restorative hip stretches, you do not grind your jaw with resistance. Let the lower jaw hang loose. Breathe in and out through the nose, deep into the belly, and watch the magic unfold with time and attention. I learned very early in my yoga work that the temporomandibular joint, the joint connecting the lower jaw to the upper jaw, is directly related to stress at the hip joint. Watch elite-level runners, and notice how their lower jaws are relaxed and even hanging in some cases. They are relaxing the jaw to achieve the ultimate range in the hips. Try this yourself: Move into a deep pigeon pose, and lock down your jaw as if you are intensely angry. Observe the effects on the hips, legs, and gut; they will likely tense up.

Armoring

Armoring is the self-protection of the injured body part, which causes stiffness in surrounding muscles and joints. It's a reflex mechanism that the body uses to tense the muscle tissue when stress or similar emotions or injury are experienced. Unexpressed emotions such as anger, fear, and grief are common causes of this armoring experience. To protect itself, the body takes a defensive stance by stiffening and tightening. The tissues enter into a muscular holding pattern that resists change and does not release. Trauma to the body, denial of injury, and even numbness are all psychological and emotional phenomena that cause the body to protect and guard an injury (often unconsciously) to allow you to live in more harmony. In fact, when you are numbed out or shut off from what your body is suffering, you are causing more misalignment, doing yourself a disservice, and inevitably causing and exacerbating crisscross effects. Watch for athletes who engage in armoring; you will see the tight areas. Be prepared to coach them in ways to decrease the stiffness so they can heal.

ASSESSMENT

There are several poses that work well for assessment purposes; from the results and visual cues, you can get a good snapshot of each athlete's needs. Assessment poses give coaches, trainers, and players a way to sideline injuries before they happen. As athletes move into and hold these poses, look bilaterally and on all planes for the following conditions to help you to assess areas for improvement:

- Are the hands fully connected to the floor?
- How are the feet positioned—do they appear symmetrical?
- Do they turn in the same direction?
- Is the athlete pronating the foot? Does it seem to have no arch?
- Are there spasms that may be causing unusual bumps and lumps?
- Is the body torqued in one direction?
- Is there tight musculature pulling the spine out of alignment?

If you have a tough time identifying these things at first, try looking at an athlete's body as more of a shape than a human form. Look at the left, right, front, back, and overall shape. Observe the negative space that the body forms; sometimes you can notice the imbalances more easily that way. For example, notice the space between the body, such as the space between the inside edge of the legs and between the arm and side body. This is negative space. It is important to get athletes into these assessment poses with only basic instructions, not too much detail, so you can see authentic misalignments. For example, when asking clients to assume downward dog, I recommend just telling them to get into the pose with the hands shoulder-width apart and the feet hip-width apart. Refrain from details like the middle finger pointing straight ahead and the tailbone directed up to the sky. When you give too many directives for assessment poses, you can inadvertently correct an imbalance and miss an opportunity to help a client.

Let's take a look at the poses I recommend for assessment purposes.

SEATED CROSS-LEGGED POSE

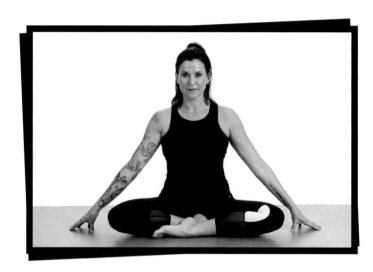

The athlete sits tall in a cross-legged position with her hands on her thighs. You can tell pretty quickly if an athlete is tight if you put her in this pose. She should be able to sit up tall, stacking the vertebrae over the hips. If the athlete is tight in the hamstrings and hips, she will be sitting behind the sitz bones, and the knees will be higher up in the air. You should also observe whether one knee is higher than the other, which indicates that on the side where the knee is higher, the hip, groin, or inner thigh is tighter than the other, and symmetry needs to be addressed.

Identifying the Dominant Eye

It is a cornerstone of the Power Yoga for Sports philosophy to pay attention to eye dominance. Observing an athlete's eyes can help to identify imbalances in the shoulders, neck, and even down to the chest. We know that open rotation of the neck can improve peripheral vision. To enable that open field of vision, an athlete should stretch the neck and shoulders in all directions of flexion, extension, and rotation. Did you know that if an athlete's eyes are of unequal size, the side of the body with the smaller eye will probably exhibit more tightness in the neck and shoulder? Notice the shape of the eyes as well: Is one eye round while the other eye is almost closed so it appears more almond-shaped? To address eye asymmetries, we want to open all the muscles surrounding the neck and shoulders in order to enable proper blood flow. This helps to prevent the muscles from pressing and impinging on the nerves.

Why are the eyes so important to performance in sports? Let's for a moment envision a right-handed batter in baseball. We have determined that the batter is right-eye dominant. Think about where a 95 mph fastball is coming from; over his left shoulder, right? If his right (dominant) eye is not clean, clear, and wide open, he is at a visual disadvantage. He already is at a disadvantage being a righty and right-eye dominant. It would certainly be better to be a right-handed batter and left-eye dominant, wouldn't it? You cannot change eye dominance that I know of, but you can change how open and clear your vision is. To make matters worse, imagine that the same player (this example is taken from an actual professional athlete I work with) tends to exhibit back and spine tension that torques his torso to the right. So now you have to make sure the spine evens out and gets back on track just so he can see the ball better. When the spine is not open, the eyes are not clear and the neck is tight; it is like driving a car without a side view mirror. We all know how uncomfortable a feeling that is—trying to back out of a parking space without the side view mirrors! Imagine doing that with a closed eye and a tight neck; that's a lot of pressure for an athlete. We want to help our athletes achieve an open neck in all directions; eyes that are wide open; even, flexible shoulders; and a supple spine in *all* directions.

To determine which is your dominant eye, hold your arms straight out in front of you at shoulder height. Bring the pointer and thumb sides of the hands together while your palms face away from you (figure 2.3). With the thumb and pointer side, bring your hands closer together until they create a small circle. Look at someone through that small circle and have him or her tell you which eye they see. That is your dominant eye.

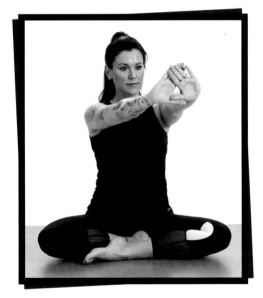

Figure 2.3   Determining your dominant eye.

SEATED TWIST

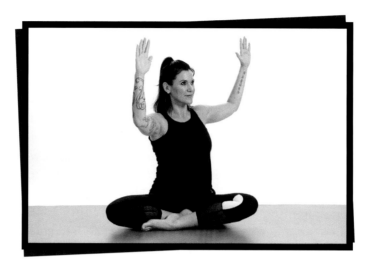

The athlete sits tall in a cross-legged position with arms in a goalpost position and twists vigorously left to right. You should be able to identify the side that is tighter. She will not twist as deeply on the tighter side; she will feel it, and you will likely see it. This is important because equal and open rotation in both directions is necessary for most sports. When one side's rotation is tighter, let's say to the left, and you happen to be right-eye dominant, you are limiting your scope of vision from a 180-degree range of vision to potentially 90 degrees or even less. This is a problem for soccer players because a limited twist to the left, when combined with right-eye dominance, can leave them vulnerable to getting their ball stolen from the left. These types of limitations, when they go unaddressed, become evident to coaches and to opposing teams when they view game films to develop winning strategies. Opposing coaches prey on the weaknesses they see. Another observation to be made here is to watch for flexibility and rotation in the shoulders. You want to see your athlete able to externally rotate the shoulder enough that the fingers point straight up to the sky when the arms are in the goalpost position.

CORPSE

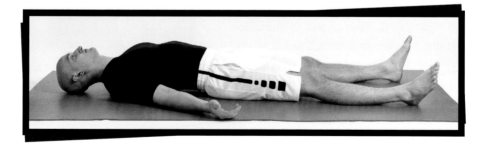

The athlete lies on his back with his legs straight and his arms at his sides in a natural position. The way the athlete lies in this position can give you valuable information without any effort from him. Look for how legs flop, and notice if one foot flops out more than the other or if they are symmetrical. If one foot flops out farther than the other, it is the other foot that is demonstrating the tighter hip or groin. You may want to pay attention to whether the head is straight, too. If the head is pointed right or left (assuming there is not a ponytail or uneven ground giving you a false read), this may indicate misalignment in the neck.

OPPOSITE-ARM OPPOSITE-LEG REACH

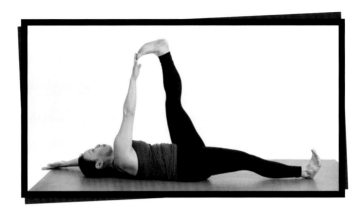

The athlete lies face-up and presses her low back into the floor to protect the spine and activate the abdominals. The arms are stretched overhead, and legs are long. The athlete brings her right arm and left leg up, touching them together and back down before repeating on the other side. The athlete continues this movement for two minutes while keeping her head relaxed on the floor. I start almost every class with this movement because it helps athletes to identify tightness in their hamstrings and hips. They can also feel which leg is tighter so that their training plan can reflect the difference and aim to evenly release that tightness. You can tell the tighter side simply by paying attention to where the hand touches the leg. Athletes with any tightness cannot touch their toes. If you observe, for example, that the athlete can only reach the left kneecap with the right hand, but can reach down to the lower right shin with the left hand, this would indicate an imbalance, specifically excess tightness on the left side, that you can correct with her training plan. The goal is to achieve even flexibility with each hand touching its opposite foot.

RECLINING COBBLER'S

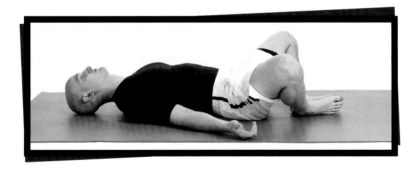

The athlete lies face-up with the knees bent and feet flat on the floor. The athlete slowly drops the knees out to each side, making sure that the bottoms of the feet line up perfectly with each other and that the seam between the feet is set perfectly in the body's center, usually aligned with the belly button. If one knee is higher off the floor, the inner thigh and hip on that side are probably tighter and need work.

Initially have the feet about 12 to 18 inches from the groin to test the inner thigh symmetry; after two minutes, move the feet about 12 to 18 more inches farther away from the groin. Asymmetry in this position, specifically a higher knee on one side, is an indication of deep hip tightness on that side.

ROCK AND ROLL

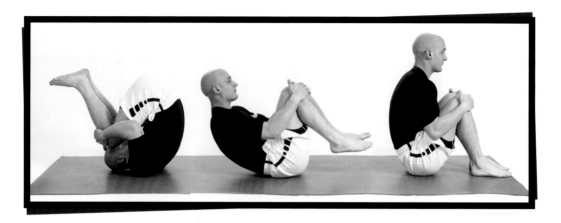

The athlete sits on the floor with his knees tucked, rolls backward onto his back, and rolls forward again to the starting position, making the rolls as big as possible. He should do this for one minute with his eyes closed. At the end of the minute, have him open his eyes and see where he ended up. There is a lot to be learned here; the side he morphs toward is usually the tighter side. For example, if you begin with your head in a 12 o'clock position and legs in a 6 o'clock position but after one minute, your head is at 3 o'clock and your legs are at 9 o'clock, it is likely that your right side is tighter than your left, due to the pulling imbalance. I have seen people finish complete circles and end up on others' mats, among other crazy things!

STANDING FORWARD BEND

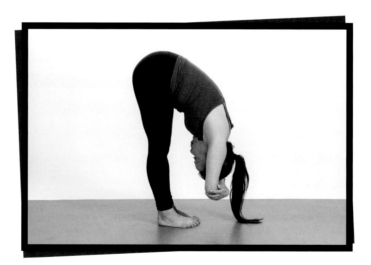

The athlete stands with the feet a little bit further than hip-distance apart and hinges forward at the hips so the upper body hangs toward the floor. The athlete holds each elbow with the opposite hand. Look at her back; signs of tightness and pulling could alter her gait, cause pain in the hips and back, and lead to an array of other limitations in rotation and flexion or extension. Observe the positioning of the feet and look for differences. Notice how the head hangs, whether it is pulling one way or the other, and notice if there are unusual asymmetrical bumps and bulges on the back.

For female athletes, look for tracking of the knees. If the knees knock in toward each other, this could present as an imbalance of tone in the leg medial to lateral. The anatomical structure of the hips puts females at a disadvantage with regard to pressure on the medial knee, resulting in a disproportionate number of ACL injuries. This forward bend is also a great position for detecting scoliosis because you can see curves and pulling.

Address Imbalances the PYFS Way

By becoming clear on how to spot imbalances using the poses previously mentioned, you will become invaluable to your athletes. A PYFS teacher can see the imbalances and is so well-versed in the poses and their effects on the body that they can instantly assess imbalances in the body. They then take action to improve the imbalances, using their knowledge of the planes of motion and overused areas of the body in relation to the athlete's sport. As stated before, the most efficient athlete is the symmetrically balanced athlete.

I once had an athlete come to me with complaints of pain in his shoulders and upper back (see figure 2.4a). After an hour of PYFS work, he looked like this (see figure 2.4b). I addressed the torque of the spine, the tightness in the right shoulder, and the length in the spine with long deep holds such as supported fish, lying spinal twist on both sides, and face-down shoulder stretch. This is a very clear example of overly developed, misaligned shoulders and the damage that can occur. You can see that he is definitely on his way to feeling better. With continued guidance and monitoring, he will be stronger and more balanced.

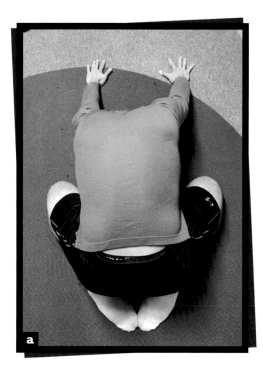 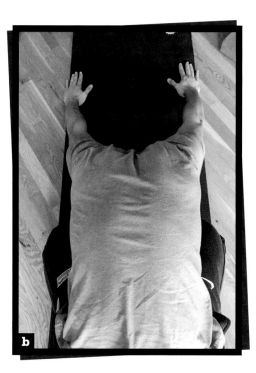

Figure 2.4 Client before PYFS protocol *(a)* and client after PYFS stretches *(b)*.

STANDING MOUNTAIN POSE

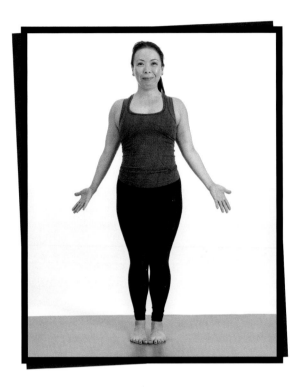

The athlete stands with her feet parallel and hip-distance apart, taking time to track the knees over the second toe. The athlete's arms hang down by her sides naturally. Observe how the head sits on the shoulders and if it pulls one way or the other and if there is any torque in the spine; note if there is a difference in shoulder height, arm length, or foot position. All of these are indications of imbalances; injuries can occur if the athlete continues to train without addressing them. If it is difficult for you to identify these types of imbalances, look at the shape of the negative space of your athletes' bodies. Note how their hands naturally fall; note specifically if one hand faces out and the other has the palm facing the thigh.

DOWNWARD DOG

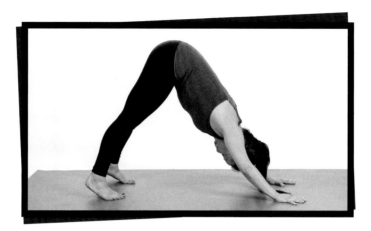

The athlete starts on her hands and knees. In this pose, the hands are approximately shoulder-width apart, and the feet are hip- to shoulder-width apart with the toes tucked and the legs straightened as much as possible. Observe how the hands line up with each other naturally before you give any alignment cues. If the athlete cannot straighten her legs or if you see a very rounded back, you know her hamstrings are very tight and need work. You can quickly assess her strength in this pose; if she gives up quickly, she may need more strength work. Look for bumps in the back that indicate a tight side.

HEAVY LEGS

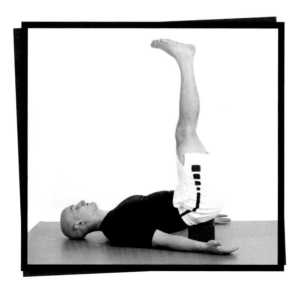

The athlete lies face up and slides his butt all the way up to a wall, straightening the legs up the wall the best he can. Arms are down by the sides. There are several things to look at here. Can the athlete actually straighten his legs against the wall? If not, he has tight hamstrings. Does the athlete have equal leg length, or is there a leg-length disparity? If there is a disparity, it could be a natural difference that the athlete has had since birth, or it can indicate asymmetrical hips and tightness in the lower back. Do the feet point evenly to the left and right, or does one foot point straight out and the other points to the side? This could indicate an imbalance in the external rotation of the hips.

CHILD'S POSE

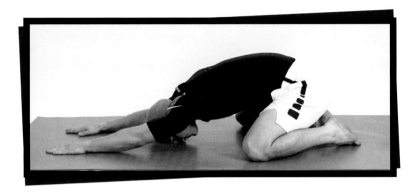

The athlete starts on his hands and knees with the knees as wide as the yoga mat and the big toes touching each other. The athlete slowly brings the hips as far back as they can come toward the heels and extends the arms straight out with elbows straight and palms flat on the floor. Look for lumps and bumps on the back, torque on the spine, and how the head is positioned, specifically if it is facing straight down or pulling left or right. Observe the hands, specifically if one hand is farther forward than the other. Also observe the hips, specifically if one hip is off the heel and one hip is resting on the heel. All of these differences may indicate critical misalignments that can lead to injury or compensation for injury. This pose is my all-time favorite for quickly determining issues in the back (see figure 2.4). Tightness on one side can cause an imbalance in strength and movement.

How do I manage the recovery process after my athlete's injury is cleared by a doctor?

Working with injuries is very common. Once an athlete is cleared to work out with you, proceed conservatively. Concentrate on the joints and muscles that surround the injury because they are likely to be tight from compensation and armoring. Remember to constantly assess your client's balance, and make daily adjustments to the training as gains occur.

Think of a great receiver and his performance requirements. In this chapter, we have shown you the process for understanding his job, his common movements on the field of play, and the way his body needs to move to be great. With your help he can move quickly downfield, sensing his surroundings, his peripheral vision like that of a bird of prey because you have released neck tension and created symmetry. He can perform deep spinal twists so that his hips and knees are ready to turn, cut, and run at any moment. No matter what sport your athletes play, achieving freedom in these movements will release their maximum potential for success, power, and longevity.

Injury Prevention and Rehabilitation Q&A

Yoga can be a vital part of training for athletes by improving their balance, strength, flexibility, mental toughness, focus, and breathing, but it can be equally important to injury prevention. When you learn the poses and what they can do for your athletes, you will be able to recommend a whole host of routines to prevent injuries or to speed their recovery from existing injuries. I have been honored to be a part of many professional athletes' rehab programs, and I have seen them experience quicker recoveries with PYFS.

Which poses to teach when student has back pain?

There is no short answer, but back pain is almost always associated with tight hamstrings. When your back is in peril, go to standing forward bend against the wall (as long as the condition is not acute), downward dog, and seated spinal twists both ways. Be sure the student is cleared by a doctor to accept your help. Perform supported fish every day for 5 to 10 minutes. These poses open the back in all directions and free the hamstrings so they do not pull on the back.

Which poses to teach when student has knee surgery/bad knees?

Always make sure students are cleared to train. Open muscles surrounding the knee with quad stretches, hamstring stretches, and hips hips hips. The best way to release the knees from strain is to open the hips as mentioned previously with pigeon, frog, hero's, and seated spinal twists.

Which poses to teach when student has had hip replacement?

Once the student is cleared to train, assign regular poses that work on hip rotation, such as pigeons (you may need to use blocks for support) and frogs, but also work on leg strength with warriors and their variations. Try spending time on standing balancing poses, like tree and king dancer, that develop more of the small muscles of the legs to improve balance.

Which poses to teach when student has spinal injuries?

Be very cautious, and proceed only if you are confident that the poses are beneficial; otherwise, wait or refer the student to the appropriate professional. This question is hard to answer without specific details about the injury and help from the student's doctor. If you want to start gently, put the student in lying spinal twist with blankets to control the depth of the pose. Stay focused on the student at all times. Conservative supported fish pose can be an effective part of a post-injury regime.

Which poses to teach when student has neck injuries?

Always get clearance from the doctor to do yoga, and avoid weight-bearing inversion until the student is cleared. Gentle plow pose with props and blankets and back-extending poses can help take up slack for the limitations on the neck. In addition, do poses that open the shoulders, chest, and back rotation. The more open these areas are, the less demand on the neck.

Which poses to teach when student has carpal tunnel?

Try table pose and wrist turns to open the carpal tunnel and release tension in the forearms and wrists. If weight bearing on the floor is too much, do wrist turns on the wall until you are ready for table pose. Once these are mastered in table pose, go to plank wrist turns.

Mindfulness Tools

3

What is mindfulness training, and why is it relevant to athletes? Well, this is your chance to train the mind to get to the next level. During a high-stakes game, you may experience an adrenaline rush—the heart pounds, the palms sweat, and butterflies flutter around in your stomach. Your brain races back and forth between past memories and concerns about today's outcome. In this type of stressful situation, the brain cannot stay in the moment, and you become more prone to mistakes and outbursts. Mental chatter makes it nearly impossible to keep calm.

It is estimated that our brains go through an astounding 800 to 1,400 words per minute, processing thoughts, sounds, and the things we see. For your athletes to perform at their peak, they must be able to make good decisions on the fly, stay composed, and rely on their training to take them to the finish line. Our bodies are equipped to handle short, infrequent bursts of stress. But in this day and age, we often live with fluctuating levels of pressure without a timeout; this is difficult for the body to manage, and we experience a stress response. We must teach ourselves and our athletes how to be calm, how to take breaks, and how to detox our minds for more peaceful living. Mindfulness quiets the noise and creates an environment where we can focus on only the things we can control, the execution of now. When you are quiet in body and mind and do not say anything, you see the unseen, become observant, and listen internally.

WHAT IS MINDFULNESS?

Mindfulness is a particular way of paying attention. It is purposefully bringing awareness to one's experience at the present moment. Mindfulness is finding presence, and it can be applied to sensory experiences, thoughts, and emotions by using sustained attention-grabbing techniques, noticing our experiences without reacting, and accepting thoughts as they come and letting them go. Mindfulness creates space and changes impulsive reactions to more thoughtful responses. Although reacting is OK, sometimes it is not OK or appropriate if your response comes from a stressed and irrational place that could affect your play or status. The best part is that it gives everyone who practices it a way to cope with the incessant storytelling our brains produce.

Some degree of stress in sports is expected, and it can help an athlete to get through the game safely. However, athletes must be able to resist internal and external distractions to make the best play, they must be able to avoid overreacting to defeats, and they must be able to turn down the stress levels when the game is over. That includes tuning out the fans, turning the page on a bad call, and forgiving themselves for botched plays. An athlete without mindfulness training may experience a stimulus and quickly, often inappropriately, react. With training, given the same stimulus, the athlete can quickly process the situation and respond skillfully. Mindfulness is rapidly catching on as an easy, user-friendly way to cope with stress and to reap additional benefits, including

- better focus and concentration,
- decreased symptoms of attention-deficit disorder and attention-deficit/hyperactivity disorder (ADD and ADHD),
- an increased sense of calm,
- decreased anxiety,
- better impulse control,
- better self-awareness,
- better conflict resolution skills, and
- a thickening of the prefrontal cortex.

Given all of these potential benefits, it is easy to understand how this type of training can help athletes to improve their performance. People of all ages are turning to these techniques to help with memorization (such as playbooks), public speaking, press interviews, competition, performance, dealings with peers, and improving family life.

Here is a great analogy to explain mindfulness training to your athletes. If you ever trained a puppy, you can understand the challenge: You have a high-energy, frenetic puppy that is all over the place. You want to train the puppy not to make a mess in the house. So you take the puppy outside on the grass and wait. The puppy is crazy and all over, jumping and running, chasing and exploring. You take the puppy back to the spot on the grass, and the puppy is crazy and all over, jumping and running, chasing and exploring. So you take the puppy and put it back on the spot on the grass, and the puppy is crazy and all over, jumping and running, chasing and exploring. Again, you take the puppy and put it on the spot on the grass, and the puppy is crazy and all over, jumping and running, chasing and exploring. Eventually the puppy starts to get the idea; with practice and diligence the puppy knows to go to his spot on the grass because running around and being crazy does not benefit him. A pattern is finally developed, and a new habit is formed. You see the pattern? It is the same process of patience and consistency that trains the mind of an athlete.

By contrast, letting the mind wander can lead to mindlessness. This can be a significant problem, especially for athletes. Mindlessness weakens performance and increases distractions. It hinders the athlete's ability to remember how to perform on the field and how to read and remember plays; thus, it influences learning and intelligence. Mindlessness hampers physical performance by detaching the athlete from the present and overwhelming him with mind chatter, and it increases anxiety, frustration, and stress.

When our thinking is clear, it feeds the creative forces in our brains. Throughout life, we learn things, and we learn to trust in what we are taught—for example, we trust that the earth is round. We begin early in life to listen to everything and everybody and to believe things because a teacher taught them or because our family has a long line of belief. Encourage your athletes to question things and to learn and experience for themselves! As they learn through their own experience, they can decide how deeply to trust in that experience, and they can recognize if it is born of jealousy, envy, greed, judgment, goodness, or truth. The brain needs assurance and repetition to relearn, so be patient. My favorite analogy of this concept follows.

Imagine a mountain that is crowded with grass, rocks, and uneven surfaces. Now, visualize what it would be like to push a large rock all the way down to the bottom of this mountain. It would take a lot of effort to push it over or around existing stones and mash down the long grass that is in the way. Suppose you continue pushing more rocks down the same pathway over and over and over again. What would happen? A groove would form. Once that groove is in place, it takes almost no energy to push the next rock down the hill. You just set the rock into the groove, and it rolls right down. This is similar to how habits are formed.

Next, suppose you want to push a rock down the hill in a new direction. That requires a change of habit. A fresh area of the mountain is rocky and grassy, and it takes a lot of effort to push the rock down to the bottom once again. Even after this is done, the old groove remains, and we must form a new one; it does not instantly disappear, and that is the key. The rock may want to roll toward the less challenging path. If we keep pushing the "rock" or new behavior down the hill over and over, a new groove eventually forms. Over time, if the old rut is not used, it will get covered over with new grass and obstructions and will become the less desirable way. The new path becomes the easier one with time, attention, and practice.

Mindfulness and Brain Health

One of the most exciting discoveries in research is that mindfulness practice stimulates the prefrontal cortex (PFC), and it may develop and thicken it, which might offer a revolutionary approach to overcoming damage caused by high-impact sports. Your prefrontal cortex is located under your forehead. In his book, *The Mindful Brain*, Dan Siegel speculates about the different aspects of well-being that are established by stimulating this area of the brain through mindfulness (Siegel 2007). Those aspects include the following qualities.

- Balance: the stop and go, high and low regulation of the nervous system. When our body is in balance, we automatically produce the proper amount of energy needed for our situation.

- Emotional regulation: appropriately regulating emotions for the current situation. When emotions are deregulated, we become overwhelmed and emotionally chaotic, and we may experience depression or a sense that our life is not meaningful.

- Fear modulation: our ability to calm and soothe or even unlearn our fears.

The PFC is responsible for executive functions, a term that represents a set of mental features that help with goal-directed behavior. We need to access the PFC to plan, organize, strategize, pay attention to and remember details (playbooks), and manage time and space. Athletes need all of these functions.

MINDFULNESS AS A LIFELONG PRACTICE

We each spend several minutes each day taking care of our physical bodies and physical hygiene with activities such as showering, brushing our teeth, eating, and getting dressed. Commit now to spending a few minutes a day on your mental hygiene. Your health and well-being are worth the time and attention. Incorporating a fluid mindfulness practice into your life can enhance your flexibility and adaptability. If you have felt stuck in old habits, mindfulness methods can retrain your brain to get off autopilot. Mindfulness enables us to put on the brakes and slow down before acting on impulse. It can help you to be present, as opposed to being overly worried about future outcomes that you cannot control anyway. You can transform a pattern of self-criticism and self-blaming to one that promotes greater patience, kindness, and acceptance of oneself and others. Your daily life will feel more fulfilled, organized, and present as you reduce negative thoughts, talk, and images. Let's take a closer look.

Thoughts

There are a few types of thought. However, when you boil it all down, many thoughts are based on lingering concerns from the past or apprehension caused by projecting those concerns into the future. Rarely are we just thinking in the now, settled in the center. Memories, worry, planning, strategy, and daydreams are all part of the endless cycle of thought, both good and bad. Trying to stop thoughts is as hard as trying to stop hearing; it's nearly impossible. This is usually what derails people from regular mindfulness practice—not knowing how to handle the thoughts. Thoughts are just thoughts, meaningless personal interpretations of experience. It is important to learn just to let thoughts be thoughts and not to allow them to become obsessions. Often the mind seems to have a mind of its own. We should strive to let our mental habits work in our best interest rather than fighting unwanted thoughts. Here we learn how.

Mental Talk

Mental talk is your inner dialogue, discussion, and debate. It is storytelling of the mind, and it includes useless chatter that is usually untrue. Sometimes it is loud and clear, at times overwhelming and judgmental. Sometimes mental talk is subtle and suggestive, like subliminal messaging or product placement in entertainment programs, and you do not even realize it is happening. Usually you do not notice all the mental talk until after it has stopped.

Mental Images

Mental images are the pictures that inundate the mind when you close your eyes. The images are based on your current mood, recent experiences, and feelings. If you are hungry, for example, your mind is bombarded with choices of food to stop the potentially uncomfortable feelings in your stomach. Your brain creates images of your most recent thinking and takes into consideration your moods, experiences, culture, and training. Most of the time, the mind is racing so much that even the images are momentary, yet still overwhelming.

Can yoga help to build mental endurance?

Visualization and mental training techniques, such as life detox, can improve your athletes' mental game. Your continual study of these techniques will equip you to help all of your athletes to find the approaches that work best for them.

Tell your athletes that the only thing they can control is the now, even if they get stuck 99 percent of the time dwelling on the past or future. I am not suggesting here that we get rid of these thoughts; they are critical to survival and the root of who we are. The positive side of reviewing past actions and thinking ahead is that it helps us to plan, to set goals, to avoid making the same mistakes over again, and sometimes to come up with creative solutions for problems. Notice that these positive forms of thinking are all goal-driven ways to plan, find solutions, and stay attentive, while negative thinking can stunt personal growth.

It is relatively simple to build mindful practices into your life while doing most of the everyday things you already do. When you are listening to someone talking, it is the perfect time to consider your own body, thoughts, emotions, and judgments. Be mindful during a conversation. Are you listening, talking, aware of when you want to interrupt or add to the conversation? Are you aware of your body? For example, is your body touching a chair? What is the sensation? When you walk, how does the ground feel beneath your feet? Choose something you do every day like cook, brush your teeth, or talk on the phone, and bring mindfulness to the activity. Easy ways to encourage your athlete to start putting these practices into play include the following tactics:

- Add it to your calendar.
- Do a different practice each day.
- Set a reminder into your phone to go device free.
- In the mornings, press snooze on your alarm and take the 10 minutes to breathe or body scan.
- Body scan as you are trying to fall asleep at night.
- When you are talking with a loved one, use the ground words technique to sharpen your focus on that person.
- Build a 1- to 10-minute seated practice into your day at the same time every day.

Mindfulness Misconceptions

As you work with athletes on becoming more mindful, make sure they understand what mindfulness is *not*.

- Mindfulness is not about forcing ourselves to be calm and conforming to a strict definition.

We expect mindfulness to bring us harmony and relaxation. We tend to want all of our experiences to be perfect and to deny anything that feels bad. We want something, we do not get it, and then we are unhappy. We think it is not working or we are doing it wrong. We start to judge our experiences and ourselves instead of just being. Although you can experience a sense of peace, calm, or relaxation while practicing mindfulness, these are not guaranteed outcomes. Mindfulness is about noticing our experiences, including all the thoughts, feelings, and physical sensations.

- Mindfulness can significantly reduce stress, but it is not about stress reduction.

- Rather than removing stress, mindfulness helps us learn to relate to stress in a different way.

- Mindfulness is not about being complacent. Acceptance does not mean complacency. It means acknowledging whatever is going on, out of kindness and empathy instead of frustration.

- Mindfulness is not religious. Mindfulness practices are useful for everyone, regardless of their spiritual beliefs.

- Mindfulness is not a magic bullet. In order to benefit from mindfulness meditations, you must view it as a new way of life, not as a two-week course that begins and ends.

MINDFULNESS TOOLS

To practice mindfulness, I have created a mindfulness toolbox. Understand the concepts, try them all, and decide what best suits your lifestyle. You do not need to practice all of them; you can pick and choose according to what you are doing at any given time, your time constraints, and what truly rings clear in your mind. These tools enable you to zero in on the now, to become fully present, and to quell the constant chatter of the mind that is preventing your success. We consider six mindfulness tools: breathing, counting breaths, body scanning, ground words, life detox, and visualization.

Breathing
Simple breathing techniques to implement are diaphragmatic breathing, three-part breathing, and alternate nostril breathing. Let's explore each one.

Diaphragmatic Breathing
Diaphragmatic breathing is simply the act of breathing in and out through the nose only and deep

into the belly. We breathe in and out through the nose because the nose has a specific function to warm or cool the breath, based on our present environment, in order to make it most amenable to the body. Also, deep breathing into the belly, not shallow breathing into the chest, tells the body to shut down the fight-or-flight response and immediately start to calm.

Here is a natural tranquilizing breath pattern to try. Breathe in for a count of four, hold your breath for a count of seven, and then slowly release the exhalation to a count of eight. Your exhalation is twice as long as your inhalation. Try this next time you are having difficulty falling asleep, and teach it to your athletes who easily become aggravated on the sidelines. It also gives the brain something to think about, so the practitioner hears less mind chatter. We tend to breathe in and out through the mouth and shallow up high in the chest when we are in high-stress situations. That is fine, and we need that at times. Diaphragmatic breath activates the relaxation system, or the air conditioning, of the body: it cools down the body and keeps the reactive core of the brain from overheating. Other benefits of diaphragmatic breathing include the following:

- Decreases in blood pressure, pulse rate, and rate of respiration; cleansing of lactate from the blood (lactate can cause increased feelings of anxiety)
- Increases in alpha brain waves, which make you calm and alert; release of serotonin into the blood, which is the feel-good neurotransmitter

Three-Part Breathing

To understand three-part breathing, it is best to try it for yourself. To prepare for the exercise, sit in a comfortable cross-legged posture, keeping the spine upright, eyes closed, and arms and shoulders relaxed. The hands are placed on your lower belly. Your belly rises on the inhale and falls on the exhale. Follow these instructions to practice:

1. Start with an inhalation, bringing the awareness to the abdomen. Consciously make a gentle effort to push the diaphragm down so the belly can fill up like a balloon.
2. Continue the deep inhalation and shift the awareness to the chest area. Expand the chest and the rib cage, filling the middle part of the lungs with air.
3. Continue the inhalation and bring the awareness to the clavicle area, lifting the collarbones upward. At the end of inhalation, take a momentary pause and begin the exhalation cycle in the reverse direction.

Allow the navel to be drawn in toward the spine as you approach the end of exhalation. That completes one breathing cycle. At the end of the exhalation, pause for a moment and begin the next breathing cycle. Continue for about four to six breathing cycles. At the end of the last cycle, keep your eyes closed and relax for a few breaths.

In this deep, three-part breathing, we engage the entire capacity of the lungs in the breathing cycle. It is estimated that we may be able to bring as much as seven times more oxygen into the system than in normal, shallow breathing. More oxygen implies that more oxygenated blood is available for circulation in the body. At the cellular level, due to the gas exchange, we can get rid of more carbon dioxide from the system. Thus, deep breathing brings in more *prana* (life force), energy, and vitality with each inhalation while providing deeper cleansing and purification with each exhalation. Deep breathing calms the nerves and reduces stress levels. That's why we may hear the suggestion to take a deep breath when we are agitated or angry!

What is prana?

Prana is Sanskrit for "vital life," and it refers to the essential, subtle energy that underlies all of reality. Pranayama is the art of breathing control.

Alternate-Nostril Breathing

To practice this breathing technique, we use deep inhales and exhales. When they devote time and practice to alternate-nostril breathing, your athletes can reestablish balance and ease in their minds and bodies. When they feel overwhelmed, stressed, and burdened from doing too many things, their internal alignment may have become out of tune. This breathing technique is great for repairing balance, and it restores stability in the left and right hemispheres of the brain. In addition to calming the mind and reducing stress levels, this breathing technique also improves focus, stimulates respiratory functions, invigorates the nervous system, and eliminates toxins.

To prepare for this exercise, sit in a comfortable sitting posture with the spine erect, eyes closed, and shoulders relaxed. Make the Vishnu Mudra where the right hand is in a soft fist, the thumb and the last two fingers are lifted up, and the middle two fingers stay at the base of the thumb. The thumb is used to close the right nostril, and the ring finger is used to close the left nostril. Follow these instructions to practice:

1. Use the right thumb to close the right nostril. Begin the first round by inhaling through the left nostril.
2. At the end of inhalation, close the left nostril with the ring finger, and open the right nostril. Then exhale through the right nostril.
3. Inhale now through the right. At the end of inhalation, close the right nostril with the thumb again, and exhale through the left nostril.

This completes one cycle of breathing. Continue for about six to seven minutes or more until you feel a sense of calm. Make sure to use deep and soft breaths for each inhalation and exhalation.

What is the best breathing technique to use with my athletes?

When in doubt, always go to diaphragmatic breathing. You can also add counting breaths to calm and comfort your players while they clear their minds of negative and unnecessary chatter.

Counting Breaths

Counting breaths is as simple as it sounds. While relaxing, or when you or your athletes feel overwhelmed by thoughts, pressure, and situations, simply start counting your breaths. Count one as you inhale, two as you exhale, three as you inhale, four as you exhale, and so on. During this practice, the mind will inevitably start to wander. When this happens, acknowledge it, push the thoughts aside, and restart the counting. Your athletes should perform this exercise until a new sense of calm spills over them. That moment when you noticed your thoughts instead of your counting was a mindful moment. Thoughts are OK, but you should not dwell on them or let negative thoughts take over your mind; acknowledge and restart your counting.

Your athletes may notice while counting breaths that even though they intend to keep their attention on the breathing, they might not make it past five or even past two. If this happens, tell them to acknowledge the thoughts, but don't give them meaning, and start over; in time, their numbers will soar.

The counting breaths exercise is a critical introduction to the way the mind works. Encourage your athletes to be kind to themselves with regard to how high they can count. They should try to accept how they do and the thoughts they notice without judgment. Nothing they do or feel is right or wrong; it just is. On some days it will be easy to focus, while on others it will be more difficult. The numbers themselves are meaningless as an indication of learning or progress; they are just a gauge as to how the mind is working at that moment. When your athletes start to notice what the mind is doing, that is mindfulness.

Body Scanning

Body scan meditation is best performed lying down. Body scanning systematically moves one's focus throughout the body, starting with the toes and finishing at the top of the head. People who do this consistently can gain a new appreciation for their bodies. Body scanning meditation has several benefits: it focuses the brain, it switches off the habit of listening to mind chatter, and it systematically relaxes the body.

Encourage athletes to find a private, quiet place to practice where they feel comfortable. They can practice body scanning at any time of day. The later in the day they do it, the more it may help with sleep. Body scanning takes between 10 and 40 minutes, depending on the intensity of the practice and how much time is available.

To begin body scanning, you should feel comfortable and at ease, either lying down or sitting upright with your feet on the floor. Close your eyes, and take a few cleansing breaths. If you feel tired but are not ready to go to sleep, sit upright in a chair and away from the backrest. Try to become aware of how you are feeling at the moment. Accept whatever happens. Let go of any ideas or goals for the session. Allow yourself to be as you are in a deep and authentic way. Follow these instructions to practice:

> Breathe rhythmically; focus your attention on your breathing for a few moments. Breathe in and out through the nose and deep into the belly, using the diaphragmatic breathing you learned previously. You are going to move your attention systematically through your whole body, step by step. First, shift your attention from your breathing down to your toes. Feel whatever sensation you can feel, whether it is profound or nonexistent. Move your attention from your feet, lower legs, upper legs, pelvic area, lower torso, upper torso, shoulders, upper arms, lower arms, and hands. Pause for a while at each area. Proceed up to your neck, face, the back of your head, and finally the top of your head. This whole process can take 10 to 40 minutes. Each time your mind drifts, notice what it was focusing on and bring your attention back to your breathing and your scan. Imagine your breath affecting each area of your body. Once you finish the full scan, take a moment to notice every part of your body. Then breathe in, imagining your breath starting at your toes on the inhale, and reaching the top of your head. As you breathe out, let the out-breath sweep from the top of your head down to your toes.

> Just be still and breathe.

There are many physical sensations, emotional reactions, and thoughts one may experience during a body scan. For instance, your athlete can feel tingly, stiff, achy, pounding, numb, itchy, tense, relaxed, cool, warm, or dry. Emotions could include joy, anxiety, disgust, contentment, sadness, anger, frustration, and happiness, to name a few. Typical thoughts may include plans, past events, judgments, wishes, hopes, and analyses, any of which can disturb one's mindfulness practice. All of these experiences are valid. Encourage your athletes to accept the thoughts, let them go, and tune back into their practice.

The body scan draws our attention to the ever-changing state of the body. Often it is not until we pull a muscle or get sick that we pay attention to our bodies and realize how good we felt before. We seldom take the time to feel our feet on the floor or the clothes on our bodies. We become detached and desensitized instead of tuning in and feeling the tiniest pain or ache before it becomes an illness or injury. Our cars have warning lights, but we do not; we have mindfulness.

With greater body awareness, your athletes will notice things that were previously just under the radar, such as discomfort in the neck or tightness in the back. This is where the body scan can provide value. That tightness or discomfort was probably there before; they just didn't notice it. They may now notice a part of the body that feels great or deeply relaxed. Others may experience more discomfort when they focus on a particular area—an itchy spot, for example.

Increased attention to a physical sensation can sometimes make it seem stronger because of the heightened awareness of it.

Ground Words

The use of ground words is a simple, yet very effective mindfulness tool. This is my students' favorite technique. Implementing ground words can instantly bring you to the now. It is best described as a narration of your day in real time. I use it most when I am driving. My work brings me to many places in one day, and driving can become hypnotic. I can get drowsy and easily lose awareness. Often I find that I do not know where I am on my journey. This is a perfect time to use ground words. While driving, I observe my surroundings—what I hear, see, feel, and smell—and describe them with a word. You can do this out loud or in your head. For example, as I drive, I see a road sign; I think "sign." I hear a horn; I say "horn." I see a blue, clear sky, I say "blue" or "sky," and so on. When you do this exercise, you stay grounded in the now and become completely aware of your being. There is one rule to the practice: You must not use any modifiers when you are narrating, such as dark sky, annoying horn. These types of modifiers can stir up emotions, causing your mind to wander. Keep the practice simple and concise. You start to see the world as you never saw it and actually enjoy the ride while wide-awake and aware. It can be practiced while doing an activity or at any time you feel disconnected or detached.

Have your athletes use this technique when they feel overwhelmed by a game situation. The fans may be agitating, a mistake may have been made, or the weather may be changing the game; now is the time to ground. Consider a basketball player, for example. Instead of listening to the fans, he may be saying in his head, "dribble, avoid, spin, step, shoot." This technique does not leave room in the brain for distractions, and it helps your athletes to perform at their best.

At first, new techniques may not always make sense or feel right. I once was teaching an NFL coach who was practicing mindfulness on an airplane. He became so acutely aware of all the people and conversations on the plane that he became agitated, and he longed for the pre-mindfulness days. He commented that he didn't like being aware now. I can understand this, but you must be aware and proactive, rather than reactive, with every situation in your life in order to stay safe and healthy, whether you like it or not. Relearning may make you uncomfortable at first, but a life of mindfulness is going to bring more positives than negatives in the long run. Stay the course. That NFL coach learned that he had numbed himself to his surroundings, and he was missing out on a lot that life had put before him. A mindful life can bring you many gifts and benefits.

Life Detox

There is a lot of negative motivation that can clutter the brains of our athletes and cause stress, therefore making them unable to be present. Deciding to live a life of mindfulness requires the support of a robust mind and a disciplined heart; otherwise, it is easier to revert to the old ways, or the old path down the mountain if you will. Think about the challenge of restructuring the way we talk and think. Dr. Wayne Dyer often said, "If you change the way you look at things, the things you look at change." Another translation of this is not to think, "Once I am debt free and a millionaire, I will be happy," but rather, "Once I am happy, I will be debt free and a millionaire."

The following approaches to being a better person can help athletes to ignore distractions and focus on the positive.

Establish Non-Harming Behavior

Non-harming means not hurting others mentally, verbally, or physically; it means avoiding anything that injures others. Violent or harming behaviors arise from fear, anger, and perhaps hatred. These powerful negative emotions can weigh heavily on a person, and they can be eliminated with careful awareness. We have all acted on them in the past, and later we feel regret and many other negative emotions.

It is hard to move on from hurting someone, and it can disable your ability to succeed in a mindful way. Encourage your athletes to pause before acting harmfully and to try to develop empathy. They can use any of the other mindful tools we've covered in this chapter before they react. Bringing goodness to others can yield tenfold returns. This type of thinking does not mean that one is weak or contented with the status quo but rather that one is pursuing overall betterment.

Practice Non-Stealing Behavior

Non-stealing behavior has many forms. It is not simply avoiding theft; when understood more broadly, it means not taking that which is not offered. That includes other people's time, energy, feelings, emotions, thoughts, and even ideas. Stealing is based on greed and envy. These types of feelings weigh heavily on you. When you steal from someone, whether the theft is large or small, it is difficult to move on. This idea includes materialism, overconsumption, hoarding, and a voracious appetite for wanting and accumulating nonessential things. Greed distorts our view of reality and leaves us unhappy. Whether or not we get what we want, selfish craving causes us to suffer, and it clouds our judgment and our clarity of mind. The Buddha said, "The greatest form of suffering is in attachment." Teach your athletes to be generous, to value simplicity, and to practice generosity. Acts of generosity can be as simple as offering a sincere compliment or giving one's time.

Train the Tongue

Training the tongue is not about censoring your words but rather about being conscious of the words that come out of your mouth. Instead of lashing out and talking senselessly with words that do not enhance lives, listen, pause, then give thoughtful responses. According to Thich Nhat Hanh, rather than simply saying "false speech," it is better to understand it as "unmindful speech" (Nhat Hanh 2007).

Words can create happiness or suffering. Encourage your athletes to be fully committed to speaking with words that inspire self-confidence, joy, and hope. Teach them not to spread news that they do not know to be true. Words can cause division and disharmony. Do not be a party to that. False speech comes from a place of needing control; these types of feelings weigh heavily on a person. When you lie to someone or are critical, it is hard to move on, and it leaves you with excessive mind chatter instead of a sense of being fully present.

Refrain from Toxins

This practice teaches your athletes to be mindful of what they are consuming. Be aware of anything that may be a toxin, literally or figuratively, including inappropriate films and TV, books, magazines, and even conversation. They should stop doing anything that does not make them smarter or better or make the world a better place. Try to recognize more than just toxic foods, drugs, and alcohol—beware of toxic overloads of media, phone conversations, the Internet, social networks, and "opinions." Toxic information dulls the minds of our athletes, affects their attention and intelligence, decreases their ability to learn, and feeds the fire of the ADD/ADHD epidemic. All of the toxicity they come into contact with clouds attentiveness and therefore their ability to focus on the current situation.

Avoiding toxins promotes clarity of mind and the ability to enjoy life with less stress and more attention. Imagine your body entering life as a pure, clear crystal, free of impurities. As the crystal comes into contact with environmental forces, toxins, and people, everything that comes even remotely close reflects off the crystal back to the world. Choose to keep your body, your crystal, clean and clear. Do not let outside influences change you unless it is in a positive way. Tell your athletes to be very particular about what people they allow into their lives, things they surround themselves with, places they go. All of these people, things, and places have a more significant effect on them than they know. They can become those things, too. To help keep the mind and body clear, they should be mindful of who they hang around with, the media they seek, and the images they see, and they should connect only with people who feed their souls.

Dangers of Outside Influences or Screen Time

One of the challenges to detoxing our lives is that many of us believe too much of what we see and hear on Twitter, on Facebook, in magazines, and in news broadcasts. We become prisoners to suggestion, losing the ability to form our own opinions based on our personal beliefs. Remind your athletes that the opinions of others, including those in the news media, are based on their upbringing and experiences, not yours or your athlete's, and those narratives may be incomplete or offered with ulterior motives.

To put it simply, the Internet is hurting all of our brains. We are continuously connected to devices. Following are some interesting facts according to a 2012 *Newsweek* article cited by bestselling author and leadership mentor Michael Hyatt (Hyatt 2012). Hyatt strives to help people win at work, achieve their purposes, and succeed at life. Followers of his philosophy can achieve success in all facets of their lives.

- On average, Americans stare at some type of computer screen for at least eight hours a day.
- When President Barack Obama ran for office the first time in 2008, the iPhone had yet to be launched. Now we apparently cannot live without it.
- More than a third of smartphone users go online before they get out of bed each day.
- The average teen processes an astounding 3,700 texts a month.

Brain scan technology tells us that our brains are being rewired and we are altering our prefrontal cortex. The brains of Internet addicts look like the brains of drug and alcohol addicts. The part of the brain accountable for processing speech, memory, motor control, emotion, sensory, and other information is actually shrinking, according to Hyatt. Research also shows that the more time a person spends online, the worse they feel mentally. Web users are using web time instead of sleep, exercise, and face-to-face interaction, which leads to loneliness and depression. There are three ways to handle this:

- Completely withdraw from using the Internet, which may not be realistic.
- Ignore the studies and go on as you have, which may not be healthy.
- Use moderation—that is, become intentional with your Internet usage, understanding that it has repercussions.

We are made to shut down for one-third of our daily cycle, meaning that we sleep for about eight hours a day. One of the quickest ways to lose the ability to be present is to cheat ourselves out of this "off switch" time our bodies need. Practicing the discipline of rest requires more than naturally induced pauses. Tell your athletes that they need to rest one day in seven and they need to take their vacations and their media fasts as well as get eight hours of sleep per night. It is essential that we sometimes pull away to a quiet place to pause and reflect, even if it is only for a few minutes to practice one of our mindfulness tools.

Also, people were made to live in relationship with others. In a world of social media and false connections, we must be intentional about building real-life relationships and real community. Deciding to live like this means making more time for our family members and trusted friends in person. In addition to cultivating relationships, we must find time for recreation. Recreation involves any activity that gives us the opportunity to express creativity. These types of activities are never urgent, but they are vital to our mental well-being, and they make us happy. It is important to teach our athletes this.

Visualization

Visualization is re-creating all the images, sounds, and feelings in your mind that are connected with an activity in order to practice in a perfect environment. It is a technique for creating a mental image of a future event.

I am fascinated with a study done years ago by Alan Richardson (1967). In this study, three groups of basketball players shot foul shots. To determine a base line count, all the basketball players shot 100 foul shots at the beginning of the study.

The foundation of this study was to prove the power of visualization and sports performance.

The first group shot foul shots for 20 minutes a day for a month. The second group did nothing related to basketball for the month. The third group was instructed to shoot by guided visualization, as though they were shooting foul shots 20 minutes a day for a month; however, they never actually touched a basketball.

After following the given instructions for their groups for a month, all the players shot 100 foul shots once again to compare the results to their baseline numbers.

The first group made a 24% improvement in their foul shots made. The second group, not surprisingly, made no recordable improvements. The final group , the visualizers, improved 23% in their foul shots. The astounding results prove the importance of adding visualization to your training regime. I love to tell my athletes about this study, especially when they are hurt and feel as though they are losing gains by not actively practicing. The positive effects of visualization could be a difference maker to getting to the next level and giving you clear guidelines to maintain your skills while healing from an injury or during the off season.

Sports visualization existed long before Alan Richardson's experiment, yet it has not gained full traction as a training technique even today. To a dedicated athlete, visualizing a sport is an anti-sport. But the opposite is true, and athletes should be doing both physical training and visualization. They are probably wary of overthinking; in the sports world, we hear expressions like "paralysis by overanalysis" or "beware the left-brained!" But visualization is not meant to replace physical training; it's meant to supplement the physical to improve even faster.

According to a *Stanford Encyclopedia of Philosophy* article on brain imagery, visualization works because our brains do not know the difference between performing an act and visualizing an act (Thomas 2014). According to this article, when we visualize an act, the brain sends an impulse to perform the movement. Cells in the brain work together to create memories and learned behaviors; as a result, the same nerves and muscles fire in the same order whether you are physically active or merely visualizing. Everybody from professional athletes to actors and successful business moguls use visualization.

Teach your athletes to practice visualization every day. This can rapidly accelerate the fulfillment of their dreams, goals, and ambitions. Actively visualizing your goals enables you to achieve a variety of things: It activates your creative subconscious, which generates creative ideas, inevitably bringing you closer to your goals. It programs your brain to more readily recognize the resources you need and the actions you need to take each day to achieve your goals. It activates the law of attraction, drawing into your life the people and resources you will need. Visualization is very specific; you must truly imagine the situation and how you will experience it through all of your senses.

You can explain visualization as it relates to the senses with a script like the one that follows.

Sight

The first thing you want to do when visualizing something is to see it as clearly as you can. Let's say you want a new car. See in your mind's eye the color and detail of the car; maybe it's candy electric blue with chrome detailing, special rims matching the chrome, and tan leather interior with a dash that glows red at night. The stick shift has roman numerals on it in black lettering. The rug is tan; the back seat is small. When you walk up to this car, the overall picture should be in your mind's eye. Be as specific as you can.

Sound

If we are using the car as our example, you might start with how it sounds when you unlock the door. Then notice the hum of the engine once you start the car. Hear the sound of your favorite song playing on your dream stereo system, the sound of the transmission shifting into gear, and the sound of the engine growling as you press on the accelerator.

Taste

You might not use this one when visualizing a new car, but for now let's say you do. Maybe you stop off at a local coffee shop while driving your new car. What are you drinking? Where will you put the cup in your car? Is your drink sweet, salty, sour, or maybe a little bitter? Really taste it.

Smell

Now back to the car. One of people's favorite things about a new car is the aroma. When you sit inside, what do you smell? Can you smell the freshness of the leather seats? Does it smell like a new car? Have you placed your favorite air freshener inside? When you roll down the window, can you smell the crisp autumn air flowing through the inside of the car and mixing with the smell of leather?

Touch

Run your hand down the side of the car. Feel how slick the paint feels under your hand. Sit in the driver's seat and feel how comfortable the seat is under you. Wrap your hands around the steering wheel and feel it. Is it soft, is it hard? Now grab the stick shift and ease it into gear. Notice how it feels in your hands.

Emotion

Now it is time to use your sixth sense, and this one is the most fun. Your sixth sense lets you know in your gut how you feel about something. Imagine now how you will feel when you drive that new car off the lot. Are you excited? Are you smiling? How do you feel when you show it to your friends? Do you feel a sense of pride? Are you doing somersaults inside your head? How do they react?

That is the complete process of visualization. Do not skip a step; believe it and do it often. For athletes, visualization increases athletic performance by improving motivation, coordination, and concentration. It also aids in relaxation and helps reduce fear and anxiety. Visualization techniques can help your athletes to train their minds to believe that what they want to have and achieve is already a reality. We already determined that, to be successful at it, you must use all six senses.

In life and work, success begins with a goal. It could be losing weight, playing professionally in a Super Bowl or a World Series, or asking for a raise. Big and small, goals give us all direction and keep us heading in that direction. It takes a lot of hard work and determination to reach your desired destination in life. Many athletes get stuck in the goal-setting state. Perhaps they start out with good intentions and a plan, but then they cannot seem to make it happen. There are many possible reasons for this, such as busyness, impatience, fear, and pressure. Before they can believe in a goal and start clearly visualizing it, they must first have an idea of what it looks like. They must create a mental image of their future as they design it. Through visualization, they can get a glimpse of what is possible. When this happens, they will become excited and motivated.

Another useful practice is to use props, which trick the mind into believing that your goal is a realized fact. A famous story that illustrates the success of this technique concerns the actor Jim Carrey, who grew up poor and who dreamed of being an actor. He took visualization seriously, and he would imagine directors coming up to him and offering him acting jobs. Jim believed in the use of props. He wrote himself a check for $10 million, dated it, and wrote "for acting services rendered" in the memo line. A few months before the date he had written on the prop check, he received a real $10 million check for his performance in *Dumb & Dumber*.

Be creative when using props, and make them as realistic as possible. For example, if your athlete is trying to play a sport professionally, encourage her to write herself a letter from a team with an offer and intent to sign her, or have her put her name on the back of a jersey of her dream team and hang it where she can see it every day.

I am known for writing up to 20 goals a year for myself each January. I carefully think about my desires for the year. I think big, and I write down dates for achieving each goal. It is important that you write the goals, that you visualize them, and that you use props, but it is most important that you take action on them each day. They will not magically arrive without an effort on your part. What happens to my goals by December? Typically I achieve at least 60 to 70 percent of them. Some I re-date because things are happening, they just have not fully appeared yet. I also find that the ones I did not act on, and consequently did not achieve, may not have been that important to me anyway, so things happened as they should have happened.

Here are some key tips for visualization to share with your athletes.

- Visualize each day, the more the better. Use any moment of downtime, even two to three minutes.
- Write down visualizations using descriptive language. The memory responds well to the written word, and this can reinforce one's ideas and increase the likelihood of achieving goals.
- Be proactive; visualization works if you work at it.

Mindfulness should be taught as a lifelong, daily practice; it should be built into our lives just as you fill in your calendar with to-do lists. There is no risk, and by adding time daily for mindfulness practice, we can become better athletes, better spouses, better sons and daughters, better mentors, and better examples for others.

The benefits of mindfulness can be very exciting, and it should be considered a necessary component of training. Your athletes should be encouraged to practice any and all of the techniques that motivate them. Remember, this is not a silver bullet but a lifelong way to exercise the mind and achieve mental well-being. It can change the way they think, move, train, and recover, and this will become evident with purposeful practice.

REFERENCES

Hyatt, Michael. "What the Internet Is Doing to Our Brains (And What We Can Do About It)." *This Is Your Life,* July 25, 2012. Podcast audio. https://michaelhyatt.com/19-what-the-internet-is-doing-to-our-brains-podcast.html.

Nhat Hanh, Thich. *Living Buddha, Living Christ*. 20th anniversary edition. 2007. New York: Riverhead Books.

Richardson, Alan. "Mental Practice: A Review and Discussion Part I", *Research Quarterly*. 1967. American Association for Health, Physical Education and Recreation, 38(1): 95-107, DOI: 10.1080/10671188.1967.10614808

Richardson, Alan. "Mental Practice: A Review and Discussion Part II", *Research Quarterly*. 1967. American Association for Health, Physical Education and Recreation, 38(2): 263-273, DOI: 10.1080/10671188.1967.10613388

Siegel, Daniel. *The Mindful Brain*. 2007. New York: W.W. Norton & Company.

Thomas, Nigel J.T. 2018. "Mental Imagery." *Stanford Encyclopedia of Philosophy,* edited by Edward N. Zalta. https://plato.stanford.edu/entries/mental-imagery.

Maximize Your Yoga Practice

4

The rules about hydration, nutrition, and other necessities for athletes practicing yoga are not hard and fast rules. I believe that people should be mindful of their bodies and how they perform best. Tune into how you feel each day, and surrender to that. If you are tired and in doubt about the day's training, don't train. If you are hungry and want to eat vegetables, have them. If the day brings you cravings for cheese, eat it. Do it all in moderation and sensibly. Here are some guidelines for optimum health and performance.

STAY HYDRATED

I have heard many rules about proper hydration, such as what to drink, what not to drink, and how often to drink. Some people find success with the standard six to eight eight-ounce glasses of nonsugary fluids per day. Others drink a number of ounces of nonsugared fluids per day equal to half their body weight. Some add that coffee should not be included when hydrating, and others live by Gatorade and other sports drinks. The problem with all of these valid techniques is that they require an awful lot of thinking, planning, and tracking every day. In my experience, this is often to no avail; many athletes still end up not being properly hydrated by the evening. I am going to make it easy for you: No thinking, no counting, and no worrying about what type of fluid to drink. You will simply go by the (for lack of a better term) "pee chart," as shown in figure 4.1.

Over the years of having the honor and privilege of working with professional teams, I have seen them achieve much success with this user-friendly guide. I have even seen teams go as far as to bench players for lack of hydration to protect them from situations that might compromise their health. Encourage your athletes to take a picture of this chart and use it until they know just by observation if they are properly hydrated. In my bathroom, the chart is framed and hung in plain sight.

EAT APPROPRIATELY

You can easily find militant nutrition guidelines that claim to contribute to the success your practice of yoga. Different forms of yoga adhere to different beliefs, from fasting to veganism and beyond. I am not going to preach what is right for you or your athletes. Everyone should practice being mindful and should explore what feels natural. Athletes from all sports must pay attention to their diets and tendencies, keeping in mind training cycles, the timing of nutrition intake, body types, the demands of a sport, and overall goals. If a wrestler needs to cut weight, many of the rules go out the door. That is an extreme example, but it is a factor to consider. It would be impossible to give a general guideline to go by because athletes and sports have specific needs. Athletes who take mindfulness to heart and practice it regularly will be crystal clear about their needs. If there are 800 million athletes on the planet, there are 800 million different ways of eating.

Simple guidelines for yoga practice include the following:

- Do not consume food or heavy drinks for two to three hours before class.
- Pay attention to how your body digests food types such as dairy, and substitute with alternatives if necessary.
- Eat good-quality whole foods as much as possible.
- Eat slowly, and chew food thoroughly.
- Eat a variety of foods from all food groups.
- Do not adhere to eating fads or trends.
- Consult with a professional about proper supplementation.
- Consider a full allergen blood panel to detect even subtle allergies that can affect wellness.
- Go with your gut; if it is not good for the body, your gut will surely tell you.

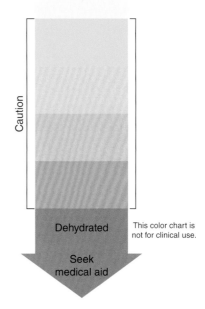

Figure 4.1   Urine color chart to determine proper hydration.

Every athlete has probably gone to practice or a game with a rumbling, empty stomach. Eating correctly on game day and beyond is essential to outstanding performance. Training and skill are of obvious importance, but the body's energy level is critical. Also, the needs of yoga practice differ from the needs of game day, training, and other activities.

You have likely heard that breakfast is the most important meal of the day, and I believe this to be true. Start the day with a well-rounded breakfast containing carbohydrates and a source of protein. My favorite book for suggested meals is *The Athlete's Plate* by Adam Kelinson. Because many athletes jam their day with as much quality training as possible, they need to plan meals ahead of time for optimum performance, and they must not skip meals. Athletes can choose whole-grain bread, crackers, cereal, and pasta for lasting energy if they need to eat well before a game or practice. Store snacks and food at proper temperatures to prevent spoilage if something won't be eaten for a while. Athletes should be careful in their choice of sports drinks that are intended to provide an energy boost for endurance sports or for training sessions lasting more than an hour; too often, these drinks are packed with unnecessary sugar and do not provide proper hydration.

Athletes love their protein and what it does for their bodies. Muscles love protein as well. Protein helps increase muscle strength, enhance recovery from exercise, and build more muscle. Athletes should spread out their protein intake throughout the day for the best digestion, and they should choose quality protein sources like lean meats, nuts, and powders. Eliminate fatty foods and protein choices, which slow digestion and cause the body to tire out quickly. The timing of eating can be everything, so athletes should be mindful of when to eat in relation to competition or training. The body may need up to three hours to fully digest, and it's important to honor that time frame. If the body is trying to digest and to train at the same time, an athlete is sure to experience cramping, illness, and other digestive issues. Nothing is worse than having stomach cramps, nausea, vomiting, or diarrhea and then having to perform on the field.

PRACTICE REGULARLY

Athletes will ask how often they should practice yoga. Again, I cannot make a blanket statement for all athletes. They must consider their training cycle first and then see how they feel to determine the frequency that works best. Most people find that yoga rewards the practitioner who does it regularly.

What if there are no mirrors where I teach my athletes?

I prefer to conduct my classes where there are no mirrors. I want my athletes to feel the experience and to be guided by my words to achieve the poses properly. Your athletes have to trust that if their poses are wrong, you will guide them properly. There are no mirrors during competition; they should not have them when they train, either.

Regular yoga sessions improve balance, functional strength, flexibility, mental toughness, focus, ease of breathing, and stress levels. Regular practice offers far greater benefits for long-term health than just improved performance in a particular sport. Many benefits are immediate, such as a reduction in anxiety; more long-term benefits include supple joints and muscles. Yoga breathing activates the parasympathetic nervous system that controls relaxation and lowers stress. The frequency of yoga practice will help determine the level of well-being, expertise, and relaxation your athletes experience.

Everyone should listen to their bodies. I often say that any amount of weekly yoga practice is better than none, and many notable teachers recommend two or three hour-long sessions per week. All athletes should know how their bodies respond. I trained an NFL player who did my yoga video before every game. Other athletes like to lay low before a game, practicing more of the mental work we learn in yoga. Still others find that the restorative styles of pregame yoga help them excel.

It typically takes two to three sessions of yoga practice a week for at least 8 to 10 weeks to see an increase in strength and flexibility from a yoga routine, so an athlete should plan for that within the training cycle. I prefer to practice later in the day, which is when I find my body responds best. For others, an evening practice can generate too much energy and make sleeping difficult, so evening mindfulness works better for them.

CHOOSE THE RIGHT EQUIPMENT

I may vary in my opinion of when to eat, when to practice, and how to hydrate, but I have clear ideas of proper equipment. For one, anyone practicing yoga should always wear clothing that is snug but not constricting. You don't want your athletes to worry about a shirt hanging improperly or shorts riding up when they should be focused on a pose.

Everyone needs a 10-foot-long strap with a quick-release mechanism with which to abort a pose at the drop of a hat or at the birth of a cramp. I suggest two three-inch foam yoga blocks and two four-inch yoga blocks for the various poses and restorative positions you will learn and teach. A timer is useful for keeping the focus on breathing without having to worry about timing the length of poses. A good yoga mat on a stable surface is needed for proper support. Practicing on artificial turf is not always optimal; I have often seen athletes get bits of artificial turf in their eyes when they do restorative poses on turf.

Is it important to do my practice on an actual yoga mat?

While sometimes I have to conduct my classes on artificial turf or outdoor fields, a yoga mat is the best surface. This promotes confidence and safety; when athletes do not have to worry about slipping, they can engage the proper muscles to execute the poses.

WARM UP PROPERLY

A warm-up is done before the main poses of your practice. The warm-up routine activates every joint in the body and get the athlete breathing and ready to stretch. Athletes who just came from the weight room or the field do not need to do the warm-up routine because they should already be loosened up and ready to go. Relax, breathe, and sink into the poses. Detailed warm-ups are included in chapters 8 and 9.

SET POWERFUL GOALS

More often than not, athletes go through life letting it happen without a plan. You would never build your dream home by hiring a builder, handing him nails, sheetrock, and wood and walking away. Amazingly, this is how many athletes approach their lives. An athlete or anyone else must meticulously think, dream, strategize, and take action each day to enjoy the desired outcome.

As you work with athletes, help them to think about the big picture, and teach them how to set goals to help them achieve both short-term and long-term success. Ask them the following questions:

Are you living your dreams?

Are you happy every day?

Are you living your best life?

What would you do if you knew you could not fail?

Is every day full of possibility?

Are you contributing to society?

Do you feel the universe is working through you to serve others?

If the answer to any of these is no, then that is the perfect time to help your athletes to be a force for change, both in their own lives and in a broader sense. When your athletes can answer yes to each of these questions, they will be well on their way to knowing exactly what they want to achieve in their careers, and they will be inspired to take action immediately. These questions can get help them develop a clear vision and a purpose for their lives.

Create a Vision

Your athletes must have a vision for what they want their lives to look like. In any sport, athletes visualize scoring that winning goal or throwing that perfect pass. Goals provide long-term vision and short-term motivation. In goal setting, we imagine exactly what we want our lives to look like in the years to come. From that vision, you can create the life that you are truly meant to live. You lead by example as a teacher, so when you have set goals for yourself, your students will want the same. Goal setting is a very compelling way to motivate people, including yourself!

When your athletes list their goals, you want them to consider all the possibilities and to think big. Ask questions such as, what is your life's purpose? What do you believe you were put on the planet to achieve? They may want to list their expectations for the future, career breakthroughs they want to accomplish, and awards or achievements they can envision earning. If an athlete says that he wants to be wealthy, ask what wealth means to him. He should be clear and concise: what is rich to one person is poor to another, and definitions of wealth vary.

You want your athletes to create the big picture, with the operative word being *big*. To create an ideal life, a person needs to start with a clear vision. You can practice the following activity for yourself and then with your athletes to help create that vision and plan for success.

1. Close your eyes and ask yourself where you see yourself in 10 years. Be as accurate as possible, down to the color of the sheets that you sleep on.

2. Open your eyes, grab a pen and paper, and begin to brainstorm. Write as much as you possibly can about what you actually want if nothing could stop you. You might not know at first, but once you start putting your thoughts to paper, ideas will come out that may surprise you. If you think that you want it, write it down. Think enormous. Write down lofty goals. If you see yourself as the next Michael Jordan or as a professional golfer even though you have never golfed a day in your life, write it down. All of this information is for you to clarify and hone. It is personal, so be honest with yourself.

3. Next, write down what you are good at. Often we are unsure how to describe our talents and skills. You should have a solid understanding of your gifts. If you cannot think of anything, ask at least three family members or friends for their opinions. It is most effective if you share the following questions in writing when you ask your supporters to answer them. They can respond in an email or on paper. They are likely to be more honest if they do not have to answer to you in person.

   ► What are my key strengths?

   ► What is unique about me?

   ► What, if anything, is bothersome to you about me?

   ► What do you or others rely on me for?

   ► Could you tell me something about myself that I do not already know?

   ► When am I most powerful?

   ► In what situation am I least powerful?

   ► When am I most inspired?

   ► If you could wish one thing for me in the next year, what would it be?

4. Analyze your results. Do you see patterns in the answers? What responses in particular surprise you or stand out to you, and why? This is the time to notice if your dreams are in alignment with what your strengths and interests are. After you start to grasp this and find direction, you are going to rehash the past. Often we are told to forget the past. However, rewinding and remembering can give you insight into mistakes you do not want to repeat.

5. In this step, write out five successes you specifically remember having that are relevant to your goals. Brainstorm ways you can duplicate them. Then, write down five failures you have experienced. These are very important to learn from. Finally, write down any past unmet goals that still linger in your mind. You need to decide either to revisit them or to move on from them.

Flip the Script on Your Thinking

Aside from material wealth, athletes may express the desire to live a full life. They can best achieve this if they avoid thinking in ways that limit their positivity. You could say that some people think sparingly, and that can be self-defeating.

Examples of thinking sparingly include assessing oneself against others, living by self-limiting standards, or engaging in "should" type of thinking. For example, someone might think, "I should have gone to school for my master's degree, but now I can't because it is too late." Others may exhibit "I"-based thinking, which is selfish and not for the greater good. It means thinking in terms of "What is in it for me?" Some people who live within this narcissistic mindset cannot find room to accept information and learn. This type of thinking is displayed as, "I am right and you are wrong; I already know." Finally, you may meet athletes who have a doomsday outlook all the time. Their typical mode of operation is, "There is no possibility, that's just the way the world works." All of these glass-half-empty types of thinking put a person in a negative state of mind and can create self-fulfilling prophecies.

Let's analyze how to shift our thinking by starting with typical phrases that already challenge us. Suggest that your athletes try thinking and seeing the plentiful side of things. They should apply this way of thinking to commitments, partnerships, and work, and they should be open to all possibilities that appear. This new attitude can propel them forward as they think. Consider the following examples of sparing thoughts and plentiful thoughts:

SPARING THOUGHTS	PLENTIFUL THOUGHTS
"It will be difficult."	"Anything is possible."
"It is going to be risky."	"I cannot fail when I plan and trust the universe."
"It will take a long time."	"There is only now; I live fully in the present."
"There will be family drama."	"I must follow what I feel so deeply."
"I do not deserve it." "It is not my nature."	"Everyone deserves the grace of truth and happiness."
"I cannot afford it."	"If I keep my faith in the universe, all I need will be provided."
"No one will help me."	"Serve others; success that is unshared is failure."
"I am not strong enough."	"If I can conceive of it, passion and the ability to create it will be given."
"I am not smart enough." "I am too busy."	
"I am too scared."	"There is nothing to fear."

Narrow It Down

Now that you have your vision brainstormed, you are ready to start breaking it down so that you can focus on your most important goals. Goals are set on different levels. First, you create your "big picture" of what you want and decide what large-scale goals you want to achieve. Second, you break these down into the smaller targets that you must hit so that you reach your goals. Finally, once you have your plan, you start working to achieve it.

You may want to start the organization process by thinking about what you would do if you knew that you could not fail. A big-picture goal might be to move to Los Angeles and become a famous actor. To do that, set a time frame for achieving the goal, such as moving to Los Angeles in six months. Without a commitment to time, it is not a goal; it is just a random thought or wish. Then you work backward, discerning things like how much money you need to move and need to have in savings so you can pound the pavement, where to find an agent, how to leave your current job, and any other details. In this example, once there's an action plan, it's time to talk to your current boss, go to a bank to start a savings account, and take on extra work to help build savings.

You might come across athletes who offer excuses for why they can't achieve their goals. They say things like, "I want to play professional baseball, but between family and school obligations, there just isn't enough time to train." In this case, you might help the athlete understand that lack of time is an illusion or a perception; we all have the same amount of time in a day. We can decide how we use our time. If the athlete is truly committed to a goal, he will put in the work to make it happen. If he wants to be a pro, he should think about things like where he wants to play, the process of training, the contacts he needs to make, and when he should make those contacts. Athletes should be specific when setting goals, and setting SMART goals is a way to do that.

SMART is a commonly used acronym that helps goal setters to organize their thoughts and structure their goals. Using this method will streamline the way you think. SMART removes the guesswork and gives you a step-by-step guide to creating success. SMART stands for *Specific, Measurable, Attainable, Realistic,* and *Time-sensitive*. Here is an example of how to establish goals using SMART:

- *Specific*: I will complete my first half marathon on July 2, 2020.
- *Measurable*: I will save $10,000 so I can move closer to my dream college by July 2, 2021.
- *Attainable*: I will complete PYFS yoga training by September 2022.
- *Realistic*: I will hike the Sedona Red Rock by December 2020.
- *Time-sensitive*: I will start a family by the time I am 30 years old.

What is the number one tip for conducting a class for athletes?

Pay attention to your voice, and structure your class. Always speak in your most confident tone to fully command your athletes' attention. Be sure about what you are teaching, and be prepared to answer questions on the fly.

Write It Down

Take time to be clear about your goals by writing them down. The things you want to accomplish that are constantly on your mind are the goals that will demand your full focus. They are the things you see others doing and excelling at and the thoughts that give you goosebumps. Sit down and first just write with a stream of consciousness; write down everything you are thinking with complete disregard for punctuation. Think about the people you admire and even find yourself a little jealous of and why you feel that way. I redefined jealousy as a way I identify the things I want most by my reaction to others who already attained them. Your reality will bubble up to the surface as you write down all of your thoughts, and then you can go back and formally re-write them as specific goals. Some additional tips include:

- Write in first person and present tense, as though the goals have already been achieved.
- Use clear, specific words that demonstrate commitment.
- Allow yourself to see pictures of your life as you dream it.
- Write goals in the affirmative.

- Include a time line with each goal.
- Time travel to the future if you need clarity.
- Begin with three domains: personal, health, and career.

Once an athlete knows her goals and has written them down, encourage her to paste them up around her home or practice space as gentle reminders of what she is working toward. She should see her goals many times each day: on a corkboard in her room, on Post-it notes on the mirror, in reminders on a smartphone, and in pop-up messages on the computer.

Follow Up

It is not enough to write your goals down and then walk away and never revisit them. To meet your goals, you must constantly revisit what goals you have written. You should make it a habit to read your list each and every day until your brain is so used to seeing them, they become solidified as reality.

Another suggestion is to write your most compelling goals on a sticky note and place it strategically where you will see it several times a day. I also suggest setting an alarm on your phone and labeling the alarm with your goal. Each day when you see your goal alarm pop up, take a deep breath and take a moment to imagine how you will feel after you meet the goal.

Here are some additional suggestions for successful goal setting:

- Accept *total* responsibility for everything that happens in your life.
- Revisit your goals often.
- Revise goals if necessary.
- Find a goal buddy so you can help each other to stay on track.
- Share your goals with people you trust for accountability.
- Create visual reminders of your goals, such as vision boards.
- If you get off track, realize it, then forgive yourself and restart the journey.
- Move forward constantly.

I have no doubt that with consistent execution of the goal-setting practice outlined here, you will not only achieve the goals of your dreams, you will also become an activist and example to your athletes about the importance of goal setting to achieve their peak performance and life's purpose and how satisfying goal setting is.

Standing Poses

5

Standing poses make up a large part of a yoga practice. In many Power Yoga for Sports classes, the first half or more of the class is done on your feet in challenging standing poses. In standing poses, you will develop better posture, improved breathing, and greater stability and balance. Demanding balancing poses also call on your abdominals for support, so a welcome side effect of practice is a better-toned belly.

Here are a few things to remember before we start:

- Always fix your gaze on a single point in front of you to maintain balance and concentration.
- You may feel soreness in your feet and lower legs as you realign and strengthen finer muscles that are often neglected. Be consistent, and you will see improvements in as little as two weeks.
- If you are unsure of what you are feeling during a pose, speak with a physician and consider working with a properly trained yoga teacher for personal instruction before continuing a yoga practice.
- If you are new to yoga, you may want to practice near a wall for a few weeks until your confidence and balance improve.
- It is best to execute standing poses on a stable surface, such as wood with a yoga mat on top. Artificial turf and rugs make balance much more difficult.

Is it OK to use the wall to assist with balance while doing standing poses?

It is OK for your athletes to use a wall if they are rehabbing from injury. Otherwise, I prefer they stand free in the center of their mats. I would rather they attempt poses that they can only hold for shorter periods at first so that they can build the balance, strength, and stamina to hold them for longer periods.

STANDING MOUNTAIN POSE
TADASANA

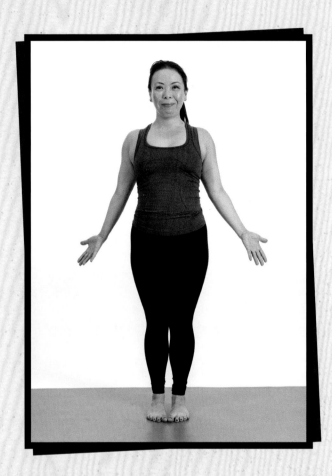

Standing mountain pose may not seem difficult, but it is the basis for all other poses, and it should be performed at the beginning of each class. This pose provides important clues for your readiness for the session and provides an opportunity to stand still and take deep, productive, relaxing breaths.

Not only is standing mountain pose a great way to strengthen the lower half of the body, but doing this pose in front of a mirror or in the presence of a yoga teacher is a great assessment tool. It is very important in the philosophy of Power Yoga for Sports and all yoga to remain constantly aware of your body as a tool. Athletes, soccer moms, and kids all need to learn about their bodies in order to sideline injuries before they happen or strengthen their bodies in the case of a jarring incident. Maintaining strength could make the difference between walking away from a hard fall and taking a trip to the emergency room.

When you practice standing mountain pose in front of a mirror or instructor regularly, you can compare one side of the body to the other, notice misalignments, identify asymmetries, and address them through training. For example, I always look to my shoulders for evidence of stress and tightness. I look to see if one shoulder is higher, how the shoulders rotate, how my hand faces forward on each side, and if my back torques to one side or the other. I then ask my yoga teacher for advice. Consider the first time you do this as a baseline test to compare to for the rest of your life. You could even take photos and archive them for comparison in the future.

BENEFITS

✓ Improves posture

✓ Strengthens legs, knees, and feet

✓ Strengthens butt and abs

✓ Helps develop arches in flat feet

✓ Provides an opportunity for full-body assessment

CONTRAINDICATIONS

This pose is contraindicated for those with low blood pressure, severe sciatic pain, or a history of recent surgery.

HOW TO

1. Stand with your feet together, heels about one to two inches apart and feet parallel, and find yourself in the center of your foot.

2. Externally rotate the thighs, and lift the kneecaps slightly to engage the legs.

3. Roll your shoulders up and gently back to open the chest, and rotate your palms to face forward, feeling the shoulder blades on your back.

4. Keep your back in a neutral position to relax the pelvis.

5. On your inhales, lengthen the spine; on the exhale, maintain the height you created.

VARIATIONS

- Do this pose while standing against a wall with the backs of your heels, your sacrum, or your lower back and shoulder blades flush up against the wall.

- Try standing crescent pose as a variation on mountain pose to elongate the side of the body and the lats and open the lungs to increase lung capacity (see variation 1). In mountain pose, inhale with the arms over your head, grab the left wrist with the right hand, and lengthen the left side of the body as you bend the body to the right. Keep the entire body facing straight ahead.

- Try standing backbend as a variation on mountain pose to train the extension of the spine and build strength in the back (see variation 2). While in standing mountain pose, bring the palms together over your head. Tuck your tailbone under to protect the back, keep the upper arms alongside your head, and begin to chest lift into a backbend. Go as far as you can without straining the back.

VARIATION 1

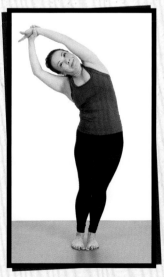

VARIATION 2

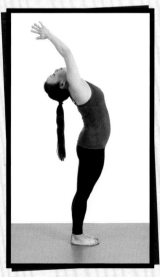

STANDING FORWARD BEND
UTTANASANA

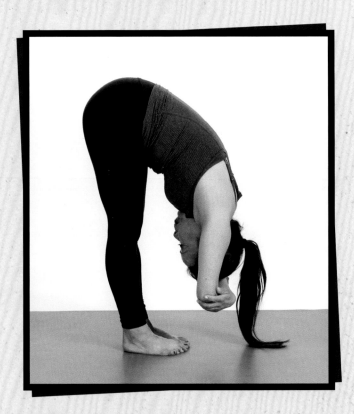

As widely recognized as downward dog, standing forward bend should be a staple pose in your yoga routine. Even if you have never stepped into a yoga studio or tried a video, chances are you have folded over into simple standing forward bend.

Standing forward bend opens the hamstrings. It is very important to keep the hamstrings open to reduce strain and tightness in the back. Long hours and hard work, long drives, and poor sleep are only a few of the many things that contribute to tight backs. Since the hamstring attaches on the lowest part of the pelvis, if the legs are rigid, it easily pulls down on the pelvis, putting unnecessary stress on the back. Over time, a chain reaction can happen: tight hamstrings, strained back, unstable hips, knee problems. When you regularly perform standing forward bend, you will not see improvements overnight, but in time your legs will loosen, and you will see a huge difference in how your body feels, so stay committed. It is a great pose for practicing visualization: seeing your hamstrings opening up. As basic as you may think this pose is, it is very important to learn proper technique in order to keep your back safe and to open the hamstrings to their fullest.

For the athlete, this pose is also important for assessing postural needs and imbalances. Athletes must constantly evaluate their bodies. All athletes can benefit from hamstring improvement. A competitor with flexible legs can improve his speed. I stress that the formula for power is strength plus flexibility. Speed and agility are always priorities for athletes. Reducing strain on the back can prevent injury and increase playing time.

BENEFITS

✓ Calms the brain

✓ Relieves stress

✓ May alleviate mild depression

✓ Stretches the hamstrings, calves, and hips

✓ Strengthens the thighs and knees

✓ Improves digestion

✓ Reduces anxiety

CONTRAINDICATIONS

This pose is contraindicated for an athlete who has had recent back, knee, or hamstring surgery. An athlete may be able to practice the pose in a limited fashion but should be observed by a trained yoga teacher.

HOW TO

1. Stand with your feet shoulder-width apart and parallel.

2. Plug your feet equally into the floor, with your weight slightly forward, but not so far forward that you grip with your toes.

3. Bend your knees a little, and fold over at your hips; never fold from your waist.

4. Touch your chest and belly to your thighs with the knees still bent. Constantly check that your knees track over your toes as you are bent forward; it is important for the safety and integrity of the knee joints to have the knees positioned this way at all times.

5. Keeping your chest and belly connected to your thighs, start to slowly straighten your knees, feeling as if you are lifting your hips up to the sky. If you feel like the chest is separating from your legs, you went a little too far.

6. If you feel stable enough, hold each elbow with the opposite hand and hang. Continue to check that your feet line up with each other and that they stay parallel. Although it is tempting to close your eyes and relax here, don't, or you will lose your balance.

7. You should not be afraid to sway back and forth and to bend and straighten the knees—anything that helps you to negotiate further into the stubborn hamstrings. I encourage my students to drape a 12-pound sandbag over their forearms while holding the pose. This method will get you to the next level faster.

STANDING FORWARD BEND AGAINST A WALL
UTTANASANA

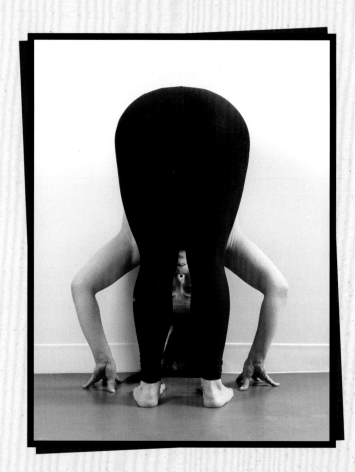

Many people want to improve the strength and flexibility of their hamstrings. My experience with this pose is that because you use gravity, you do not have to worry about falling over. I love this version of standing forward bend to fully release with the support of a wall and to increase flexibility more quickly and safely. You can release and relax in the pose faster, therefore increasing the flexibility of the hamstrings faster. You can also let the head go as you relax the neck, which helps to reduce any strain in that area.

Tight hamstrings not only slow an athlete's game; they can cause pressure in the lower back and decreased rotation of the spine. Tight hamstrings put unnecessary demands on the knees and negatively affect the hip flexors and power. With all that said, improving flexibility in the hamstrings is not easy; it takes time and dedication due to the thickness and size of the muscle group. With this version of standing forward bend, you will see faster results, and you will not have the added worry about overstretching the back that you may have with other versions of forward bending. Flexible hamstrings can provide a greater range of motion in the spine and can lessen the low back load. This pose can also help to maintain the proper lumbar curve, which offers better shock absorption when landing on courts or turf.

BENEFITS

✓ Lengthens the hamstrings

✓ Places traction forces on the neck

✓ Stretches calves

✓ Relieves stress on the back

CONTRAINDICATIONS

This pose is contraindicated for those who have had recent back surgery, a history of vertigo, or glaucoma.

HOW TO

1. Find a safe, smooth wall that does not have pictures or obstacles on it.

2. Stand facing the wall with your feet approximately hip-width apart and parallel.

3. Bend your knees a lot, and carefully (without bumping your head on the wall) bring your chest and belly to your thighs.

4. Let the hands hang down to the floor, and keep the eyes open for balance. Make sure your feet are approximately 12 inches from the wall.

5. Lean your back and the back of your head against the wall to let the wall support you. The floor keeps your feet flat and in alignment, and gravity deepens the stretch.

6. Gradually straighten the legs as much as you can while your weight remains against the wall. Your tailbone should feel as if it is lifting up.

7. Hang, breathe, and hold this pose for about two to three minutes as you let your upper body sink down toward the floor.

8. If your heels come off the floor, reposition your feet so they stay flat. Some people are so tight that only the back of the head touches the wall. In time and with practice, your head will drop further down, and your mid-back will be touching.

9. To come out of this pose, bend the knees, and drop the butt down to the floor. You may experience some dizziness as you stand, so stand up slowly and with caution.

CHAIR
UTKATASANA

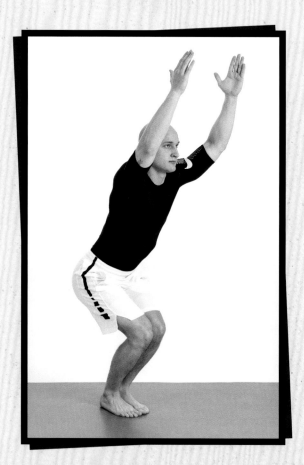

Sometimes known as fierce pose or powerful pose, this pose is part of the yogi's beloved salutation to the sun B. Chair pose is a relatively easy pose for most people to learn, but do not let its simplicity fool you into thinking it is easy. Some of the best thigh or quadriceps training comes from long chair holds.

Chair pose elongates the back and energizes the anterior and posterior spine. Since the pose opens the chest and builds power in the spine, it is a great pose for people who have breathing issues. Opening the rib cage and chest gives the lungs more space to breathe and opens the spaces between the ribs (intercostal muscles) for additional lung potential. Chair pose is also great for people with knee problems because it builds strength in the quadriceps to support the vulnerable knee joint.

Athletes will notice that chair pose is similar to the position taken in skiing and the ready position for a fielder in baseball. It is an awesome pose for those who play hockey as well and for all sports positions that require strong quadriceps, such as that of a lineman in football.

Chair pose also strengthens the vulnerable Achilles tendon because it gently stretches the tendon, giving the ankle more flexibility and range of motion. The more open and strong the muscles of your ankles and feet are, the more power you will have to run. This pose will also help athletes open the shoulder joint and elongate the side of the body, making it useful for sports like basketball, where greater range of motion in the shoulder makes it more comfortable to reach the arms overhead when playing defense.

BENEFITS

✓ Strengthens supporting muscles of major joints such as shoulders, hips, knees, and ankles

✓ Develops core strength

✓ Strengthens the quads and gluteal muscles

✓ Helps protect the knee joint by building stability

✓ Builds heat in the body

✓ Opens the shoulders and chest

✓ Improves ease of breathing

CONTRAINDICATIONS

This pose is contraindicated for those with severe back problems or recent ankle surgery. Those with knee problems should begin against a wall.

HOW TO

1. Begin in standing mountain pose, with the feet together and equal weight in both feet.

2. Lengthen and contract the muscles in the legs as you gently tuck the pelvis to avoid overarching the low back.

3. Lift the spine, open the shoulders and chest, and take a few deep breaths.

4. Lower your hips as if you were sitting on a chair behind you. Sit as deep as you can while keeping your feet flat. It is imperative that you keep your spine neutral and your back flat. At first, you can practice chair with the knees together; in time with practice, you can keep a one- to two-inch space between your knees.

5. Keep the knees pointed over the feet, the breath steady, and the chest open, with the chin parallel to the floor.

6. Raise your arms overhead without lifting your shoulders. Extend the arms and rotate your palms to face each other.

7. Drop your shoulders away from your ears, and draw your shoulder blades down your back. From a side view, there should be one line from your hip joint up through your torso, beyond your shoulder joint to your fingertips. As you sink your tailbone on the exhales, extend your body and arms on the inhale. Become aware of this dynamic opposition.

VARIATIONS

- Beginners can start this pose against a wall or lift the arms parallel to the floor rather than overhead.

- Try chair twist as a variation on chair to realign the spine and challenge balance at a different angle (see variation 1). While in chair, bring the left elbow to the outside of the right thigh. Pushing the back of the left upper arm against the outer thigh will enhance your ability to twist. While in chair twist, make sure your knees stay aligned with each other and point straight ahead.

- Try flat-back chair as a variation on chair to activate the abdominals and back muscles and at the same time to further challenge leg strength (see variation 2). In chair pose, extend the back halfway up until it becomes parallel with the floor, then hold.

(continued)

- Try figure-four chair as a variation on chair to further challenge balance and ankle strength and stability (see variation 3). In chair, place the outer left ankle against the right thigh above the knee.

- Try toe balance for further balance training (see variation 4). From figure-four chair or half lotus chair, slowly bend the knee of the supporting leg (e.g., the right knee) deeper until you can fold over and bring your hands to the floor. Lower yourself enough that you are sitting on your right heel. Your hands are alongside you on the floor or in prayer heart center for ultimate balance training.

- Try half lotus chair as a variation on chair to open the hip more deeply (see variation 5). This variation is similar to figure-four chair except the left foot would be all the way up into the right hip crease instead of against the left thigh. This variation makes it easier to fold over and then move into toe balance.

- Try half lotus chair twist as a variation on chair to add further balance challenges and a deep spinal twist (see variation 6). Twist to the right, bringing the left elbow to the outside of the right thigh, then press and twist, bringing the heart to the right.

VARIATION 1

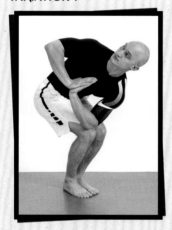

VARIATION 2

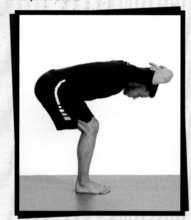

VARIATION 3

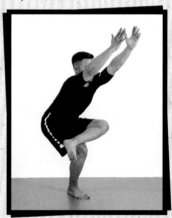

VARIATION 4

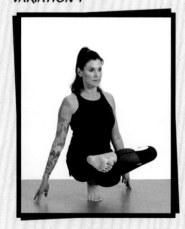

VARIATION 5

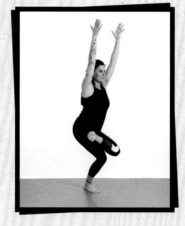

VARIATION 6

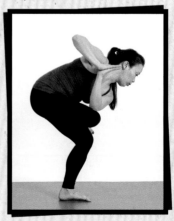

TRIANGLE
TRIKONASANA

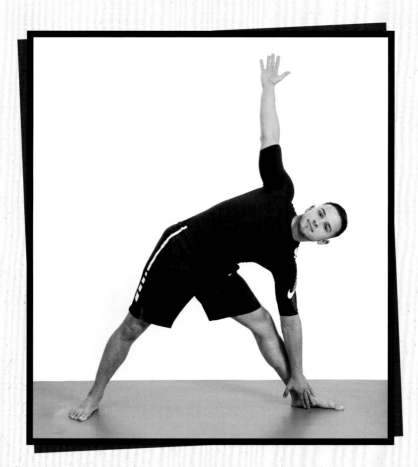

Tri means three and *kona* means corner or angle in Sanskrit, thus triangle pose, a popular pose in many styles of yoga. It can be a therapeutic pose, and, for the athlete and yogi alike, this pose is great for strengthening the core and back.

The rigors of everyday life tend to weaken our backs. This pose strengthens the back and core at the same time so they can support each other. Because it is also a gentle twist, it helps the back to stay supple and flexible as well, therefore helping to stave off the detrimental effects of arthritis and osteoporosis. It works the spine from the sacrum (base) all the way to the top of the neck. The twisting action also acts like a massage for our internal organs, helping them to remain in top function and to maintain their ability to rid us of toxins more efficiently.

Many sports require a strong yet flexible core and back. Think of the actions of a soccer player, changing direction on the field every second. Visualize a hockey player, whose continuous changes of direction require not just physically powerful abs, but an equally strong back and flexibility to match. Another reason athletes should practice triangle is because of its ability to open the muscles of the groin area. This is a spot of great vulnerability to any athlete, so it is a good idea to keep the groin area flexible. Since this is a standing pose, it also challenges balance, which is an obvious benefit to athletes. Finally, the positioning of the legs in triangle requires sturdy ankles. Positioning your ankles with the right balance of stretch and openness can decrease the likelihood of twists and sprains.

(continued)

BENEFITS

✓ Stretches the legs, especially the muscles around the knee, ankle joint, hips, groin muscles, hamstrings, and calves

✓ Stretches the shoulders, chest, and spine

✓ Strengthens the legs, knees, ankles, back, and abdominals (especially the obliques)

✓ Stimulates the abdominal organs

✓ Relieves stress

✓ Improves digestion and helps to relieve constipation

✓ Helps to alleviate back pain and symptoms of menopause

✓ Used therapeutically for anxiety, infertility, neck pain, and sciatica

CONTRAINDICATIONS

This pose is contraindicated for those who have diarrhea, eye strain, varicose veins, extreme fatigue, low or high blood pressure, heart conditions, or diagnosed neck problems.

HOW TO

1. Starting from standing mountain pose, turn sideways on your mat.

2. Walk or jump your feet apart approximately the length of one of your legs. It is very important to start this pose with perfect alignment so you can get deeper into the pose. Look down at your feet; you should be able to draw a straight line from your left big toe to your right big toe.

3. Turn your left foot out 90 degrees, and turn your right foot in about 45 degrees. Make sure you have a full external rotation (turn out to the left) of the left thigh so the left knee is aligned directly over the left foot. This means that the rotation of the left leg comes from the hip joint, not the ankle or knee joint.

4. Lift your arms up, and extend them out directly from your shoulders, parallel to the floor with the palms facing the floor. Take a deep breath, and drop your shoulders away from your ears.

5. Extend your torso to the left directly over the left leg, bending from the hip and not the waist. Imagine your body is between two panes of glass. Keep activating and pressing down through the outer right foot to secure your pose and lengthen the body.

6. Keep pressing your whole left foot down, being careful not to roll off your big toe connection to the floor. You should imagine that the left side of your body is just as long as the right; do not crunch up the left side, just go deeper.

7. Slide the back of the left hand down the inner left shin until you feel resistance in the leg and inner thigh, then stop and hold.

8. Do not hold onto your ankle; doing so deactivates your abdominal muscles and causes you to sink your left shoulder into your left ear. You want to maintain a feeling of pressing the back of your hand against the inner left leg and at the same time pressing slightly back against the hand with the left shin.

9. Drop your left side (shoulder and torso), and open your right side.

10. Your head should be held neutral. Don't let your head drop out of alignment. If you want to go deeper, you can turn your head to gaze at your right hand.

VARIATIONS

- Try revolving triangle pose as a variation on triangle pose to add a deeper focus on balance and to create an intense stretch in the IT band (see variation 1). From triangle pose (left foot forward), square the hips to the front of the mat, rotate the torso until it is square with the left leg, and soften the left knee. Place a block on the floor inside the left foot, and put your right hand on the block. Start to extend your spine and rotate it to the left, keeping your hips square. When you cannot twist any farther, straighten your left leg, and straighten your left arm up to the sky.

- Try reverse triangle as a variation on triangle pose to further strengthen the legs and open the side of the body for better respiration (see variation 2). From triangle pose, come up to standing (right foot forward), and start to slide the right hand down the back of the right thigh. Keep the heart lifted, and bring your left arm up and over your head.

VARIATION 1

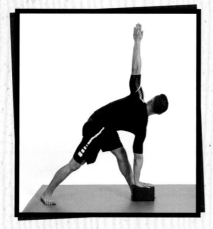

VARIATION 2

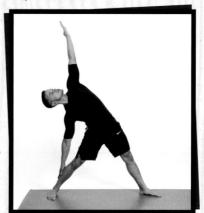

PYRAMID POSE
PARSVOTANASANA

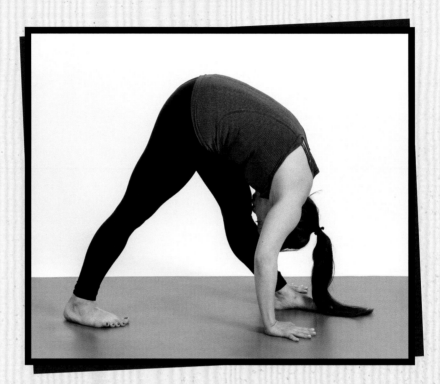

This pose is recognizable to both yogis and nonyogis. You can often see this pose being done instinctively by runners and team sport players during their warm-ups. Pyramid pose should be a staple for all who desire more open, flexible hamstrings.

For the beginner, pyramid pose elongates the back and lengthens the hamstrings. Tight hamstrings for most people result in changes in the angle of the pelvis. When the pelvis tucks too much, the result is stress and strain on the back. Everyone should stretch their hamstrings to preserve back health for life. When your back is aligned and strong, your gait and your entire body are more at ease during everyday chores. This results in less stress on all of your joints, especially on the vulnerable knee joint.

Athletes need open hamstrings for all of the reasons described, but in addition, their jobs often depend on the flexibility of their legs. Good posture and healthy joints are critical for athletes of all ages, but let's not forget the golden rule of Power Yoga for Sports: Strength + Flexibility = Power on the field of play. When athletes focus not only on doing the squats and lunges that fortify their legs but also on lengthening their leg muscles, the results are huge increases of power. Consider gymnasts—who generates more power during competition than they do? Whether you are a soccer player who must run eight to nine miles per game and create forceful kicks or a basketball player who must combine catlike agility with flying leaps, it is critical to devote time and attention on your hamstrings.

BENEFITS

✓ Mild inversion calms the brain and flushes the sinuses of congestion

✓ Stretches the spine

✓ Strengthens the legs and spine

✓ Improves posture

✓ Aids digestion

✓ Elongates hamstrings

CONTRAINDICATIONS

This pose is contraindicated for those who have had recent back surgery.

HOW TO

1. Start with your feet three to four feet apart with the feet parallel, toes pointed toward the long side of the mat.

2. Turn your left foot out 90 degrees to point directly to the front of your mat.

3. Turn the back foot in about 45 degrees. If you drew a line from the left heel back to the right foot, the heel would bisect the right foot. Firm your feet, and feel a slight external rotation of each thigh.

4. Take a deep breath, and elongate your spine. Put your hands on your hips, and be sure to square the hips to the front of your mat, swinging the right hip forward and pressing the left thigh back.

5. Start to fold your torso, from the hips, over the left thigh. Keep folding over with a flat back until your back is parallel to the floor. Without rounding, bring your fingertips to the floor. If you cannot reach, stack blocks on each side of the left foot so your hands can rest comfortably.

6. Inhale and elongate the back. Exhale as you deepen the stretch. If your hamstrings allow it, you can continue to fold with a flat back until your forehead touches your left shin, at the same time maintaining the strong feet, externally rotated thighs, long back, and active core.

7. Stay for several breaths, allowing the hamstrings to open and elongate.

EXTENDED SIDE ANGLE
UTTHITA PARSVAKONASANA

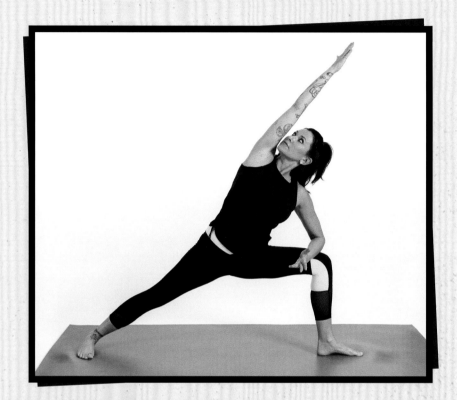

This pose is very familiar even for the nonyogi. Most people who have worked out have done this move or seen it done by others.

This is a great pose for building critical strength in the legs. This is important for building your practice into more challenging holds. It is a great transition pose when you are planning a flowing vinyasa practice. Extended side angle helps the practitioner to build enormous strength in the spine. A stronger, more stable spine helps to avoid slipped discs, herniation, and chronic pain. All these ailments can be experienced by repetitive movements during a typical day, such as driving, computer work, getting walked by your dog, and constant poor posture. Feel the extension and increased feeling of height this pose can give you, and breathe a sigh of relief, literally.

For the athlete, this is a great way to open the groin and inner thigh. Keeping the hips and thighs open and supple results in less stress on the knees. Athletes ask me about ways to relieve pressure on the knee joint. If the inner thigh is taut and pulling, it causes the placement of the foot to change, perhaps pronating or collapsing inward, and it subsequently puts pressure on the medial knee. Also, for athletes in cardio sports like soccer and basketball, it keeps the rib cage open to maximize space for your lungs to work. When you can breathe efficiently, you can stay on the field longer, experience less anxiety, and perform at your best.

BENEFITS

✓ Strengthens and stretches the legs, knees, and ankles

✓ Stretches the groins, spine, waist, chest and lungs, and shoulders

✓ Stimulates the abdominal organs

✓ Increases stamina

✓ Increases breath capacity

✓ Builds stability in the legs

CONTRAINDICATIONS

This pose is contraindicated for those who have had recent spinal, ankle, or knee surgery.

HOW TO

1. Start with your feet about three to four feet apart. Anchor your heel, and turn your right foot in about 45 degrees, as long as it can remain flat and plugged into the floor. Turn your left foot out 90 degrees. Feel the external rotation of your left thigh.

2. Tuck your hips under slightly to avoid putting unnecessary pressure on your low back.

3. Slowly bend your left knee to form a 90-degree angle.

4. Keep your knee tracking directly over your left foot to avoid injuring the knee. Feel the connection between both feet.

5. Lift your torso; be long and extended. Bring your arms up to shoulder height, palms facing down, much like a warrior 2 pose.

6. Exhale, and bring your right hand to the floor on the inside of your right foot. If this is too far to reach, bring the left elbow to rest gently on your left thigh. If placing the hand on the inside of the foot is too easy, bring your left hand to the floor on the outside of your left foot.

7. The key to this pose is to avoid collapsing the left side of your body while positioning yourself; keep the left side just as long as the right side.

8. Extend your right arm, and bring it up over your head. The angle of the right arm should be a continuation of the angle you have created with your extended right leg, one nice, long line.

9. Hold and breathe, extending as the name indicates.

VARIATIONS

- Try right angle pose as a variation on extended side angle to open the shoulder at a different angle to get a better feeling of your chest opening (see variation 1). While in extended right angle with your left hand to the floor, straighten the right arm up to the sky. The arms should now be in one line from right wrist to left fingertips.

- Try right angle bind as a variation on extended side angle to add extra challenges to leg strength and shoulder flexibility and to increase demands on balance and focus (see variation 2). While in right angle with the left leg bent and forward, bring the right arm up to the sky and behind your back. You can tuck the left hand in the left hip crease, or you can then move the left hand under the left hamstring and behind the back to connect left and right hands. Then you extend the back and open the heart.

VARIATION 1

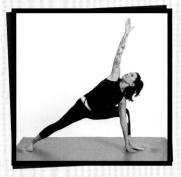

VARIATION 2

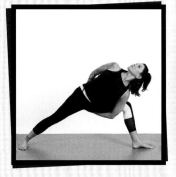

VARIATION 3

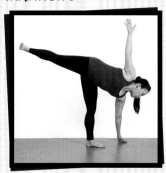

HALF MOON

ARDHA CHANDRASANA

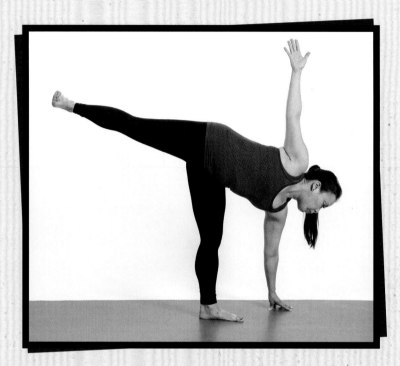

This pose adds a deeper level of balance and focus to your practice. It is set up to challenge your focus; if you lose focus, you will fall. It strengthens the legs, core, and back.

For the athlete, this pose is a nice way to pause and work on your mental toughness. Athletes who must repeatedly make diving plays and reaches will benefit from this pose because it trains you to extend, reach, and breathe. In addition, athletes like basketball players, runners, and cyclists who need strong, stable ankles should practice half moon.

BENEFITS

✓ Strengthens back, legs, ankles, and core   ✓ Improves balance   ✓ Improves focus

CONTRAINDICATIONS

This pose is contraindicated for those who have had recent knee or ankle surgery.

HOW TO

1. From right angle pose with the left foot forward, look down. Place the left fingertips on the floor or on a block approximately 12 to 18 inches from your left toes.

2. Place your right hand on your hip, and slowly begin to put all your weight into your left hand and left foot while lifting the right leg off the floor. Ultimately, your right leg should be parallel to the floor.

3. Extend your right hand straight up to the sky so that there is a straight line from your right fingers to your left fingers.

4. Radiate out from your center, and eventually move your gaze over the right shoulder up to the sky. Be sure to keep the neck extended.

CRESCENT LUNGE
ASHWA SANCHALANASANA

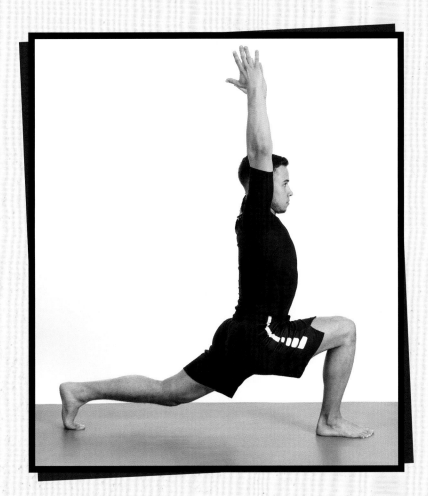

This is a very familiar pose. Most of you have done it without even knowing its roots are in yoga. It is many stretches in one, which makes it a great stretch for athletes to incorporate into their routines. Be sure to maintain perfect alignment.

This pose is a great choice for helping improve balance. Any time you are working with balance in a pose, you are using the abdominal muscles. It is very subtle but effective. When you achieve balance, you are in a more focused state, clearing your mind and deepening your breath.

For the athlete, the lunge is a perfect choice to open the hip flexors and the front of the thigh. We focus a lot on the tightness of the hamstrings; the truth is, you need to address the complementary muscles just as much to increase flexibility. When an athlete opens both the hamstrings and the hip flexors, it becomes easier to run and jump and recover. You lower the risk of injury by being more symmetrical, so there is less stress in one direction. You also reduce the pressure on the knee by opening and releasing the hip joint more deeply.

(continued)

BENEFITS

✓ Strengthens the support muscles of the knee

✓ Strengthens and aligns the legs and hips

✓ Opens the hip joint in extension and flexion

✓ Helpful for sciatic problems

✓ Strengthens the abs

✓ Opens the quadriceps and hip flexors

✓ Stretches the calves

✓ Opens the bottom of the foot and toes to reduce symptoms of plantar fasciitis

✓ Helps athletes increase speed

CONTRAINDICATIONS

This pose is contraindicated for those who have had recent knee or neck surgery and for those with acute foot pain. Those who have hip or low back issues should use modifications, such as putting the knee to the floor and holding it for a shorter amount of time.

HOW TO

1. Begin the pose on your hands and knees in tabletop pose.

2. Bring the right foot forward between the hands so the right knee is directly over the right ankle or heel and forms a 90-degree angle. This creates a strong base with the least amount of strain and effort.

3. Tuck the left toes under, and straighten the left leg.

4. Peek down, and make sure your left heel is straight up to the sky and you are on all five left foot toes. This guarantees the safety of the knee.

5. Lift up onto the fingertips, and start to extend the spine and elongate the neck. You can place blocks under the fingers if you need more room.

6. Square the hips and shoulders to the front of the room. Make certain that your knee always tracks directly over your foot to secure the safety of the right knee.

7. Tuck the tailbone under to increase the stretch to the left hip flexor. Press all the way back through the left heel and feel the energy all the way through the top of your head.

8. Stay here for several breaths, or climb your hands onto your right thigh and hold. Another option is to bring your arms up to the sky, palms facing each other with length in your side, and hold. Whatever variation you choose, think as much about length in your spine as you do about the depth of flexion in your right knee.

VARIATIONS

- Try knee-down crescent lunge as a variation on crescent lunge by lowering the back knee to the floor if you are not strong enough to straighten the back leg or if you are having low back issues (see variation 1). This variation enhances the stretch in the straight leg's hip flexor.

- Try crescent lunge twist as a variation on crescent lunge to add a deeper level of focus on balance and to increase spinal rotation (see variation 2). While in crescent lunge right leg forward, bring the hands into heart center, twist to the right, and place the left upper arm on the outside of the right thigh. Twist as deeply as you can until your chest faces right.

- Try lizard as a variation on crescent lunge to increase leg flexibility and mental toughness because this pose is often held for a longer period of time (see variation 3). From crescent lunge, bring both hands to the floor on the inside of the front foot. In time, you will be able to rest on your forearms here. Until then, use blocks.

- The ultimate expression of a crescent lunge is to prepare your body for a split (see variation 4). In knee-down lunge, you place two or more blocks under your right hip (if your right leg is forward). Continue to inch your right leg forward and your left leg back until you can settle in a split preparation with your hip on the blocks. Hold there and breathe. With time and attention, you can eventually perform this pose without blocks under the hip.

- In crescent lunge, push off the back foot moving the body forward toward the front of your mat and back to neutral again. The lunge push-off stretches and opens the bottom of the foot and toes and adds stability in the ankle.

VARIATION 1

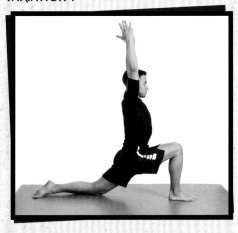

VARIATION 2

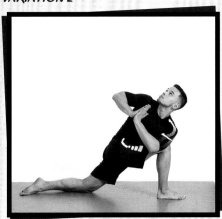

VARIATION 3

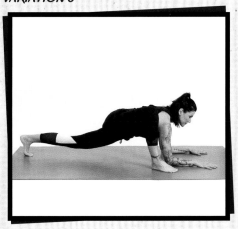

VARIATION 4

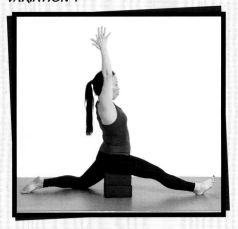

GODDESS POSE
UTKATA KONASANA

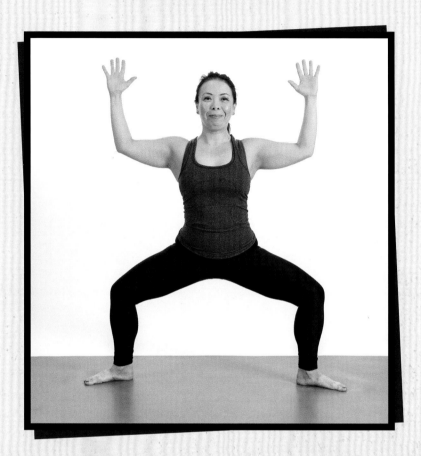

While not a widely used pose in vinyasa flow or power yoga classes, goddess is a common pose for practitioners of Kundalini yoga. It's a great blend of strength, stretch, and mental toughness.

Goddess pose does a lot to strengthen the legs and to help train you to get a sense for a long, strong back. I find this a great pose to hold while I perform a long series of breath of fire breathing. It also helps to identify which joints are weak and tight for assessment purposes.

For the athlete, this pose can help to open the groin and protect the knees, stretch the hips and Achilles tendon to decrease the risk of injury, and increase speed on the field. Holding this pose for a little longer develops core strength. The longer hold will challenge an athlete's focus and mental toughness. Finally, holding the arms in alignment will build functional strength in the shoulders without building bulk that can impede range of motion.

BENEFITS

✓ Opens the hips, legs, and chest

✓ Strengthens the legs, calves, abs, and knees

✓ Stimulates the urogenital system and pelvic floor

✓ Strengthens and stretches the shoulder joint

CONTRAINDICATIONS

This pose is contraindicated for those who have chronic knee problems or who have had recent knee surgery.

HOW TO

1. Start standing, and separate your feet approximately the distance of the length of one of your legs. You can turn your feet out to a comfortable degree, usually about 45 degrees.

2. Raise your arms out straight from your shoulders, and bend them at your elbows to form a 90-degree angle. Your palms are facing forward, fingers energized and extended.

3. Slowly bend your knees until they also reach a 90-degree angle, and hold the pose.

4. Be very careful that as you bend your knees, they do not knock inward; be sure that the knees always track directly over the toes, even if that means modifying the angle of your feet. This is important to building leg strength correctly and to protecting the very vulnerable knee joint.

VARIATION

A great challenge to balance and leg strength is to vigorously twist left to right in this pose.

STRADDLE FORWARD BEND TWIST

PARIVRTTA PRASARITA PADOTTANASANA

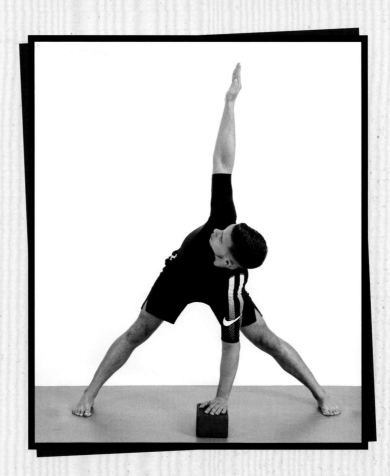

Considered by some to be in the beginner's category of poses, this pose can prove to be very challenging for most, especially for people who experience tightness in their trunk rotation and hamstrings.

This twist is a great combination of balance, strength, and stretch. The triple threat always improves the body, mind, and spirit. The pose opens the legs and decompresses the spine for greater vitality and energy. The pose teaches you to open and let go but to remain in control and present so that you do not topple over.

For the athlete, this pose is amazing for opening the hips and hamstrings. You can surrender to the pose without the force and constant yanking of a seated forward bend. It is extremely effective for maintaining the strength and stability of the ankle joint. It's great for people who play on unstable surfaces or for those who require great agility on the field, such as soccer players or racket sport competitors, who need strong ankles to support quick moves. This pose helps athletes to improve trunk rotation, which is a huge advantage to players like wide receivers, soccer players, hitters at home plate, and golfers who depend on power in the twist. This pose, coupled with deep hip openers like pigeon pose, creates superior power in play.

BENEFITS

✓ Increases flexibility in the back of the thigh and leg

✓ Opens the hips

✓ Lengthens the neck

✓ Strengthens the back, legs, and ankles

✓ Increases lung capacity by opening the ribs

✓ Improves the trunk's rotation ability

✓ Stretches the inner thigh

✓ Calms the brain because it is a mild inversion

✓ Fights headache, fatigue, and mild depression

CONTRAINDICATIONS

This pose is contraindicated for those with lower back injury, herniation of the spine, concussion, or glaucoma.

HOW TO

1. Start with your feet apart; the distance between your feet should be approximately the length of one of your legs. Make sure your feet are on the same line and that they are parallel.

2. Take a deep breath in; on your exhale, fold yourself over from the hip joint. You are folding your pelvis over your legs. It is very easy to fold from the back, but you should not do this. No matter how tight your hamstrings are, you can get the fold you need and a proper stretch in the backs of the legs without overstretching the back.

3. Hang here for several breaths, stabilizing yourself and focusing on the feel of the stretch.

4. With both hands on the floor in front of your feet, take a deep breath in, and come halfway up with a strong, flat back. The flat back is critical for proceeding to the pose's twist action. When you come up halfway with the flat back, extend out through the top of your head; do not lift your chin, and stay neutral in the neck, your two feet, and your right hand.

5. Continue to extend the back flat; rounding here restricts the twist.

6. Twist your chest open to the right. Drop your left shoulder, and open the right chest and shoulder. On every inhale, get longer and flatter; on every exhale, twist deeper.

7. Keep your hips squared. Avoid the desire to drop your right hip into the twist.

8. The whole time you are holding this pose, keep in mind that you are keeping your feet flat and strong, pushing into the floor. Feel a connection at all times at the base of the big toe, the base of the pinky toe, and inner and outer heel. The temptation is to release all your energy to the outer ankle, but over time that can fatigue and strain the ankle.

VARIATIONS

- If you find your hamstrings are too tight, modify the pose by allowing a bend in the knees to provide some laxity in the hamstrings and to allow you to feel how you should fold properly.

- Try straddle forward bend as a variation to enhance the hamstring stretch and to allow you to hold the stretch for a longer period of time (see variation). Use the same setup, but forward fold the body in the center.

VARIATION

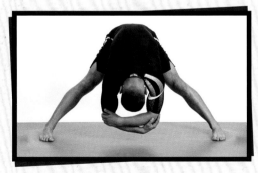

EAGLE POSE
GARUDASANA

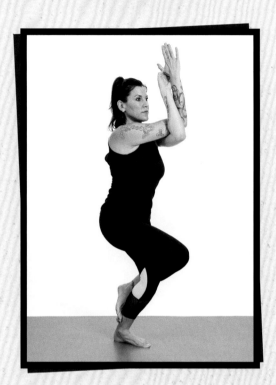

Eagle pose generates great stability in the joints and balance in the body. This pose demands your full attention for its success. Eagle pose requires you to focus equal attention on the upper and lower body at the same time. The more you release your muscle tension on your exhales, the better.

Eagle pose offers many therapeutic applications. Almost every joint of your body is affected in this pose. Since it opens the back, it is an important pose for people who suffer from asthma. It helps to open the rib cage and intercostals, therefore improving your breathing. Eagle opens the hips, legs, calves, and knees and in doing so, it has been known to significantly improve symptoms of sciatica. When you sit deeply in this pose, it releases all the gluteal muscles as well as the piriformis. The piriformis is a pear-shaped muscle that lies deep in the glutes. There is a hole in this muscle that the sciatic nerve passes through. Releasing the piriformis can relieve tension on the nerve and bring relief for nagging pain. Many people find that they have low back and gluteal stiffness after long days of driving or sitting at their desks. Eagle pose will lengthen the back and release the hips to undo those stresses.

For the athlete, this pose is great for maintaining the strength and integrity of the ankle joint. Many sports such as soccer, football, and tennis rely on a grinding, running, and cutting game. The ankle can take a beating. Athletes must take time to keep the joint open, clean, and strong for power and longevity. They also need to address the needs of the Achilles tendon to avoid a blowout, and this pose helps to do that, too. Your ankle joint must be strong and agile, but flexibility is crucial to avoiding injury. Say a football player makes a successful tackle, but at the end of the play another player lands on his ankle. It may hurt to be landed on, but a properly trained ankle will bounce back immediately or very quickly without long-term damage. Also, any pose that helps keep the hips open contributes to a healthy knee. It is the athletes with the greatest range of motion in their hips who avoid major damage or injury to the knee.

BENEFITS

✓ Strengthens arms, legs, knees, and ankles

✓ Opens the shoulder joint and creates space between the shoulder blades

✓ Opens hips and IT band

✓ Increases circulation to all joints

✓ Improves digestion and elimination

✓ Improves balance

✓ Improves focus

CONTRAINDICATIONS

Those with a history of low back, knee, or hip problems should begin with modifications such as leaning against a wall, not tucking the toes of the raised leg behind the calf, and lying on the floor.

HOW TO

1. Begin this twisted pose by putting all your weight on your left leg.

2. Bend your knees as though you are about to sit in a chair.

3. Keep your spine extended. Lift your right leg, and place it over your left leg. It should start to look like you are sitting in a chair with your legs crossed.

4. If it is possible, your right thigh should be above your left knee. In time and with practice, you will be able to hook your right ankle behind the left lower calf. If that is not possible right away, place the top of the right foot on the left calf or press it against the inside of the left calf. Squeeze the inner thighs together; this will bring you into a more solid center.

5. Keep your hips squared to the front of the mat, and try to bend the left knee even deeper.

6. Bring your arms out to the sides, as if you are walking a tightrope and need them for balance. Open and expand your chest.

7. Cross your right elbow over the left in front and at the center of your body. Wrap and twist your arms until the palms come together. This full expression of the pose may take time and practice to open the shoulders enough to perform.

8. Relax your shoulders away from your ears, and keep the shoulders squared to the front of the mat just like your hips.

9. Raise your elbows to shoulder height, and press your hands toward the front of the mat until you feel an opening between your shoulders and deep in the joint.

10. From the waist down, feel your body sink deeper into the floor. From the waist up, lift and lengthen.

(continued)

VARIATION

Try sleeping eagle to use the abdominals more deeply, to further challenge your balance, and to train the supporting leg (see variation). Once you become well acquainted with eagle, you can take it to the next level by slowly folding over. The ultimate sleeping eagle is done with the eyes closed in total concentration.

VARIATION

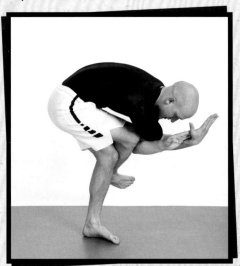

Several of my athletes seem to get frustrated when they are fatigued in standing poses or lose balance often. Should I continue to teach or bring them to the floor?

If you have carefully crafted PYFS routines for them with standing poses that make sense to do, then keep on keeping on. If they are unsuccessful, chances are these are exactly the poses they need to be working on. Your athletes do not need to spend a lot of time on poses they can already do easily. Be encouraging, and continue to motivate them to try again.

SQUAT
MALASANA

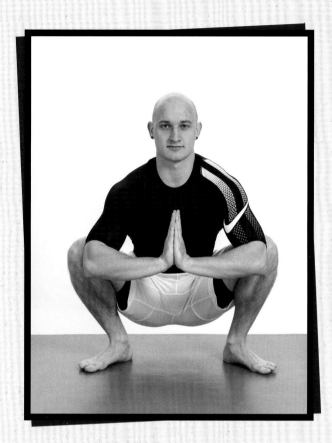

Squat pose is a pose of grounding and centering. It affects the internal organs as well as the hips. It represents the epitome of balance, strength, stretch, focus, breath, and internal change. It is touted as a relaxer and purifier of the entire body.

Squat elongates the spine and builds strength in the back. Today's world contributes to back problems. We must continue to work our abdominals to support the anterior (front) spine and our back muscles to support the posterior (back) spine. Total back health comes when there is a balance between the anterior and posterior spine. Most daily activities have us leaning forward, weakening the abdominals and overstretching the back, which leads to imbalance and injury. Squat is one pose you can do daily to open the hips and focus on the balance of the spine. Also, the invention of the chair and high-heeled shoes has led to the demise of the Achilles tendon because they cause significant shortening of the vulnerable tendon. Shortened Achilles bring more stress to the knees and destabilize the ankles, leading eventually to tweaks and tears.

For the athlete, this pose is critical for Achilles tendon health. Once you have pain or aggravation in the Achilles, you risk inefficient or slower running. Pain in the Achilles increases the likelihood of unconscious changes in your gait and can lead to knee and ankle issues as well as strain on the shins. You will unknowingly change the way you land on your feet to decrease the pain. Another vital reason for the athlete to practice the squat is to achieve deep hip opening. Sinking into the pose opens the hips intensely. Keeping the hips unlocked also notably reduces pull and torque

(continued)

on the knee joint. Any time the hip is tight and limited in its range, extra tension goes to the most susceptible place, the knee. You can clearly see the connection between this pose and a catcher's stance in baseball or an infielder's defensive stance. You can see the importance of this pose for offensive linemen in football and for goalkeepers in soccer. It is similar to a primary ready position in many sports.

BENEFITS

✓ Builds strength in the legs, feet, calves, and ankles

✓ Excellent for people with low back pain

✓ Opens the groin, hips, ankles, and Achilles

✓ Stimulates abdominal internal organs

✓ Stabilizes the spine

✓ Stimulates the sex glands and spleen

✓ Helps to relieve pressure on the lumbar nerve plexus

CONTRAINDICATIONS

This pose is contraindicated for those who have had recent knee surgery, have severe back pain, or have an acute herniation.

HOW TO

1. Stand with the feet approximately shoulder width apart.

2. Bend your knees, and drop your hips toward the floor. Go as deep as you can with your heels staying flat on the floor. If your heels come up, you went too far for now.

3. Initially, the feet could be significantly turned out; in time, you will try to bring them to a parallel position. You never want to force the feet into parallel until they are ready. Doing so puts undo strain on the vulnerable knee joint.

4. Keep your gaze ahead of you, and bring your hands into the heart center in prayer position. The backs of the upper arms gently press against the knees; this encourages the pelvis and hips to open further. Make a clear and full connection from one hand to the other.

5. Bring your attention to the feet. There must be a full foot connection to the floor. Do not roll to the outer or inner edge of the foot.

6. Focus on the base of the big toe, the base of the pinky toe, and the inner and outer heel engaged with the floor. You can eventually lift your toes off the floor in squat.

7. Think of dropping the tailbone and lengthening the spine. With time and practice, your back will be very upright and flat as if you were leaning against a wall. Think of the skull ascending and the sacrum descending.

VARIATIONS

• Try squat turns to build additional strength in the legs and hips and to develop more flexibility in the hips and back (see variation 1). While in squat, turn 360 degrees to the right and 360 degrees to the left, returning to squat center.

- Try squat pike to pursue the ultimate balance and leg strength (see variation 2). From squat, extend one leg out in front of the body. The arms can be by your sides, held out like you are walking a tightrope, or extended to hold the foot of the straight leg. If you are very advanced, try to stand up from the squat pike. This is a great addition to squat, and a good time to execute this is at the end of the rock and rolls in your warm-up.

- Try squat twist for a deep spinal twist that is extra challenging because you are also in a deep squat (see variation 3). While in squat, lean forward slightly and slide the back of your right shoulder to the right as far in front of the right shin as you can. Place the right hand on the floor out in front of your right foot, extend the left arm up, and gently exhale as you twist your torso to the left.

VARIATION 1

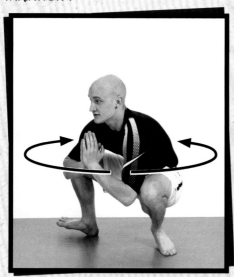

VARIATION 2

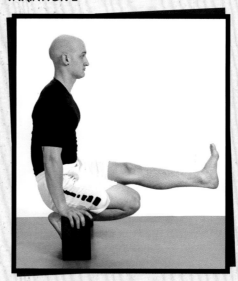

VARIATION 3

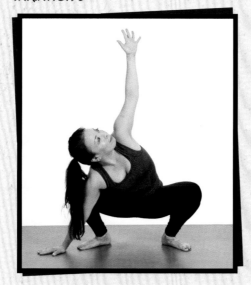

WARRIOR 1
VIRABHADRASANA I

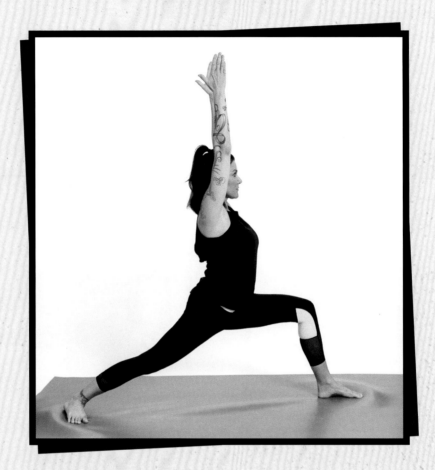

Warrior 1 focuses on the hips and lower body, and it is commonly used to connect poses within a yoga flow. Warrior 1 is a powerful pose that should begin from the body's center and radiate out through the limbs and head.

When emphasis is given to the back leg, the practitioner can get great results opening the corresponding hip flexor. This pose is dependent on proper alignment to open the body appropriately. It is a multipurpose pose. You should always feel from the waist down that you are sinking deeply and strongly rooted, while the upper body is lifted and elongated, stretching further on every inhale. This pose can give you a clear idea how open the shoulder joint is; when the arms are extended up to the sky, you should notice the upper arms right alongside the head. Pay attention to the feet being plugged fully into the floor. Squaring the hips forward brings you into balance; once you are aligned, it can build great strength. It is important to be in alignment before practicing deeply and especially before holding poses for longer amounts of time.

Athletes who need long strides for speed and power can benefit from this pose, especially when it is held for one to two minutes. Warrior 1 opens the hips, which is important for batters in baseball, receivers in football, soccer players, basketball players, and especially pitchers in baseball who rely on explosive power generated from the lower half of their bodies.

BENEFITS

✓ Elongates and strengthens the leg muscles

✓ Stretches the calves and Achilles tendon

✓ Opens the hips and shoulders

✓ Lengthens the torso and sides, which allows freer breathing

CONTRAINDICATIONS

This pose is contraindicated for those who have had recent or chronic injury to the hips or knees. If you have neck problems, you should keep your head in a neutral position and not look up at the hands.

HOW TO

1. Stand sideways on your mat, and step your feet wide apart, about four to five feet.

2. Turn your left foot out 90 degrees.

3. Pivot your right foot inward at a 45-degree angle.

4. Align your front heel with the arch of your back foot. Keep your pelvis turned squarely toward the front of your mat.

5. Press your weight down through your right heel. Then bend your left knee until it is over your left ankle, to 90 degrees. Your thigh should be parallel with the floor.

6. Reach up strongly through your arms. Lengthen the sides of your waist, and lift through your chest.

7. Keep your palms and fingers active and reaching, facing each other.

8. Let your shoulders drop away from your ears.

9. Press down through the outer edge of your back foot, keeping your back leg straight.

VARIATION

While in warrior 1, tuck the tailbone under to increase the hip flexor stretch and lift the heart to the sky, adding a slight backbend. This variation opens the anterior spine further, challenges the balance, and increases the flexibility of the legs.

WARRIOR 2
VIRABHADRASANA 2

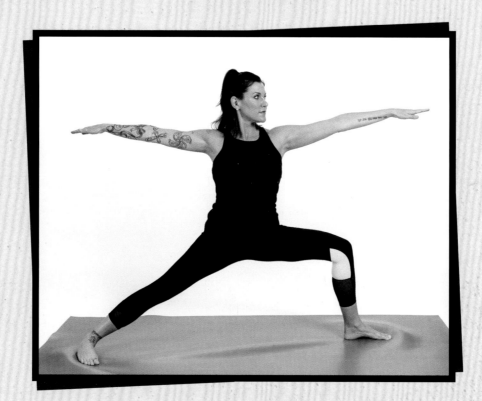

Just like warrior 1, holding warrior 2 for one to two minutes puts demands on you that help improve your focus, breathing, and mental toughness, the perfect formula for a great pitcher and an extraordinary athlete. This is a deep hip-opening pose that strengthens the muscles in the thighs and glutes. It tones the abs, ankles, and arches of the feet. This pose also opens the chest, heart, and shoulders, improving breathing capacity and increasing circulation throughout the body. It is known to be therapeutic for flat feet and sciatica.

For the athlete, strengthening the back in warrior 2 ensures that the spine is aligned and healthy. It allows for fuller rotation and quicker reactions on the field of play, court, or course. Incorporating and keeping your mind open to alternate positions with your arms while you are in warrior 1 and 2 enables you to explore shoulder stiffness and connect better to your needs. Try moves like swimming strokes with your arms in all directions and even trunk twists. Flex, extend, and rotate the wrist joints. Be creative, never stay inside the box, and find ways to open every joint in every pose in traditional and nontraditional ways.

Something Power Yoga for Sports stresses a lot is training for the mental game. It is a gift to practice a pose that can train all aspects the athlete needs: balance, strength, flexibility, mental toughness, and focus. Warrior 2 does it all. Athletes who particularly need to develop great functional shoulder strength and flexibility include those who participate in swimming, racket sports, soccer, cricket, basketball, and water polo. This pose is also good for athletes who need lower-body strength and balance in a stance: hitters in baseball, football players of all sorts, soccer players, basketball players, and lacrosse players, among others. There is hardly anyone who wouldn't benefit from warrior 2.

BENEFITS

✓ Opens the hips

✓ Strengthens the legs, thighs, and glutes

✓ Builds strength in the core

✓ Strengthens and stabilizes the shoulder

✓ Hones discipline and focus

✓ Sharpens focus and breath

CONTRAINDICATIONS

This pose is contraindicated for those who have had recent or chronic injury to the hips or knees.

HOW TO

1. Stand sideways on your mat, and step your feet wide apart, about four to five feet.

2. Turn your left foot out 90 degrees so that your toes are pointing to the front edge of the mat.

3. Pivot your right foot slightly inward. Your back toes should be at a 45-degree angle.

4. Raise your arms out to the sides to shoulder height so that they are parallel to the floor. Your arms should be aligned directly over your legs, with your palms facing down, reaching actively from fingertip to fingertip.

5. On an exhalation, bend your front knee. Align your knee directly over the ankle of your front foot.

6. Your front thigh should be parallel to the floor. Create a 90-degree angle with the front knee.

7. Press down through the outer edge of your back foot, and keep your back leg straight.

8. Keep your torso perpendicular to the floor.

9. Turn your head to gaze out at the tip of your left middle finger.

10. Drop your shoulders and lift your chest.

11. Draw your belly in toward your spine.

VARIATION

Try reverse warrior to open your back at a different angle, to open the ribs to improve lung activity, and to further strengthen the legs and abdominals (see variation). While in warrior 2 with the left foot forward, maintain the pose and slide the right hand down the back of the left thigh as you raise your left hand up to the sky.

VARIATION

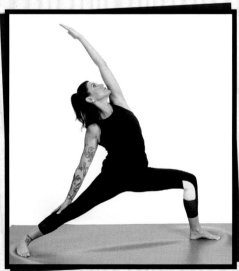

WARRIOR 3
VIRABHADRASANA 3

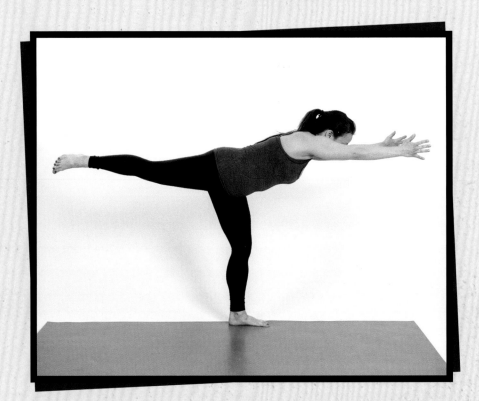

This pose is unique in that it puts demands on one leg at a time. Warrior 3 demands total focus and concentration, and it brings your awareness to small fluctuations in the ankle.

This pose will develop balance and focus a step further than warrior 1 and warrior 2. You move from using the strength and stability of two legs to depending on one leg, which is a more demanding pose to execute. Your gaze has to be fixed, and your mind has to be present, or else you will tumble. Reaching the arms strongly over your head gets deep shoulder joint muscles working their hardest. At the same time, the supporting leg is working hard to stabilize the body. This is a great transition pose to make students hold a little longer, challenging them to face the commitment it requires.

This pose is identical to the follow-through position for a baseball pitcher (visualize moving from warrior 2 or warrior 1 to warrior 3 to standing split). If you can hold this pose for a minute on your mat, you will surely ace it on the mound. This pose is important for athletes like basketball players, volleyball players, runners, cyclists, soccer goalkeepers, and any athlete who needs vertical jumping skills. The more durable, stable, and strong your ankle is, the better your performance. There is hardly a sport where this does not apply; even swimmers must work on the strength and flexibility of their ankles.

Warrior 3 strengthens the legs, core, and ankles perfectly. This pose also helps athletes to build the strength they need around the knee. You want to be sure you are balanced on the lower leg without pushing too hard and hyperextending the supporting knee. This pose is also one of a few that strengthen the neck muscles, and this helps protect the shoulders and head from the shock of impact sports.

BENEFITS

✓ Strengthens the legs and core

✓ Stretches the hamstrings

✓ Improves balance and posture

✓ Develops keen focus

✓ Stabilizes the ankle

✓ Strengthens the whole backside of the body, including the shoulders, hamstrings, calves, ankles, and back

✓ Tones the abdominal muscles

CONTRAINDICATIONS

This pose is contraindicated for those who have had recent or chronic injury to the hips and knees and for those who have serious neck issues.

HOW TO

1. Stand sideways on your mat, and step your feet wide apart, about four to five feet.

2. Turn your left foot out 90 degrees so your toes point to the front of the mat.

3. Pivot your right foot inward at a 45-degree angle, and square your hips to the front of the mat.

4. Bend your left knee.

5. Align your knee directly over the ankle, and keep your thigh parallel to the floor.

6. Raise your arms overhead with your palms facing each other, imitating a warrior 1 shape.

7. Pour your weight into your left foot, and lift your right leg as you hinge your torso, bringing your body parallel to the floor. Your arms, still extended, now reach forward.

8. Activate your right foot, pointed or flexed, and straighten your standing leg as you continue to lift the right leg.

9. Feel a dynamic opposition from your stretched fingers against the lifted back leg.

10. Work toward bringing your arms, torso, hips, and raised leg parallel to the floor.

11. Gaze at the floor a few feet in front of your body.

STANDING SPLIT
URDHVA PRASARITA EKA PADASANA

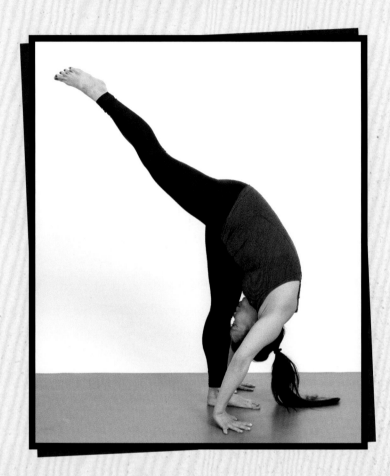

Standing split pose offers preparation before performing handstands or while you are learning such inversion poses. It also is a great choice for focused ankle work. There are a lot of creative moves to be considered while in the standing split. For example, you can practice leg kicks for glute strength, or you can perform the pose without the support of your hands.

With the variations of this pose, you can significantly increase your focus, breathing, and mental toughness, but those are not the most important benefits of this pose. The standing split develops the hips, spine, and glutes while changing your perspective and challenging your orientation and balance. Practicing this pose is a great way to make a smooth transition into handstands. Once you practice and can execute the pose with one or no hands, you incrementally increase the demands on focus and breathing, and you develop all the very tiny finesse muscles of the ankle. The legs are well developed in this pose, using its burdens to increase strength and flexibility at the same time.

For the athlete, the ankles seem to bear most of the load of the cutting, twisting, and pounding in sports. Fields of play are seldom smooth and perfect, so finely tuned ankle joints are useful for dealing with changes in topography. An open, strong ankle produces a powerful push-off for jumping, swimming, and any sport that involves speed on the run. While practicing this pose, you strengthen the ankle, increase the flexibility of the calf, and load the hamstring. The shape of this pose makes it easy to see its utility for figure skaters, speed skaters, and skiers.

BENEFITS

✓ Elongates the neck

✓ Decompresses the back and spine

✓ Improves balance

✓ Improves strength and flexibility of the legs

✓ Increases abdominal strength and glute power

✓ Stretches the groin

CONTRAINDICATIONS

This pose is contraindicated for those with glaucoma, those with a tendency toward vertigo or dizziness, and those who have had recent or chronic hip or knee injury.

HOW TO

1. Start in a standing forward bend; be sure you are bending from the hips and not from the low back.

2. Claw the floor with both hands. If you cannot touch the floor, consider using a block under each hand.

3. Let your head hang, and keep your hips squared to the front of the mat.

4. Slowly shift your weight onto your left foot, and start to raise your right leg to the sky. Keep the hips squared; do not open the right hip to the sky.

5. Once you meet resistance, stop and hold the pose.

6. Direct your energy through your right leg and foot, pressing it high to the sky.

7. Let your head hang. You can do variations using one hand or no hands.

VARIATIONS

- Once you master standing split, you can experiment with releasing the hands from the floor and grasping the lower leg (see variation). This variation creates the ultimate balance and concentration pose.

- While in standing split with the left leg up, continually raise and lower the left leg in a kicking motion. This variation of the pose can greatly increase leg and glute strength. You can also alternate split kicks for an added bonus.

VARIATION

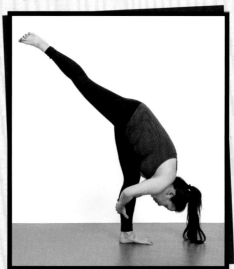

TREE POSE

VRKSASANA

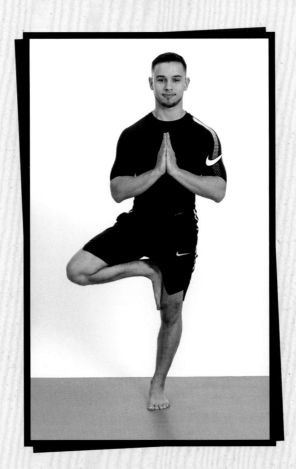

Tree is a great pose to practice even while waiting in line at a store. It's a fun way to continue to work on focus, mental toughness, breathing, and ankle stability. Tree will develop a solid body center and a strong spine.

Tree pose is a great way to find a moment of center in your practice. It helps build stamina in the practitioner, and it focuses breathing. If you are concerned with balance, practice this pose for a minute or two and feel the subtle changes and fluctuations of the lower leg and foot. If your concentration wavers for a second, you will lose the pose. A great lesson to take from tree pose is to accept the changes that are constantly happening in your mind and body and make quick, nonjudgmental adjustments on the fly to maintain the pose.

Athletes should consider using this pose to train and strengthen the ankles and calves. If you need to perform and have super concentration at the same time, tree is for you; arguably, this describes all athletes. In tree you also train the core, so if you need strength in your center as well as balance for racket sports, volleyball, basketball, and many more, you need finesse in your lower-body movements and control of the upper body. Practicing this pose will make you aware of your weak side and will help you to build its strength and flexibility to the same level as on the other side. I recommend athletes challenge themselves to hold this pose for one to two minutes. If you are feeling really spot-on, the ultimate quiet tree is done with the eyes closed.

BENEFITS

✓ Increases leg strength

✓ Improves balance

✓ Improves focus

✓ Strengthens the core, calves, and ankles

✓ Stretches the groin and inner thigh

✓ Helps flat feet

CONTRAINDICATIONS

This pose is contraindicated for those who have had recent surgery or injury to the ankles.

HOW TO

1. Start in standing mountain pose.

2. Start to shift your weight onto your left foot.

3. Reach down and grab your right foot. Plug the bottom of the right foot (especially the heel) into the left upper inner thigh, as high as your body will allow. If you cannot put the right foot up all the way, bring it as far up the inner left leg as possible. The only exception is never to plant the right heel against the inside of the left knee. Anywhere above or below the knee is acceptable.

4. Feel your right heel press in against the left thigh, and at the same time feel the inner left thigh push back against the right heel.

5. Firm up your left supporting leg.

6. Lift tall through the top of your head, with the core firm and strong.

7. Bring your hands to heart center, or extend the arms straight up to the sky.

VARIATIONS

- Try half lotus tree to increase ankle strength and stability while challenging your balance and focus (see variation 1). While in tree, bring your right outer ankle to the left upper hip crease as far up as you can. To maintain the pose, press the outer ankle against the left front thigh and the left front thigh back against the right outer ankle.

- Try extended leg tree to increase ankle strength and stability and core and leg strength while challenging balance and focus (see variation 2). While in tree pose, whichever leg is bent, slowly extend it straight out in front of you and hold.

VARIATION 1

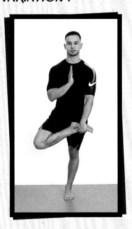

VARIATION 2

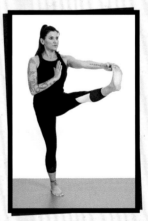

Is there a simple standing pose to improve balance and ankle strength?

Nothing is better than a simple tree pose. While in the pose, feel the small fluctuations of the muscles in the ankle and foot to understand how your body compensates and builds stability. If your athlete is more seasoned, have her do tree pose with her eyes closed to really increase the ankle work.

KING DANCER
NATARAJASANA

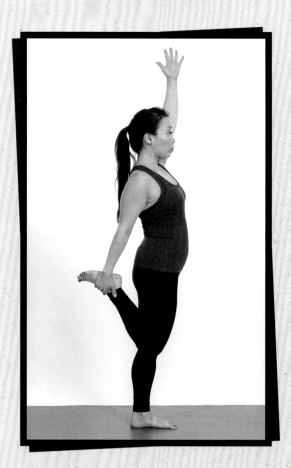

King dancer is a more advanced pose that develops great balance and focus. You will improve your ability to set your body in center with this pose and to strengthen the abdominals and legs. You are stretching your energy in all directions with king dancer in order to maintain balance.

For the athlete, this pose comes in handy for agility sports. It helps create great lower leg strength and ankle stability. For athletes who must start and stop on a dime at full speed—infielders in baseball, receivers and defensive backs in football, tennis players, and soccer players, for example—practicing this pose can help develop the smaller muscles in the legs for more finesse on the field and less injury.

BENEFITS

✓ Increases leg, abdominal, back, and ankle strength

✓ Increases flexibility of the hip flexors and back

✓ Develops strong ankles and lower legs

✓ Encourages better focus and breathing

CONTRAINDICATIONS

This pose is contraindicated for those who have had recent back or leg surgery.

HOW TO

1. Stand tall in mountain pose, and shift your weight onto the left foot.

2. Bend your right knee, and grab the big toe side of your right foot with your right hand.

3. Lift your left arm straight up to the ceiling.

4. Lift your right leg behind you as you bring your torso forward to counterbalance.

5. The energy of your right leg should be pressing back into the hand toward the back of the room and up to the sky at the same time.

VARIATION

Release the top leg and extend the foot straight out in front of you as parallel to the floor as you can and hold (see variation). This greatly challenges balance and focus while building leg and ankle strength and stability.

VARIATION

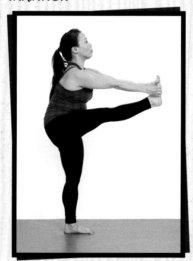

THREE-LEGGED DOG
EKA PADA ADHO MUKHA SVANASANA

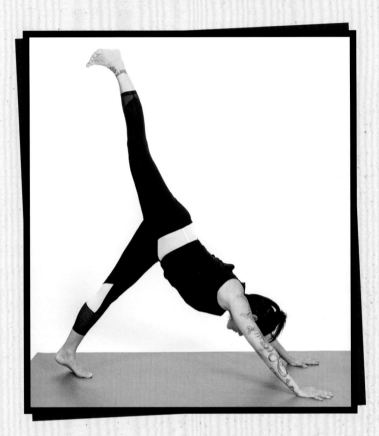

Starting in your basic downward dog, doing these variations helps to train more areas of the body and to improve balance on each side of the body as well as on the front and back. You will increase the strength of the back and tone in the arms.

I love to use the three-legged dog variations when teaching my athletes. It works many body parts at once while also calling for focus and breath. It is a gentle inversion, so it can help with sinus headaches and pressure. This pose tones the arms and strengthens the shoulder joint at a different angle than the typical bench press and shoulder press angles. If you hold this for one to two minutes, you are challenging your strength as well as any bench press competition. This pose looks easy, but it is not. It tones and flattens the back, undoing the constant forward slouchy posture most of us take on during our day. Three-legged dog variations open the wrists and prepare them for falls while releasing the tightness and stresses that lead to carpal tunnel syndrome. This condition is very common nowadays because we spend so much time on computers and devices, overworking all the small carpal muscles.

Any athlete who is susceptible to falls in sports such as soccer, football, basketball, and hockey should practice poses like this that focus on strengthening and stretching the wrist joint. This could prevent some serious injuries. If you are in a sport that requires overhead strength and flexibility in the arms, you should take advantage of the many benefits of this pose. Hold it and breathe through it. If you are afflicted with tight hamstrings, holding this pose and focusing on the sinking of the calves will subtly stretch them without force. The angle of the calf and the stretching effects on the Achilles are exceptional. Hang on and work the variations for minutes on end. Opening the ankles makes you more elusive to your opponents, and the wrist work gives you more agile hands.

BENEFITS

✓ Increases core strength

✓ Improves body awareness

✓ Improves flexibility of hamstrings and shoulders

✓ Strengthens and stretches the wrists

✓ Stretches the calves and opens the Achilles tendon

✓ Strengthens the shoulders and spine

✓ Relieves neck pain and decompresses the neck and spine

CONTRAINDICATIONS

This pose is contraindicated for those with recent injury or surgery on the wrists or glaucoma.

HOW TO

1. Starting in downward dog, feel the connection of both hands to the floor, fully connecting them and plugging them in.

2. Sink your weight into the left heel slightly more than the right heel.

3. Start to lift the right leg up to the sky, keeping the hip squared to the floor, foot flexed or pointed, and leg straight.

4. Lift the leg as high as you can, and then stop.

5. Keep both arms strong and straight; sink the left heel while you lift the right leg.

VARIATIONS

- Start in downward dog, sinking both heels into the floor and firming up the legs. Shift your weight onto the right hand and slowly bring your left hand to your low back, or perform any variation that makes sense to you.

- Try three-legged dog twist to build a different angle of strength in the shoulders and to deepen the spinal twist (see variation 1). With the right leg up to the sky, bend the right knee and twist and open the chest. Keep your hands firmly grounded, and fix your gaze under your right armpit up to the sky.

- From three-legged dog twist, you can keep twisting until the top leg drops you open, bringing you into the flip the dog variation (see variation 2). This helps open the wrists, increases the suppleness of the spine, and strengthens the shoulder joint in all directions.

VARIATION 1

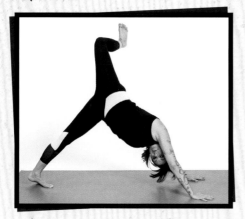

VARIATION 2

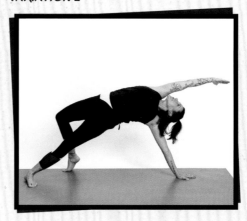

HALF SIDE SQUAT
SKANDASANA

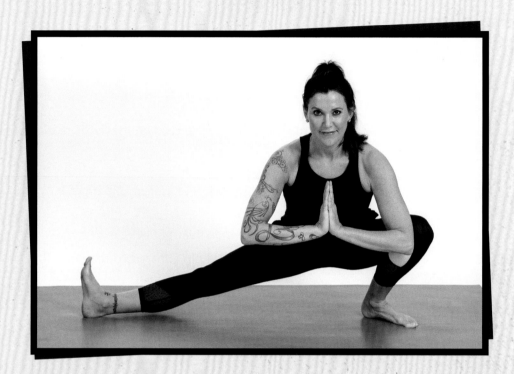

I love half side squat for a multipurpose stretch because it allows you to zone in on each side individually for imbalances and tightness. It can also challenge your balance and overall flexibility.

This pose stretches and strengthens many parts of your body at once, saving time and energy. This pose can be good one day and feel tight the next. Since this pose is so driven through the hips, your clarity of mind or stress level on a given day can affect how well you can perform it. You should always sink in slowly and breathe deeply. Be very precise when aligning your bent knee directly over the toes as doing this yields the safest results for the knees. Push through the heel of the straight leg, release deep through the hips, and extend and flatten the back. A simple tip for success is to keep your chin neutral.

Success in many sports depends on flexibility in the hips in order to be fast and elusive on the field of play. The beauty of this pose is that you are targeting different angles of the groin, hips, and inner leg. If your sport depends on quick footwork and perhaps even jumping ability, you should always target the range of motion in the ankle, Achilles tendon, and calves. You will have to do other poses to add plantar fascia and toe stretches, but this is a great start.

BENEFITS

✓ Stretches the inner thigh and groin

✓ Releases the hips

✓ Lengthens the Achilles tendon and calves

✓ Strengthens the back

✓ Opens the hips

✓ Challenges your balance when you are deep in the pose

CONTRAINDICATIONS

This pose is contraindicated for those who have had recent knee surgery or labrum surgery and for those with hip displacement or medial knee pain.

HOW TO

1. Starting in downward dog, bring the left foot forward between the hands; slowly turn the body to the right.

2. Your left knee is bent as deep as it can go as long as the foot is flat and the knee can track over the second toe. Some will have the hips high and some will be deep in left leg squat, while the right leg is long and stretched out, knee straight.

3. The right foot should point straight up to the sky. If your flexibility allows, place your hands at the heart center.

4. Lift up out of the pose, and shift to the other side.

VARIATION

If your flexibility doesn't allow you to place your hands at heart center, you can place the hands on the floor and breathe deeply.

VARIATION

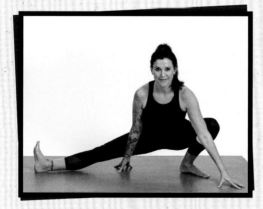

LUNGE TWIST
PARIVRTTA ANJANEYASANA

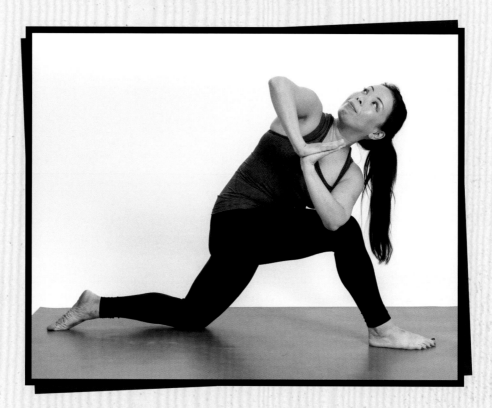

The lunge twist encourages you to align the spine while testing your ability to focus and challenging your balance. Precision and dedication are essential to executing this pose.

The twisting lunge is a well-rounded pose that illustrates the essence of Power Yoga for Sports, which is our equation, Strength + Flexibility = Power on the field of play. Not only does this pose challenge you to dig deeper with each breath and stretch further on each exhale, it demands your attention in order to hold your balance. Lunge twists lengthen, strengthen, increase respiration, and make you reach in all directions at the same time.

For athletes, we stress the development of strength and flexibility to get to the next level. However, if the athlete cannot breathe and manipulate the body at the will of the breath, this pose teaches that. This pose is great for receivers and for athletes who need eyes in the back of their heads. It helps them by increasing the rotation in the entire spine, primarily in the neck. Once you increase neck rotation, you will open your field of vision and be unstoppable. This pose also teaches you to be in the moment and in your center; otherwise, you will fall flat on your butt. It's a great pose for sports that require great spinal rotation like swimming, soccer, basketball, field hockey, lacrosse, golf, and tennis.

BENEFITS

✓ Aligns the spine

✓ Stretches the hip flexors, ankles, toes, and feet

✓ Increases rotation in the entire spine

✓ Helps to develop better balance

✓ Strengthens the legs

✓ Develops quality of mind

✓ Focuses the breath

CONTRAINDICATIONS

This pose is contraindicated for those who have had recent back surgery or those who have severe neck issues.

HOW TO

1. Starting in downward dog, bring the right foot forward between the hands, and form a perfect 90-degree angle with the right knee. In the beginning, you rest the left knee on the floor. As you progress, work to keep the left knee up off the mat and the left leg straight.

2. Reach the arms up to the sky, and straighten them.

3. If your shoulder flexibility allows it, turn the palms to face each other.

4. Bring your hands into prayer in heart center.

5. Keep the length in your back, and rotate the spine to the right as the armpit tries to cup the right knee.

6. Place the left arm against the outer right thigh to help deepen the twist on the exhales.

7. Lengthen out through the top of your head, and, at the same time, extend back through the left heel. Split yourself apart from the center and twist, twist, twist.

8. On good balance days, you rotate your head so your chin is over your right shoulder and you are looking up to the sky.

9. If you experience low back strain, focus on tucking the tailbone under to lengthen the back further so you can twist more deeply.

Seated Poses

6

Seated poses add a lot of value to your practice. These poses do not require intense balance and focus to perform, which makes it the best time to sink in deep and hold poses for extended periods to improve flexibility. While seated, you can evaluate for imbalances by tuning into the way your body is connected to the floor and noticing if you feel weighted on one side and disconnected on the other. This type of yoga work is particularly beneficial for recovery days for athletes: the lower functional strength demands and longer holds tend to help eliminate soreness in the body to prepare them for the next game or practice.

Performing these poses in front of a mirror will help athletes to spot imbalances and asymmetry.

Should I limit the amount of seated poses because they are so relaxing so my athletes will not zone out?

To the contrary, many seated poses are the most challenging, and it is your job to keep the athlete engaged and aware in each pose. This is a great time to cue breathing, to talk through a guided visualization, and to encourage them to share what they feel in their body at the moment of executing the pose.

EASY CROSS-LEGGED POSE
SUKASANA

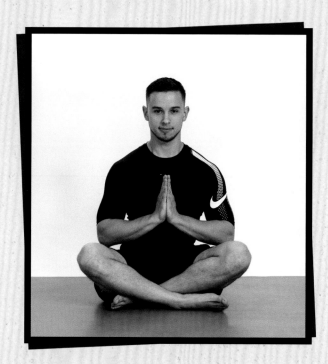

Sukasana, easy cross-legged, crisscross applesauce—these are all familiar names for one basic pose. The most widely recognized yoga pose and home to most meditators, this pose is a building block as well as an assessment staple.

You can free your mind with this easy-seated pose and focus on the lift of the spine while at the same time expanding the chest and belly with breath. It seems the perfect pose to feel the stacking of the spine without the worry of having to balance or hold a complicated pose. This frees the mind to develop a meditation practice.

For the athlete, easy cross-legged can often be difficult. I insist that athletes who are new to yoga sit on a sturdy yoga block or two. This will allow the back to lengthen to its capacity without hip tightness inhibiting the pose. For the athlete, it is a serious pose of assessment. At first, most people will not be able to sit up tall, and they will find that they are sitting behind their sitz bones. This is a great clue that your hamstrings need more flexibility. As you hold the pose, you will find there is nothing "easy" about it—the groin grips, the hips shake with exhaustion, the back aches. With constant practice and attention, this pose will get easier, and you will master being still.

If you are recovering from knee surgery, you may want to place blankets under your knees for support or place your feet farther away from your body at first. Even the most seasoned athlete can find this pose to be a challenge.

BENEFITS

✓ Stretches hips, knees, and ankles

✓ Calms the mind

✓ Increases blood flow to the abdominal organs

✓ Strengthens the back

CONTRAINDICATIONS

This pose is contraindicated for those who have had recent knee surgery, recent serious hip injury, or ankle difficulties.

HOW TO

1. Sit with your hips propped up on a folded towel, bolster, or pillow so that your hips are slightly higher than your ankles.

2. Stack your spine on top of your sitz bones, and elongate on every exhalation.

3. Fold one leg in so your heel is tucked in up to your groin, then fold the second leg. It does not matter which leg folds in first, but you should switch sides every now and then.

4. Place your hands on your knees.

VARIATIONS

- Easy cross-legged twist is a staple move for Power Yoga for Sports warm-up sequences. Begin in easy cross-legged pose with the arms in a goalpost shape, and vigorously twist the torso left to right (see variation 1). Not only does this help realign the spine, but this move is also perfect for identifying imbalances in the rotational ability of the spine.

- Try arm-ups while in easy cross-legged pose to bring tremendous heat to the shoulders quickly (see variation 2). In easy cross leg, extend the arms straight out to the sides; on the inhale, lift the arms all the way up, with the palms facing up; on the exhale, lower the arms to the floor, palms facing down. The endurance needed to complete two minutes of this calls for the athlete to focus and breathe and demonstrates mental toughness.

- Try seated cat and cow to warm up the flexion and extension of the spine and bring heat to the body (see variation 3). In easy cross-legged position, place your hands on your shins. On the inhale, lift the heart, shoulders back, chin up, and exaggerate the arch in the spine. On the exhale, round the back, slump the shoulders forward, and press the chin to the chest.

VARIATION 1

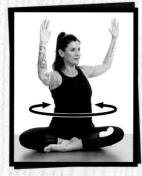

VARIATION 2

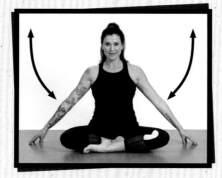

VARIATION 3

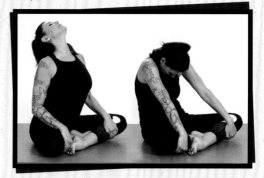

COBBLER'S POSE
BADDHA KONASANA

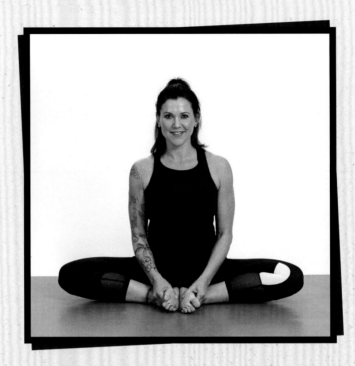

Most athletes have performed this pose at some point. In sports, it is fondly known as the butterfly stretch. It is useful for every sport and recreational activity, and it should become part of every warm-up or cool-down from a workout.

Cobbler's pose helps tone and strengthen the thighs, which can help you improve your yoga technique. Strong legs are useful for many of life's daily activities in addition to sport. The more you practice this pose with a sturdy, tall back, the more you can ease your breathing and reduce daily anxiety.

For the athlete, cobbler's pose is incredible for releasing a tight groin and inner thigh before or after a game. Taking the time to open the hips in all directions is a sure way to reduce stress on the vulnerable knee joint. Setting yourself up in this pose is a perfect way to observe if one hip or side of the groin is tighter, indicating which side needs more work. Observe which knee is higher; that is the stiffer side. This pose is a must-do for all athletes.

BENEFITS

✓ Stimulates the abdominal organs, ovaries and prostate gland, bladder, and kidneys

✓ Improves circulation

✓ Stretches the inner thighs, groin, and knees

✓ Helps relieve fatigue

✓ Soothes menstrual discomfort and sciatica

✓ Therapeutic for flat feet

✓ Consistent practice of this pose until late into pregnancy said to help ease childbirth

CONTRAINDICATIONS

This pose is contraindicated for those who have had recent back surgery. If you have had a groin or knee injury, only perform this pose with blanket support under the outer thighs.

HOW TO

1. Sit on a stable, even surface. Regardless of your level of expertise in this pose, I recommend that you fold a blanket or towel to sit on. This keeps your hips higher than your heels and places you in the pose with less force. With your hips propped up, you will have a slight feeling of going downhill in the pose, which makes it easier to sink into.

2. Bend your knees and bring your feet together. Take some time to perfectly align the bottoms of your feet, and gently press them together.

3. Hold onto your lower leg or foot. Do not hold your toes unless you are very flexible or familiar with the pose. When you grab the toes, you tend to pull your ankle and foot out of alignment, which can stress the knee and encourage an improper stretch. Begin to let your knees drop toward the floor.

4. Position your heels as close to your body as you can without strain on the knee.

5. You can hold here, focusing on breath and a tall, straight back, or you can begin to fold forward. If you fold over, use your elbow on the inside of your legs to help encourage the knees to drop down further, never forcing or bouncing. Take it slow.

6. Fold forward with a flat back, aiming to feel that your chest would touch the floor before your forehead would.

SEATED MOUNTAIN POSE
DANDASANA

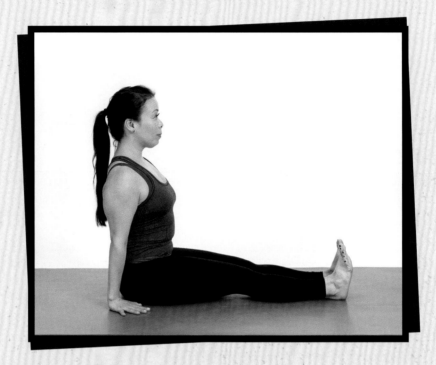

A starting pose for many advanced poses, dandasana is a great place to set your intention, ground yourself, and begin holds or other vigorous practices.

Seated mountain pose strengthens the muscles that are responsible for perfect posture. Once perfect posture is achieved, then you can also benefit from increased oxygenation and blood flow to the abdominal organs, important for optimum functioning. This is a suitable pose for assessing asymmetry in the hips, legs, and feet, giving you an opportunity to prevent injury. Awareness is the key, and as the Power Yoga for Sports philosophy teaches, you should be proactive to health and not reactive to injury.

For the athlete, this pose strengthens the back and improves abdominal strength. From agile soccer players to acrobatic hoops stars, it is always important to spend time on these areas to optimize performance. Seated mountain pose also strengthens the hip flexors and quads. After holding this position for several minutes, athletes will likely know if they need to work on strengthening these areas even more.

BENEFITS

✓ Stretches the hamstrings and back

✓ Strengthens the back and legs

✓ Improves posture and digestion

CONTRAINDICATIONS

This pose is contraindicated for those who have had recent back surgery or those who have serious neck problems.

HOW TO

1. Sit on your mat, legs extended out in front of you.

2. Inhale and lift yourself up tall, sitting directly on your sitz bones.

3. If your hamstrings are too tight to sit with a tall, straight back, sit on a block or two, or slightly bend the knees until you can achieve the lifted feeling. Imagine your back is straight up against a wall. As a variation, you can sit actually sit with your back to a wall.

4. Create a slight internal rotation of the thighs to engage them. The feet should look as though they are pressing against an imaginary wall in front of you. Scan your body for asymmetries that may indicate tightness or impending injury.

5. Inhale and lift your spine. On the exhalation, remain lifted through the top of the head.

6. Stay here for several minutes if you can. Although the pose sounds easy, it may prove to be challenging.

SEATED FORWARD BEND
PASCHIMOTTANASANA

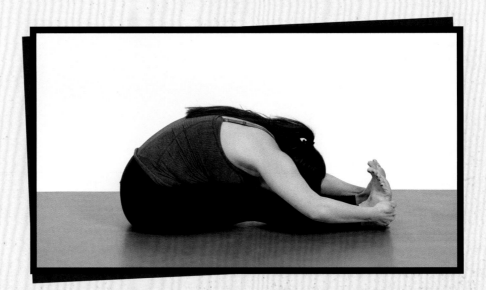

Most every athlete has experienced seated forward bend. People are often frustrated by the slow progression they make in this pose, but it should be considered a daily practice.

Seated forward bend opens the hamstrings. It is very important to keep the hamstrings open to reduce strain and tightness in the back. Long hours spent sitting at desks and driving vehicles help to create tight hamstrings, which in turn put strain on the back. Since the hamstring attaches on the lowest part of the pelvis, if the legs are rigid, it pulls down on the pelvis, putting unnecessary stress on the back. If this is not addressed, over time a chain reaction happens: tight hamstrings, strained back, unstable hips, knee problems. Increasing flexibility in the hamstrings takes commitment and constant practice because they are a large, dense muscle group, which makes them difficult to change.

For athletes, this pose is important for assessing postural needs and imbalances as well as for the benefits just mentioned. All athletes can benefit from hamstring improvement. A competitor with flexible legs will improve her speed. Many athletes want to improve their speed and agility, and it is always good to reduce strain on the back to lower injury risk and increase playing time.

BENEFITS
✓ Calms the brain

✓ Relieves stress

✓ May alleviate mild depression

✓ Stretches the hamstrings, calves, and hips

✓ Strengthens the thighs and knees

✓ Improves digestion

✓ Reduces anxiety

CONTRAINDICATIONS

This pose is contraindicated for an athlete who has had recent back, knee, or hamstring surgery. One may be able to practice the pose in a limited fashion, but a trained yoga teacher should observe.

HOW TO

1. Sit with your feet shoulder-width apart and parallel.

2. Align your feet as though they were square to a wall in front of you with the toes pointing straight up to the sky.

3. Bend your knees a little, and fold over at your hips; never fold from your waist.

4. Touch your chest and belly to your thighs with the knees still bent.

5. Keeping your chest and belly connected to your thighs, start to slowly straighten your knees. If you feel like the chest is separating from your legs, you went a little too far.

6. Once you meet resistance in the hamstrings and feel a challenging stretch, then you can rest your head on your thighs or position a block under your head. Continue to check that your feet line up with each other and that they stay parallel.

7. I encourage my students to drape a 12-pound sandbag over their backs while holding the pose. This method can help get you to the next level faster.

8. I also suggest for people with very tight hamstrings to start by practicing this pose while sitting up on blocks, bolsters, or blankets. This gives the feeling of folding downhill, and the body releases more quickly.

VARIATIONS

- Try one leg seated forward bend to focus on one hamstring at a time (see variation 1). Sit and extend your left leg out and bend your right knee, placing the bottom of the right foot against the inner left thigh. Lengthen the back and fold from the hips square over the left leg.

- Try seated forward bend with legs crossed to stretch the hamstrings somewhat differently than the traditional seated forward bend (see variation 2). In seated forward bend, cross the right ankle over the left ankle and fold. Do this on both sides.

- In seated forward bend, separate the legs into straddle as wide as you can and then fold over (see variation 3). It is nice to rest your head on stacked blocks and sink in. For this variation, I recommend you sit on blocks or bolsters to make the pose easier to perform. From this straddle position, you can also slide your left hand down the left leg as far as you can toward the left foot. On an inhalation, lift the right arm up to the sky, turn the palm toward the left, and side bend, bringing your right hand as close to your left foot as possible (see variation 4). This variation increases lung capacity for better respiration and changes the angle of the stretch in the legs.

(continued)

VARIATION 1

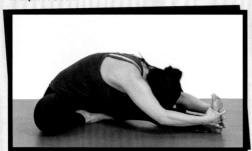

VARIATION 2

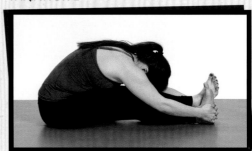

VARIATION 3

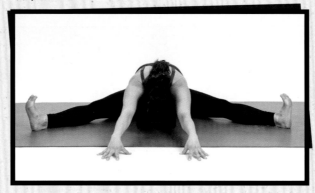

VARIATION 4

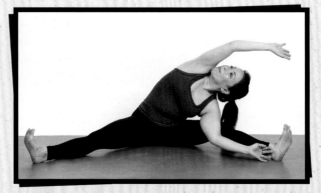

What if I am doing a seated forward bend and my back hurts more than my hamstrings?

Your back should never hurt in this pose. Slightly bend the knees, flatten the back, and lengthen the spine before you fold over until you become more flexible. This should ease the back discomfort. You can also prop your hips up on a folded towel or blocks so when you fold, you feel as though you are going downhill, thus making the pose more effortless.

BOAT POSE
NAVASANA

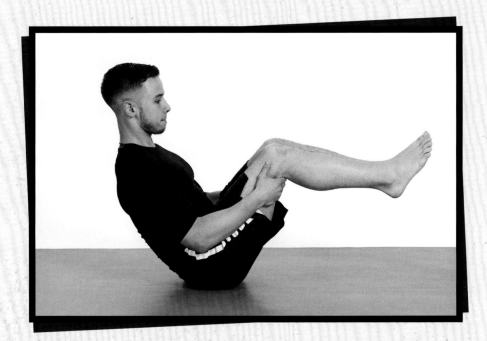

Boat pose is recognizable to workout enthusiasts as well as yogis; it is a staple pose to help strengthen the abdominal muscles. This pose resembles the letter V, and it can be an important addition to everybody's workout or yoga routine. I recommend boat pose because it works many areas at once. For example, holding this pose for several deep breaths will help to undo the forward bend we all suffer from throughout our daily routines. The pose also works the abs; opens the chest to increase lung capacity; stimulates the thyroid due to the position of the head to increase metabolism; and strengthens and tones the legs, quadriceps, and deep hip flexors such as the psoas. Increasing the power of the psoas/hip flexors helps the pelvis stay in a better position, making strides more efficient.

For athletes, it is important to find various ways to strengthen the abdominals. I challenge you to find any sport or athlete who does not rely on a strong core. A strong core also helps support the spine. This type of work is great for swimmers, cyclists, runners, and rowers, to name a few.

BENEFITS

✓ Strengthens the abdominals, hip flexors, and spine

✓ Stimulates the kidneys, prostate, thyroid, and intestines

✓ Relieves stress

✓ Improves digestion

(continued)

CONTRAINDICATIONS

This pose is contraindicated for those with diarrhea, low blood pressure, neck issues or injury, or hernia or for those who are pregnant.

HOW TO

1. Sit on your mat with the knees bent and feet flat on the floor. Place your hands behind your knees.

2. Slowly lean back, slightly rolling your tailbone under so it does not grind into the floor. As you lean back, lift your legs off the floor and balance. Your lower arms and lower legs are parallel to the floor.

3. Lengthen and flatten your back, trying to eliminate any roundness. Lift through your sternum or upper chest. Slide your shoulder blades toward each other behind you, and keep lifting long through your neck and head.

4. Keep your energy flowing in all directions, and breathe calmly and deeply. Hold for several breaths, challenging your abdominals, legs, hip flexors, and back.

VARIATION

While in boat pose, inhale and open the V shape of the body, then exhale and draw the knees close into the chest. This yoga move will deepen the ab work and also help strengthen the back.

PROGRESSIONS

Once you have mastered the pose with the arms and lower legs parallel to the floor, you can develop the pose. The first progression is to keep the lower legs parallel to the floor, releasing your grip on the legs and energetically reaching your hands toward your feet (arms still parallel to the floor), at the same time keeping the shoulders back so as not to round the back (see progression 1). The next progression is to straighten your legs to about a 45-degree angle to the floor so the feet are at about eye level, maintaining a flat back and a lifted chest (see progression 2). The final progression would be knee-ins, and this is to bring the knees in and out with your breath to further challenge the core muscles (see progression 3).

PROGRESSION 1   **PROGRESSION 2**   **PROGRESSION 3**

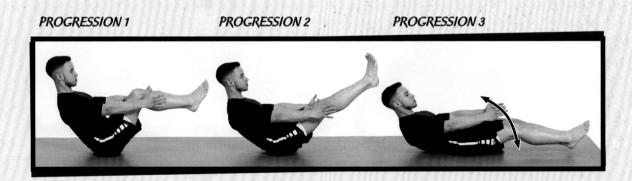

HERO'S POSE
VIRASANA

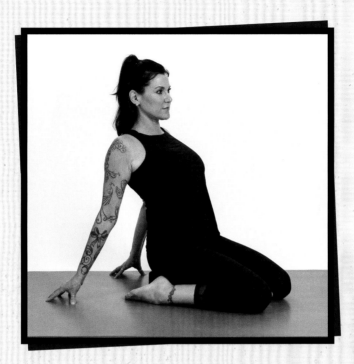

Hero's pose may seem like a great position in which to watch TV or just sit, but there are many requirements for executing this pose safely. It requires proper attention and a strong foundation in order to maximize the benefits and avoid discomfort or pain.

Hero's pose is a great pose for aligning the body and settling in for meditation. It strengthens the back and spine. At the same time, it opens the chest and helps increase lung capacity. It is a cooling pose to find your center. It stimulates and brings blood and oxygen to the lower organs, which is beneficial to people suffering from reproductive problems or sexual issues, past or present.

For athletes, I teach this pose either as described or with a toes-tucked variation. This helps those who need speed and agility to open up the plantar fascia of the foot. Most importantly, it stretches and keeps the vulnerable Achilles tendon supple. This pose is a must for soccer players, runners, wide receivers, tennis players, and basketball players who need explosive feet. Another huge benefit of hero's pose is that it can help athletes avoid the dreaded turf toe. Turf toe is a compression injury to the joint at the base of the big toe, also known as the ball of the big toe. It is categorized as a sprain to the big toe joint. By keeping the toes as flexible as possible, the impact of repetitive plays on hard surfaces is lessened.

BENEFITS

✓ Increases flexibility in the hips, legs, ankles, and knees

✓ Encourages proper alignment in hips, legs, and knees

✓ Opens the hips

✓ Stretches the quads

✓ Encourages and trains internal rotation

✓ Strengthens the low back while lengthening the spine

(continued)

CONTRAINDICATIONS

This pose is contraindicated for those who have had recent ankle surgery. Modifications should be made if you are currently suffering knee pain or have recently had knee surgery. If you have pins and plates in your knees, you should avoid this pose altogether unless you are closely monitored.

HOW TO

1. Start on your hands and knees, and slowly sit back onto your heels while lengthening the upper body into a tall, seated position.

2. The most important part of this pose is to ensure that the tops of your feet press into the floor and the bottoms of your feet face up. Pull the thighs together unless you feel strain in the knees; in that case, allow for a comfortable space between the thighs.

3. Ground through the little toe side of the foot. Lift both sides of your rib cage and lengthen through the crown of your head. Relax your shoulders. Rest your hands on your thighs, and relax into your breath.

VARIATIONS

- For some, just sitting back on the heels can be painful. If this is the case, place a block or two on the floor between your feet and sit back on the block until you are secure and open enough to take it away. If you are extremely tight or recovering from knee surgery, place a rolled-up towel behind your knees before sitting back. This will reduce the risk of overflexing the knee.

- Try half hero's pose to allow you to focus on one quadriceps at a time. Sit in hero's but with one leg extended straight out in front of the body (see variation). You can also fold over the straight leg to add more hamstring work.

VARIATION

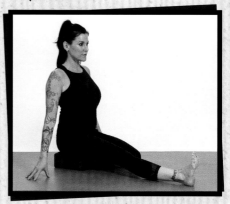

PROGRESSION

As a progression, you can move deeper into the pose by trying to sit on the floor between your feet (see progression). It will take time and practice to deepen this pose. Try to remain tall and lifted without rounding the back. Eventually the legs will open enough that you can start to sit further back into reclining hero's pose. First, the hands go on the floor behind you, and eventually you will be lying flat on your back here.

PROGRESSION

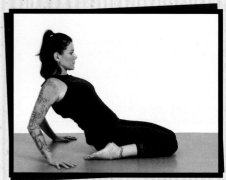

HERO'S POSE WITH TOES TUCKED
VIRASANA VARIATION

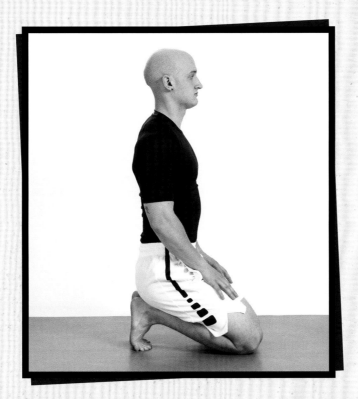

This pose is one of the most challenging for my athletes. They find it difficult to breathe and concentrate here, but the benefits far outweigh the two minutes of discomfort felt.

Whether you are in high heels for much of your day or simply on your feet in work boots, you can suffer great pain and stiffness in the ankles and feet. Taking time to sit in this pose and allow muscles you wouldn't normally think of to stretch will increase the range of motion in the ankle and foot. Better movement of the ankle and foot makes it easier to walk and reduces foot cramping.

Athletes must pay particular attention to their feet. They must stretch their toes, ankles, and lower legs for greater ease of movement, for quickness, and for greater jumping ability. So for basketball players, volleyball players, and goalkeepers, you would consider this for improving their vertical leap. For runners, soccer players, and outfielders who run a lot, you would consider this to increase their finesse and ease of motion while running. Athletes who often need power to push off and go uphill, such as hikers, should also make the time for this pose. Perfecting this pose can greatly reduce the likelihood of serious injury if an athlete rolls his or her ankle while playing.

BENEFITS

✓ Stretches the plantar fascia and the bottoms of the toes

✓ Relieves foot cramping

✓ Opens the Achilles tendon

✓ Stretches the calves

✓ Slows the progression of bunions

(continued)

CONTRAINDICATIONS

This pose is contraindicated for those with acute turf toe, those with calf problems, or those who have had recent foot or Achilles tendon surgery.

HOW TO

1. Start on your hands and knees, and tuck your toes under.

2. Be sure that your heels are pointing straight up to the sky. If they are not, you could be putting undue stress on the knee joints.

3. Slowly sit back onto the heels; you may need to lean forward with your hands on a block until you are open enough to sit straight up.

4. Hold this pose for two minutes.

5. It is a good idea to do a traditional hero's pose after this to open the ankle in both directions.

VARIATION

If it is too difficult at first to sit on the heels, you can come to standing on the knees to reduce the pressure in the foot until you are ready to engage in a full-seated position (see variation).

PROGRESSION

Once you feel comfortable in this pose, consider bringing the hands behind you on the floor to add a deeper progression to the foot and ankle stretch (see progression).

VARIATION

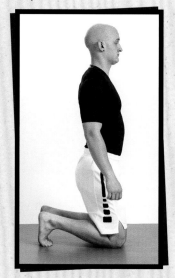

PROGRESSION

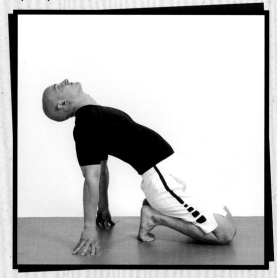

CAMEL POSE
USTRASANA

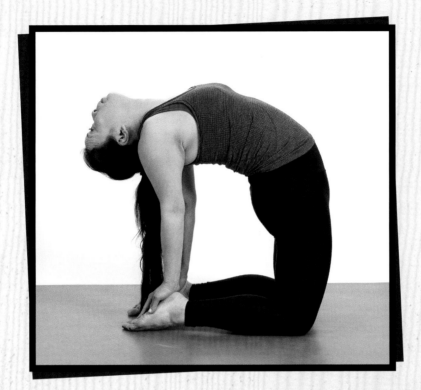

Camel pose is a great front body opener. The more elongated the front and back of the spine are, the deeper and more powerful your rotation will be. Rotation is king for golfers and for increasing the authority in their swing. Most people slouch through their daily routines whether they are at a desk, driving, or walking. Camel is key to opening the front of the spine, extending the back, and opening the lungs.

For athletes, the more back extension they have, the less the demand on their shoulders. For sports such as tennis, lacrosse, and wrestling that require power in the shoulders, the shoulders can get overextended and become stressed. If the back can go with the shoulder movement, it will absorb some of the shock and depth of stretch, many times preventing injury.

BENEFITS

✓ Stretches the front of the body, the chest, abdomen, quadriceps, and hip flexors

✓ Improves spinal flexibility and posture

✓ Strengthens the back muscles

✓ Creates space in the chest and lungs, increasing breathing capacity and helping to relieve respiratory ailments

✓ Stimulates the kidneys, which improves digestion

✓ Energizes the body and helps to reduce anxiety and fatigue

(continued)

CONTRAINDICATIONS

This pose is contraindicated for those who have had recent back surgery or spinal herniation.

HOW TO

1. Start on your knees with your knees hip-distance apart. Press your shins and the tops of your feet into the floor. For this version, start kneeling with your toes tucked to help keep the feet open and cramp free, a bonus to this pose.

2. Tuck the tailbone under to protect your low back from too much pressure.

3. Reach back and rest your right hand on your right heel. Once you are open enough, rest the left hand on the left heel at the same time.

4. The action in the pose should feel like you are lifting the heart to the sky, pressing the hips forward; if your neck is OK, drop the head back.

5. Hold the pose for three to five breaths and release to rest. Repeat it three or four times until your spine feels supple and your abdominals feel a good stretch.

VARIATION

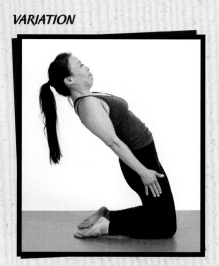

VARIATION

Try camel leans to increase the flexibility in the hip flexors and quads and to strengthen the legs (see variation). From camel pose, place the arms alongside your outer thighs and hinge from the knees, leaning back as far as you can without breaking the line of the body from shoulder to knee.

Does it matter if I do seated poses first or last in my allotted teaching time?

It does not matter. In fact, there are deep restorative sessions I do where the athletes never stand at all. You must use your knowledge and experience to make the proper decisions each day you teach.

COW FACE POSE
GOMUKHASANA

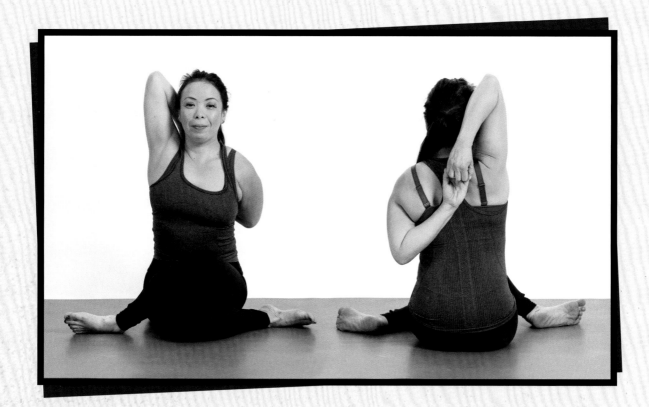

Cow face is a challenging seated pose. It is a deep hip opener, as well as being famous for its difficulty for those with tight shoulders. Although it is a seated, deep hip stretch pose, it is noted as being a restorative one as well for its ability to allow you to sit and go inward in order to get a full muscle release.

Cow face pose opens the shoulder joint, giving a wider range of motion. It is a key pose for opening the hips. Hips are the known storage depot for stress, anxiety, and fear. Sitting in this pose for several minutes while concentrating on your breath helps to release these deep muscles. Cow face pose improves your posture because of the intense focus on the lift of the spine.

For the athlete, cow face pose tests the ability to stay tough in a difficult situation. Working to open the shoulder joint, this pose is an obvious choice for pitchers, quarterbacks, or any position that depends on powerful, accurate arm movements. It opens and clears the rotator cuff while strengthening the supporting back muscles to add power. Stretched and strengthened hips and thighs equate with power and speed in running games from tennis to basketball. Opened glutes give more power to push for speed. Improved posture for athletes translates into more space in the chest cavity, improving lung capacity and breath control for runners, wide receivers, basketball players, and any others whose aerobic capacity is key to success and longevity in their sport.

BENEFITS

✓ Deeply stretches the hips, ankles, thighs, shoulders, armpits, chest, deltoids, and triceps

✓ Aids chronic knee pain

✓ Strengthens the spine and abdominals

✓ Helps decompress the low spine (during folded variation)

✓ Clears the hip joint

(continued)

CONTRAINDICATIONS

This pose is contraindicated for those with neck, knee, or shoulder problems and for those with untreated herniation of the spine. If you have sciatica, the use of a prop under the hips or while folding forward could aggravate the condition.

HOW TO

1. Start in a seated position with the legs crossed. Align the bent left knee over the bent right knee, stacking them directly on top of each other and under your center (chin). The heels are equidistant from each hip.

2. Fully plug into the floor through both hips. Lift your sternum and achieve a flat, tall spine.

3. Reach your right arm up to the sky. Bend the right elbow so that the left palm rests on the upper back. Bring the left arm out to the side, palm facing back and thumb down. Bend the left elbow, and move the left hand behind your back, palm facing out. The left forearm is parallel to the spine, and the hand is between the shoulder blades.

4. Hook the fingers together behind your back. Energetically lift your right elbow toward the ceiling, keeping the elbow close to the right side of your head, and lower the left elbow toward the floor while keeping it close to the body.

5. Sit straight and tall in the back, keeping both hips in contact with the floor. It is easy to overstretch your left side (top arm side) and collapse your left side; keep both sides of your body equally long.

6. Hold for the desired time, and then switch sides. The emphasis on this side is the right anterior shoulder; therefore, this side is more difficult for right-handed people. The reverse is true when switching to the other side. This pose may be frustrating in the beginning; however, the shoulders tend to open quickly, so stay focused and determined, and results will come quickly.

VARIATION

If both hips aren't evenly on the floor, sit on a blanket or block to place equal weight on both sitz bones. If one hip is higher than the other, you are starting the whole pose off crooked, and this will dramatically change the back and shoulder positions, causing potential harm. If it is not possible to connect your fingers, place a strap in the left hand. Let the strap hang behind your head and grab the other end with the right hand, working the fingers closer and closer to each other until eventually they connect.

PROGRESSION

Once you have mastered this pose, if you feel you can go deeper, fold from the hip joint as you extend over the left thigh. Do not round your back.

PROGRESSION

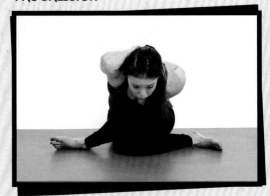

7

Floor Poses and Inversions

Practicing floor poses and inversions are essential when teaching athletes how to hold poses longer so they can move into a deeper stretch. This is a good time for you to focus on breathing and mental toughness while utilizing visualization techniques to get athletes through the tough moments of wanting to stop the pose before time is up. Athletes tend to over-relax in these poses, so it is important for you to make sure they maintain proper form and structure in each pose for the duration of the hold. Floor poses will significantly increase the degree of flexibility your athletes have. For some of the prone floor poses, your focus will be on alignment and functional strength building instead of flexibility. The demands on the body are clearly geared toward stability and muscle building rather than increased suppleness.

OPPOSITE-ARM OPPOSITE-LEG

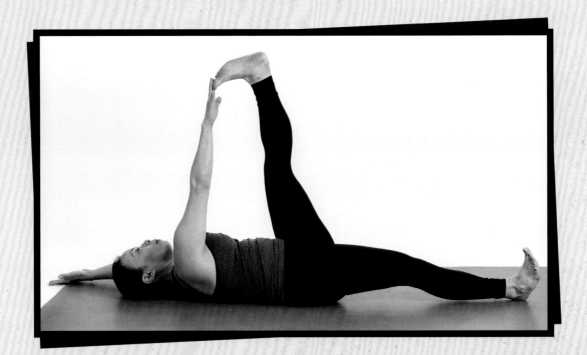

This is not exactly a yoga pose; it is more of a centering warm-up yoga movement that I start all my yoga classes with. This movement is a great habit to get into before starting your yoga practice. It is a perfect way to disconnect from the outside world and center your breath and your thoughts to prepare for a more focused practice. This is the time to tune into your body and identify any tight spots or misalignments to focus on during the practice. For example, notice which hamstring is tighter during this movement.

For athletes, opposite-arm opposite-leg is also an opportunity to tune into misalignments and imbalances and to synchronize the breath with the movement. Too often, athletes hold their breath during workouts. This exercise helps them get into the habit of breathing when they move. It is an amazing way to warm up the whole hip joint to prepare you for a grueling day on the field of play. The more open the hip before taking to the field, the less the pressure on your knee joints and the quicker and more agile you will be right from the get-go. Every athlete wants to explode on the field. This move also warms up the whole shoulder joint. This big motion is done deliberately to warm the joint before it has to bear weight, catch a pass, or throw a fastball. Finally, it is a gentle way to engage the abdominals, creating more strength and stability in the core.

BENEFITS

✓ Lubricates the shoulder and hip joints

✓ Stretches the hamstrings

✓ Opens the shoulder joint and hip joint

✓ Strengthens the abdominals

✓ Allows you to practice syncing the breath with movement

✓ Centers the mind and body

CONTRAINDICATIONS

This pose is contraindicated for those who have had recent shoulder surgery, those who are in the late stages of pregnancy, and those who have a low back injury. Those who have pins in their shoulders may use modifications, such as performing the move without using the arms or taking a wider angle with the arms.

HOW TO

1. Lie on your back, arms stretched overhead and toes pointing to the front of your mat.

2. Reach overhead and arch the back; this move will almost send you into a big yawn.

3. After taking a few breaths, inhale as you press your low back into the mat while you engage your abs.

4. As you exhale, leave your head on the floor as you lift your right arm and left leg up to touch your fingertips to your leg. In a perfect world, the fingertips touch the toes. This means that your hamstrings are nice and open. I often hear athletes say, "My arms are not long enough!" That is not the case. Some people start out only able to touch their knees. With time and practice, this will gradually improve.

5. Repeat with the opposite arm and leg, and continue this alternating motion.

6. Pull your knees into your chest when you are finished.

Supine Floor Pose

RECLINED BIG TOE POSE

SUPTA PADANGUSTHASANA

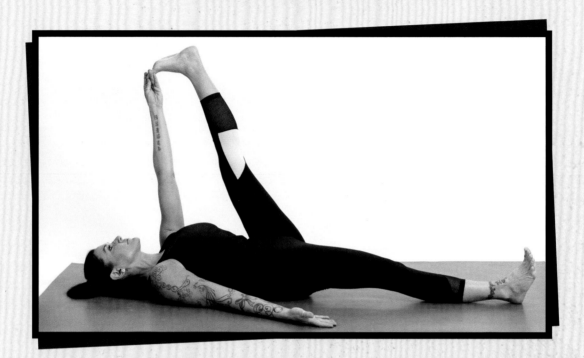

Reclined big toe pose is exactly what its name suggests, and it works to deeply open the legs. You may have done this pose without even knowing its name or seen this pose done on the sidelines by coaches and trainers with their athletes.

This pose improves the flexibility of the hamstrings, groin, and calves. It gives you the opportunity to see the differences in each leg and to address serious issues before they cause injuries. It is the pose to prepare you for utthita hasta padangusthasana, which looks like the same pose except that you perform it standing up, and it is much more challenging. Once you create the muscle memory of the pose while you are lying down, adding the standing balance element becomes easier.

For the athlete, this pose is essential for the health of the hamstring. I find it a better choice than seated forward bend because athletes with tight hamstrings tend to overpull their backs while doing seated forward bend. This lying pose makes injuring the back a nonissue. It's a great pose for athletes who need their legs to be open and agile. Once you've mastered the pose, you can ask a partner to carefully help you push the stretching leg farther and farther.

BENEFITS

✓ Stretches the hips, hamstrings, calves, and groin

✓ Helps strengthen the knees

✓ Improves digestion

✓ Helps the athlete to become aware of asymmetries in the legs

✓ Helps relieve back pain and symptoms of sciatica

CONTRAINDICATIONS

This pose is contraindicated for those with high blood pressure, those with serious neck issues, and those who have had recent knee surgery.

HOW TO

1. Lie on your back, and draw your left knee into your chest.

2. At the same time, extend the right leg on the floor, and reach through the heel.

3. Slowly straighten your left leg toward the ceiling, pushing through the left heel. Always be mindful of pushing through both heels, creating a strong dynamic opposition.

4. Aim for a 90-degree angle with the legs, and grab your left big toe with your left first two fingers and thumb.

5. While pulling the left leg in, be sure not to pull so hard that you lift your shoulders off the floor.

6. Keep your shoulders broad and flat on the floor. Press the right thigh down, and try not to arch your back.

7. Keep both hips on the floor and square.

8. Hold for one to three minutes, then switch to the other side.

VARIATIONS

Place a strap across the arch of the left foot if you cannot reach the toe. In time and with practice, you will be able to pull on the strap to draw your leg closer to your face and to open the left hamstring further. Eventually, you will not need the strap. To challenge yourself even more, let your right leg hover about two to three inches off the floor.

How do inversions affect athletes with high blood pressure?

First, be sure your athlete is cleared by a doctor to do inversions. Standard medical advice for people whose blood pressure is controlled by medication is to engage in exercise and other healthy activities that a person with normal blood pressure would do. Therefore, it seems reasonable that you can safely introduce inversions if you do so gradually. In fact, inversions trigger several reflexes that temporarily reduce blood pressure.

LYING SPINAL TWIST
SUPTA MATSYENDRASANA

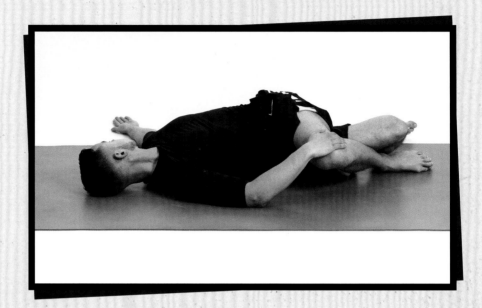

Lying spinal twist is a master pose that opens many parts of the body at the same time. It is best saved for when you can devote a longer period of time to it.

Many people find themselves slouching and holding poor posture in the spine over the span of a day. This creates restricted breathing, weakened abdominals, and overstretched spines. Seated spinal twist supported by the floor allows the back to lengthen again and deeply realign. Any twisting pose is considered a pose of detoxification due to the literal wringing out of the internal organs.

For athletes, adding spinal twists becomes critical for those engaged in agility-focused, high-speed, moving sports. Athletes in lacrosse, soccer, tennis, and golf should add this pose to their regimens. Note whether it is more difficult to perform on one side of the body than the other, and spend more time on the side that holds more tension. In this pose, you are stretching the spine, chest, anterior shoulder, and hips all at the same time.

BENEFITS

✓ Stretches the spine, chest, shoulders, and neck

✓ Aids digestion

✓ Improves respiration

CONTRAINDICATIONS

This pose is contraindicated for people who have had recent back or shoulder surgery.

HOW TO

1. Lie on your back, and draw both knees into your chest.
2. Cross the left thigh over the right thigh, and slowly drop the legs to the right, resting the legs on the floor.
3. Use the right hand to weigh down the knees to the right.
4. Extend the left arm to the left with the palm facing up, and turn the neck to the left, aligning the chin over the left shoulder.
5. On the inhale, press the knees further into the floor; on the exhale, press the back of the left shoulder closer to the floor. Eventually, you will be able to press the knees and the back of the shoulder flat on the floor at the same time.
6. Release in the belly and breathe deeply.

VARIATION

Try lying spinal twist with a block between your thighs to engage the legs and lower abdominals. Extend the arms out on the floor, palms facing down. With the knees into your chest, drop your legs all the way to the right (see variation), then return to center and drop to the left. Repeat this yoga move for two minutes to warm up the spine, hips, and shoulders and to bring heat to the body.

VARIATION

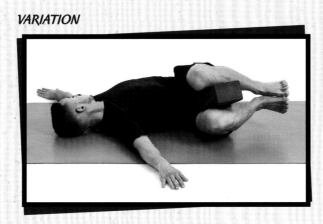

SEATED SPINAL TWIST
ARDHA MATSYENDRASANA

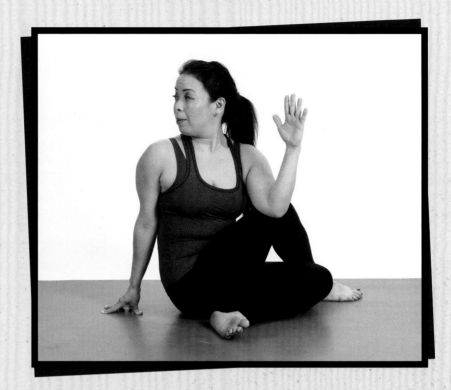

Seated spinal twist has many of the same benefits as lying spinal twist. The added bonus of being seated is that you are strengthening the back and core muscles. This pose also allows you to twist more deeply than lying spinal twist. The lying version is limited to the knee touching the floor, whereas in seated you can twist deeper and deeper without restrictions. All twists are detox poses because they seem to "wring out" the organs; they are also great for aligning the spine. If you find yourself slouching at a desk all day or enduring long hours in a car, it would do you well to sit and twist, taking time to realign, stretch, and lengthen the spine.

This pose is particularly important for athletes who lunge, twist, run, and are very acrobatic on the field of play. Soccer players, hockey goalies, wrestlers, lacrosse players, receivers in football, and infielders in softball and baseball are examples of athletes who should be taking time to improve their spinal flexibility. This will make their reactions on the field more fluid and effortless and will protect the back from injuries.

BENEFITS

✓ Stimulates the liver and kidneys

✓ Stretches the legs, back, shoulders, hips, and neck

✓ Stimulates the digestion

✓ Relieves menstrual pain and fights fatigue

✓ Alleviates sciatica and backache pain

CONTRAINDICATIONS

This pose is contraindicated for athletes with herniated disks and those who have had recent back surgery.

HOW TO

1. Sit on the floor with your legs straight out in front of you.

2. Slide your left foot under your right leg to the outside of your right hip. Lay the outside of the left leg on the floor. Both hips should be firmly plugged into the floor.

3. Place the right foot over the left outer thigh, and be sure your right foot is flat on the floor. The right knee should point directly up at the ceiling.

4. Exhale and twist toward the right. Press the right hand against the floor just behind your right buttock.

5. Your left upper arm should be on the outside of your right thigh near the knee. Pull the right thigh in toward your chest.

6. Lengthen the torso on an inhalation; on an exhale, twist deeper and turn your chin toward your right shoulder.

ROCK AND ROLL

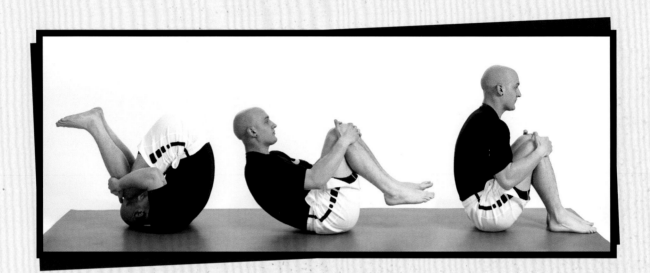

Rock and roll is part of the typical warm-up, and I do it before every class starts. It is a great way to help align the spine, warm up the body, and analyze your athlete. This move is a good icebreaker because it is easy and it is fun, reminiscent of younger days.

For the athlete, I find this move critical. Athletes and the coaches can instantly identify imbalances in the back that may need further help. This movement is especially good for swimmers because they need to be aligned in the spine. If they are pulling to the right or left even a centimeter, it can cause them to work less efficiently and ultimately can cost them a race.

BENEFITS

✓ Aligns the spine

✓ Stretches the posterior spine

✓ Can be used for assessment

✓ Aids digestion

✓ Eases abdominal cramps

CONTRAINDICATIONS

This pose is contraindicated for those who have had recent back or neck surgery or spinal herniations.

HOW TO

1. Start by lying on your back, drawing the knees into your chest. If your athlete has knee issues, they should always grab behind the thighs, not over the shins; this will avoid the possibility of overstretching the knees.

2. Inhale and exhale while tucking your chin to your chest, then start to get momentum, and rock and roll.

VARIATION

For the twisted root abdominals variation, while you are on your back, bring your hands behind your head as though you were going to do an abdominal crunch. Wrap your right thigh over your left thigh and your right foot behind your left calf, if possible, as though you were performing eagle legs. Crunch your forehead to your knees and at the same time bring your knees to your forehead (see variation). Do this repeatedly for deep core work.

VARIATION

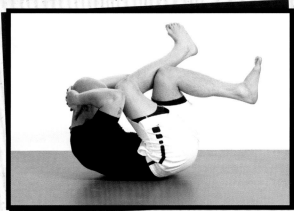

Supine Floor Pose

PLOW
HALASANA

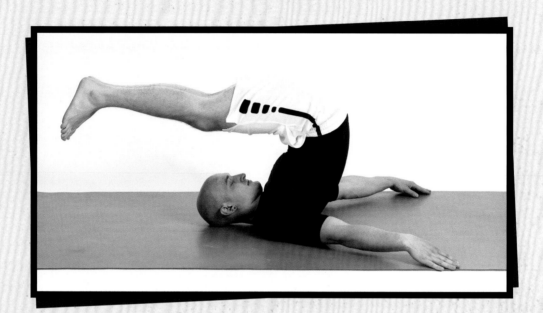

Plow is the go-to stretch for the posterior spine, releasing tension. For allergy sufferers, it is a perfect choice to open the neck and squeeze the glands in that area to help them drain. Plow pose enables practitioners to reap the benefits of a mild supported inversion without stressing the neck as in headstand. When you focus, you will feel an amazing, itchy type of feeling in your muscles and a deep stretch from the base of your skull down to the heels.

For athletes, this is a targeted pose to release, de-stress, and feel your breathing. I recommend this pose to athletes such as wrestlers to prepare their necks for awkward positions they find themselves in during matches. I have also seen soccer players and football receivers playing at top speed lose their footing and fall; because they have so much momentum, they end up doing a backward somersault. If they prepare their bodies with plow holds, they lessen the chance of suffering a neck strain.

BENEFITS

✓ Stretches the spine, shoulders, and back

✓ Calms your nervous system, reduces fatigue and stress

✓ Improves digestion

✓ Massages and stimulates the thyroid and lower organs

✓ Detoxifies the lungs

CONTRAINDICATIONS

This pose is contraindicated for those who have had neck surgery or spinal fusion or for those with neck pain.

HOW TO

1. Start by lying down on your back. Arms should be down by your sides, palms flat on the floor.

2. Draw your knees into your chest, and press down into your arms.

3. Bring your legs up and over your head. If your flexibility allows, straighten your legs and allow your feet to touch the floor over your head. Reach the legs long.

4. Snuggle the shoulder blades closer to each other, then interlace your fingers, extending the arms long along the floor. When you snuggle the shoulder blades under, it lifts C6 and puts less pressure on the neck.

5. You should feel a back stretch, a hamstring stretch, and a gentle stretch to the back of the neck. The deep stretch to the whole back of the spine and body here will help release tension in the back and in the neck.

6. Hold and breathe.

VARIATION

If you are less flexible, you may have a slight bend in your knees, and your feet will not touch the floor. Snuggle the shoulder blades close together under your body, bend the elbows, and place the hands flat on your back (see variation photo). In this way, you support your body in the pose.

VARIATION

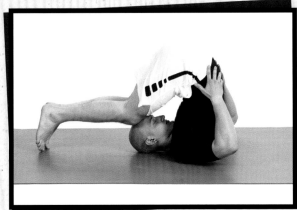

FACE-UP SHOULDER STRETCH

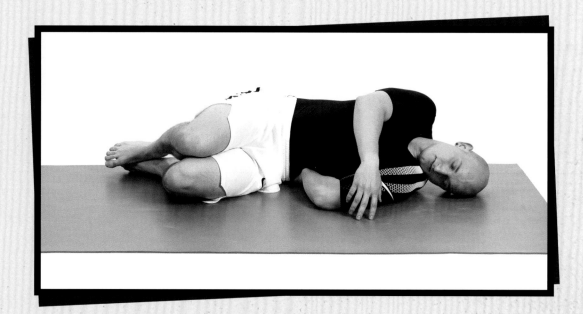

This pose is a very localized stretch, but it offers big benefits. If you suffer from bursitis pain in the shoulder, face-up shoulder stretch targets the muscles that overlay the bursa, which can bring relief or even help to prevent the bursitis altogether.

Even though face-up shoulder stretch seems to be stretching a small area, the results are huge. When you can release the chest and front shoulder, you will increase the range of motion in the shoulder joint. Since it is a shallow ball-and-socket joint and vulnerable to injury, when it is not too rigid you have more give and therefore can absorb more shock with larger movements. Many people collapse the chest and shoulders with poor posture and decrease their depth of breathing. This pose will help you to stand taller and breathe easier. Great posture not only looks better but also promotes better organ function and overall health.

For the athlete, keeping the shoulder joint supple yet strong is important to its health and longevity. Also, shoulder mobility lessens the strain on the back. Sports like swimming, racket games, softball, and many more use the shoulder to the utmost. Stretching the shoulder in all directions while maintaining strength in all directions will give you great power. For cyclists, this pose is crucial to release a tight anterior deltoid and chest.

BENEFITS

✓ Releases tension on your bursa sac

✓ Stretches the anterior shoulder

✓ Increases range of motion in the shoulder joint

✓ Improves posture

CONTRAINDICATIONS

This pose is contraindicated for those with a history of shoulder dislocation or those who have had recent shoulder surgery. Also, never allow anybody to adjust or push you in this pose. For this reason, be sure small children or large dogs are not in the area while you perform this pose.

HOW TO

1. Start by lying on your back, knees bent and feet flat.

2. Bend your left elbow so your arm in relation to your back creates a figure-four shape, and place the left hand palm-side down, hand flat, and fingers spread underneath the small of your back. Note that if you place the hand under your butt, you will crush it; the slight arch of the low back is the place to settle the hand. The right arm is relaxed at your side.

3. Slowly drop your knees to the left, stacking the legs as they drop over. If it feels too deep at first, place a block under the legs.

4. Breathe and sink into the pose.

5. Eventually, you will start to roll the back to the right, too, instead of lying on your back. You can bring the left arm across your chest. Feel the deep front shoulder stretch. Try to release and relax with every exhale.

Supine Floor Pose

BRIDGE
SETU BANDHA SARVANGASANA

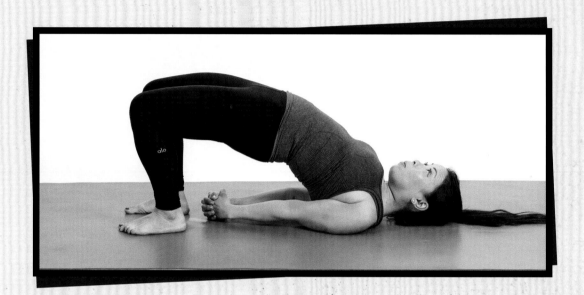

Bridge pose is classified as a backbend, but it should be considered an assessment pose as well as a therapeutic pose. Bridge is accessible to practitioners of all levels, and it should not be overlooked by advanced yogis and athletes.

Bridge pose lengthens the front of the body as well as the back of the body, creating space between your vertebrae and relieving pressure on the disks. For people who are concerned about thyroid function, the bend in the neck and holding of the pose for lengths of time is believed to stimulate a sluggish thyroid. The thyroid is responsible for stoking your calorie-burning fire. In addition, bridge pose supplies the posterior neck with an awesome stretch. It also holds you (especially if you use blocks for support) in a gentle backbend.

For the athlete, this pose is a great tool for assessment. You have a bird's-eye view of your chest and sometimes the abdominal area to observe any imbalances or asymmetry. This will give you a clue about what poses you will need to improve your game. Bridge pose also gives the practitioner an easy way to open the hip flexors and psoas, which is essential for keeping the back healthy and strong. It gives the athlete a pose to assist in opening the chest, which creates lung space and increases breathing capacity. When you snuggle the shoulders under, it gives an amazing stretch to the chest as well as to the anterior deltoid. When practicing this pose, be careful not to sink into it too much, but remain very active in it at all times. Finally, holding this pose without block support strengthens the hamstrings.

BENEFITS

✓ Strengthens the back, glutes, legs, and ankles

✓ Opens the chest, heart, and hip flexors

✓ Stretches the chest, neck, shoulders, and spine

✓ Calms the body and alleviates stress and mild depression

✓ Stimulates organs of the abdomen, lungs, and thyroid

✓ Rejuvenates tired legs

✓ Improves digestion

✓ Helps sinus health

CONTRAINDICATIONS

This pose is contraindicated for those with neck injuries, unless they are supervised. Those with low back pain or knee pain should use modifications. Also, it is important that you get your shoulder blades under you as much as you can. The further they go under, the more they lift your spine off the floor, creating a canal underneath you. This canal keeps the spine from grinding into the floor. Cervical vertebra number six sticks out a little more than the rest, so if you are not properly set up in this pose, it is easy to bruise it or feel too much weight.

HOW TO

1. Start by lying on your back, knees bent, feet flat and hip-width apart.

2. Feet should also be parallel and the ankles directly under the knees. It is important to have the feet parallel to reduce pressure on your low back. When the feet are turned out, they close the space in the sacroiliac joint and create more stress on the joint and back than necessary.

3. Begin to tilt the pelvis and raise your hips off the floor, pressing down through the feet and arms.

4. Once your hips are as high as they can get, snuggle your shoulders underneath your upper back, and try to interlace your fingers under you. In time and with practice, your fingers will be interlaced, and your arms will be extended fully on the floor, palms connected. If you tend to hyperextend your elbows, be cautious here.

5. Try to get your chest to meet your chin, and press your shoulders down and away from your ears.

6. Relax and release into the pose, holding for several minutes. You should feel a dynamic opposition of pressing down with your arms and feet while lifting the pelvis and chest.

VARIATIONS

- It can be helpful to place a light, soft block between your knees to help engage your inner thighs in this pose. It is also an amazing therapeutic pose if you put two blocks together, on their highest side, directly under your sacrum and clasp your hands beyond the blocks. Also, consider sometimes interlacing your fingers the opposite way than you usually do. This places your shoulders in a slightly different position and minimizes the effects of habit and stagnant practice.

- Try bridge lifts to increase the flexibility of the hip flexors and quads and to strengthen the glutes and hamstrings. In bridge pose, lift and lower the hips.

- Try figure-four bridge to add load to work the hamstrings and glutes (see variation 1). In bridge pose, flex your right foot, and bring your right knee into your chest. Rest the outer right ankle against the left thigh, resembling a figure-four. You may need to center the left foot for better alignment. Keep the hips square. Hold this pose, or raise and lower the hips.

- Try reclining pigeon if you are recovering from knee issues and the traditional pigeon pose places too much pressure on the knees (see variation 2). From the figure-four bridge, lower the hips. Reach and grab your left thigh with both hands, and draw the thigh in as tight to your chest as needed to feel a deep hip and glute stretch. Use your right elbow to guide the right thigh in an external rotation.

VARIATION 1

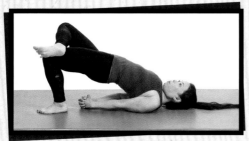

VARIATION 2

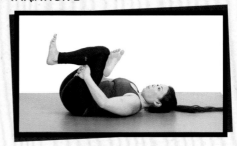

INVERTED PLANK POSE
PURVOTTANASANA

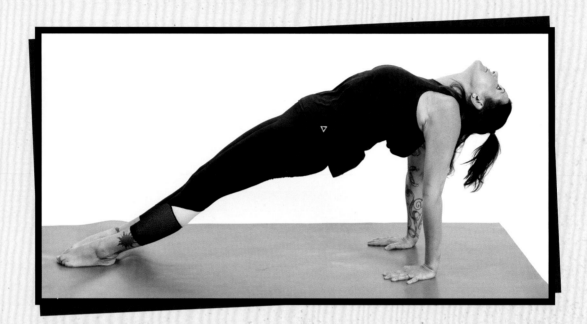

Inverted plank is a stabilization and back-bending pose. It affects several glands in the body, including the adrenals, thyroid, and thymus. The pose stimulates the organs of the abdominal cavity as well as the diaphragm and breath. This pose is also a powerful pose of purification because it stimulates the kidneys.

Most people hunch forward much of the day: desk jobs, driving, and taking care of little ones encourage a forward posture. We would all benefit from stretching, strengthening, and lengthening the front of the body. In addition, strengthening the back of the body—which becomes overstretched from our day-to-day grind—is a great relief to the internal organs and abdominals. Inverted plank also opens the wrist joint, which can help to prevent carpal tunnel syndrome.

For athletes, this pose is a great pelvic stabilizer. Pelvic stabilization and suppleness are important to lessen the strain on knees. More importantly, it is superior for building strength, stability, and openness in the wrist joint and shoulders, as described for the plank and side plank poses. Inverted plank also extends the elbow joint. This is important because many athletes have very developed biceps muscles, leaving the elbow with less range of motion. This can decrease power, especially for a baseball pitcher or a football quarterback who needs a powerful throwing arm. Finally, inverted plank pose decreases the anterior rotation of tight shoulders, which lessen range of motion and can even torque the trunk out of alignment.

BENEFITS

✓ Stabilizes the pelvis

✓ Strengthens the buttocks, back, legs, arms, and shoulders

✓ Increases oxygenation by opening the chest and ribs to allow for greater lung capacity

✓ Massages the abdominal cavity

✓ Stimulates the glands

✓ Stretches the shoulders, arms, and hip flexors

CONTRAINDICATIONS

This pose is contraindicated for those who have had shoulder pain or a history of injury and those with high blood pressure, stroke, or heart disease. Modifications, such as keeping the chin tucked into the chest, should be made for those with back and neck issues.

HOW TO

1. Sit on the floor with the legs extended straight out in front of you, back tall, and arms down by your sides (seated mountain pose).

2. Bring your arms behind you about 12 inches, shoulder-width apart. The correct distance will place the wrists directly under the shoulders when you are fully expressing the pose. Make sure your fingers are spread wide and the hands are completely plugged into the floor. Lean back into your hands, and slowly pour your weight into them.

3. Expand your chest with breath, and feel the shoulder blades come closer together.

4. Press equally into the hands and heels, and raise your hips off the floor until your body makes a long line from your toes up your legs and through the torso, chest, and head. Reaching that point takes diligent practice.

5. Press equally and firmly through both heels. Elongate the top of the foot as you extend the foot so the toes touch the floor. Keep a strong line of energy up the legs. Internally rotate the thighs slightly to help you in getting and keeping the big toes connected to the floor. Do not lift the hips too high or let them sag. Beginners can keep the chin tucked into the chest; as you progress, drop your head back, opening your throat.

6. Press the hands down into the floor, getting full extension of your arms and elbows. This will strengthen the wrists, which should be at a 90-degree angle. Continue to open the chest with your breath, expanding and lifting it. Keep your pelvis and low back neutral. Feel the torso and legs stretching away from each other.

VARIATION

Try inverted table pose if inverted plank pose is too difficult or if you want a deeper hip flexor stretch or wrist challenge (see variation). Bend the knees to 90 degrees, supporting the lower body with both feet on the floor.

VARIATION

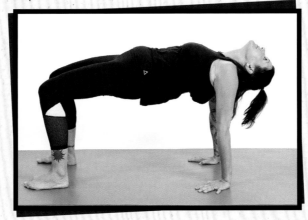

HEAVY LEGS
VIPARITA KARANI

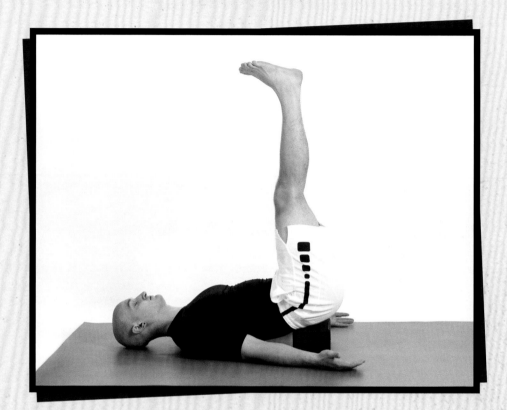

This is a therapeutic yoga pose and one that is highly touted in the yoga community as the "destroyer of old age" because it is said that it can rid you of all that ails you. This pose is easy to perform for people of all levels and all ages.

Heavy legs is considered an excellent restorative pose. It is usually practiced at the end of a class or instead of final resting pose. People who experience leg edema find that lying in viparita karani eliminates the painful "full" feeling in their legs and feet. Also, anyone will benefit from the lymph drainage promoted by this pose. Lymphatic system flow, unlike the blood flow, is blind-ended in the hands and feet, so when we are too sore to run or to go about our normal activities, the lymph collects in the extremities, causing feet and hands to swell. Sitting in heavy legs is much more effective and relaxing than just putting your feet up.

For athletes, this pose is great for soreness 24 to 48 hours after a tough game or workout. Many athletes, especially those who depend greatly on the strength and stamina of their legs, will benefit from this pose. Often athletes complain of the heavy or dead feeling they get in their legs after grueling days on the field. This will alleviate that feeling. I do not have to describe to you how critical fresh legs can be to winning championships. I also do not have to explain the importance of quickening your step and lightening your load to making game-winning plays. All athletes can do this pose without compression equipment or wraps. You can do it either before or after games. In fact, this is a great pose to do for three to five minutes before a game while you visualize your game-winning strategy.

BENEFITS

✓ Believed to help relieve anxiety, arthritis, headaches, insomnia, digestive problems, mild depression, varicose veins, menstrual cramps, PMS, and menopausal symptoms

✓ Regulates blood pressure

✓ Relieves tired, cramped legs

✓ Stretches the hamstrings, low back, and back of the neck

✓ Calms the mind

✓ Lightens the legs and quickens the step

✓ Drains sluggish lymph

✓ Relaxes the body and eases the mind

✓ Improves deep breath and focus

CONTRAINDICATIONS

This pose is contraindicated for those with a history of serious eye problems such as glaucoma, serious neck issues, or very high blood pressure. Those who have had recent back surgery should perform the pose with bent knees.

HOW TO

1. Lie on the floor and simply walk your buttocks all the way up against a wall, or if a wall is not available, you can put your low back on a block as shown.

2. Extend your legs straight up the wall. If you have very tight hamstrings, you may walk your hips about six inches away from the wall, or you can have a bend in the knee. In time and with consistent practice, you will be able to straighten your legs.

3. Arms can be out to your sides, palms face-up, or extended straight out from the shoulders with a 90-degree bend in the elbows, palms facing up.

4. Tuck the chin to the chest to extend the back of the neck.

5. Soften your eyes, and be very heavy on the floor. Stay in the pose from 1 to 15 minutes.

6. To come out of the pose, slowly bend your knees and roll over onto your right side, curling up into a fetal position. Linger for a few breaths, and then press up to a sitting position.

VARIATIONS

• The use of a block and a strap is recommended if you do not have an available wall for support (see variation 1). Adding the strap also helps deepen the stretch in the calves and Achilles tendons.

• Try straddle heavy legs to increase the flexibility of the groin and inner thigh (see variation 2). From heavy legs, open the legs as far as you can into a straddle position.

(continued)

VARIATION 1

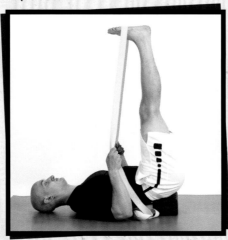

VARIATION 2

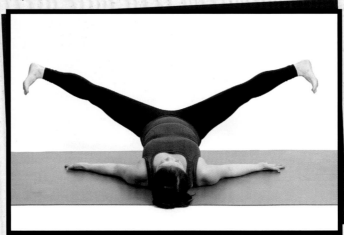

I heard the heavy legs pose is good for lymph drainage. Can you explain what that is and how it helps athletes?

Yes! Lymph is not circulatory like the blood, so it depends on the contraction of muscles and movements to get flushed out of the toes and fingers. Has your athlete ever gone for a run and couldn't take his rings off when he was done? That is because they forced the lymph into the fingertips. After a game or when your athletes are sore, their muscles are less efficient at flushing the lymph, and therefore they experience a heaviness, a cement-like feeling in the legs. To get the "fresh legs" trainers and coaches strive for, have your athletes lie in this pose for three to five minutes.

HAPPY BABY POSE

ANANDA BALASANA

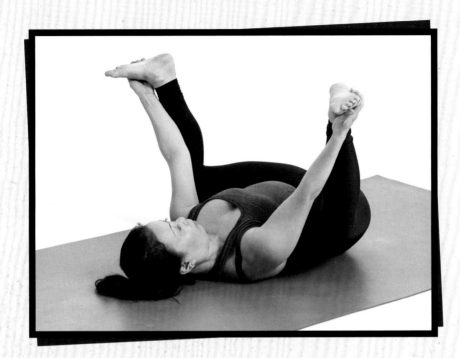

You can probably imagine what this pose would look like by its title. I often tell my students that if they are in a good mood, it is happy baby pose; if they are not feeling so great, it is dead bug!

Happy baby pose elongates and lengthens the back. The pose offers a safe way to release low back tension as well as neck strain, such as that which we get from long hours at the computer. This pose is also a great way to open the hips and groin. It is a good warm-up pose to perform before a workout.

For the athlete, this pose should be considered before the start of any training or workout. It offers an easy groin and inner thigh stretch without placing a strain on the back or a demand on the legs. For basketball players, it is an all-encompassing stretch not only for the groin but also for the Achilles tendons and calves. Teach this to athletes such as soccer and tennis players because along with the stretching, it is a great pose for identifying asymmetries in hip flexibility. When the feet are pulled toward the armpits in this pose, it will become clear which hip is tighter, and this can indicate what needs to be done to avoid potential injuries. For example, if the right knee does not come nearly as close to the armpit as the left, it is an indicator that deep hip openers such as pigeon pose (see page 178) need to be done on the right side.

BENEFITS

✓ Relieves stress

✓ Increases vitality

✓ Stretches low back and calves

✓ Opens groin and inner thigh

✓ Releases neck strain and tightness

(continued)

CONTRAINDICATIONS

This pose is contraindicated for those with a serious neck injury or herniated disks, those who have had recent surgery, and those who are pregnant.

HOW TO

1. Lie on your back, and draw your knees into your chest.

2. Grab the outsides of your feet, and square your feet to the ceiling.

3. Your ankles should be lined up directly over your knees, with the knees forming a 90-degree angle and the thighs perpendicular to the floor.

4. On your exhalations, move your knees in toward your armpits. If your flexibility allows it, bring the knees closer to the floor alongside your body.

5. Lengthen the neck, and lower the tailbone to the floor, releasing the low back.

VARIATION

If you cannot reach the feet, hold a strap that is draped across the balls of the feet.

RECLINING COBBLER'S POSE
SUPTA BADDHA KONASANA

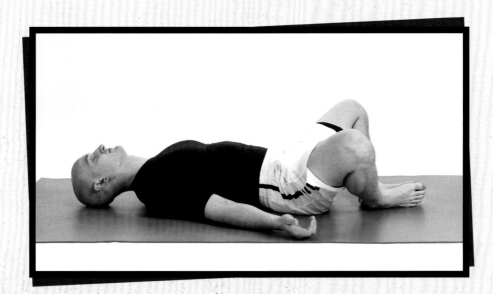

This pose, also called diamond pose, is a nice alternative to corpse pose or a final resting pose. While you fully surrender here, you are pulling double duty, opening both the groin and the inner thigh. I prefer to do this pose as part of my warm-up routine in class; it is beneficial whenever you fit it in, even as a stand-alone pose. Make sure you concentrate on fully letting go. Pushing the feet a little farther away from you in this pose while forming the diamond shape will shift the intensity of the stretch for most people from the deep groin and inner thigh area to the outer glutes and hips. It can feel very satisfying, especially when paired with a pigeon pose.

Since training time is so precious to athletes, I can kill two birds with one stone with this pose. That is why I like to have my clients hold this pose as a final resting position or in the beginning as a body scan. You can gently rock left to right with the legs so that you know that you are not holding lower body tension. While holding the pose, lift your head up, and look at your knees. If one knee is higher than the other, you probably have a tighter hip and groin on that side, so you need to stretch to that side more. You see this type of imbalance a lot with kickers, punters, pitchers, and even soccer players who have favored plant legs and kicking legs. Finding time for mindful breathing is difficult, but if you are coupling that time with a focused stretch, it is time well spent. For athletes who depend on healthy knees—and what sport doesn't—this pose will open the hips at a different angle, relieving some pressure on the medial knee especially. Cyclists also tend to overuse their adductors to find balance on their bikes; this is a good pose to sit in and allow the opposite movement.

(continued)

BENEFITS

✓ Stretches the groin, inner thigh, and outer hips

✓ Releases pressure in the low back

✓ Increases depth of respiration

✓ Induces feelings of calm

✓ Releases deep tension in the body

✓ Lengthens the low back

✓ Settles the mind

✓ Increases mindfulness

CONTRAINDICATIONS

This pose is contraindicated for those who have had recent knee or low back surgery.

HOW TO

1. Start by lying on the floor with your knees bent and your feet flat.

2. Drop the knees open, one in each direction.

3. Slide your feet forward about 12 inches from your bottom so that the inner edges of your legs form a diamond shape. Make sure your feet are in alignment with each other, toes against toes and heels against heels. The seam between your feet should align with your body center, sternum, and nose.

4. Hold and surrender to gravity for one to five minutes.

VARIATIONS

• Try reclining cobbler's pose with a block with athletes who are already flexible in the groin and are looking for a deeper option or for athletes with very well-developed thighs (see variation). When the thighs are very muscular, they inhibit the full stretch because the outer part of the thigh will touch the floor before the deepest stretch is reached. In the same position as reclining cobbler's, simply put your feet on a yoga block.

• Diamond Pose: Maintain the same positioning except move your feet forward toward the front of your mat an additional 18 inches (see variation photo). The inner edges of your legs should resemble a diamond shape. This variation changes the focus of the stretch from groin inner thigh to deep outer hip.

VARIATION

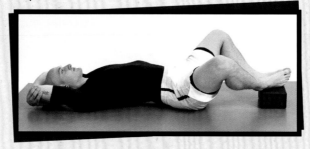

PLANK POSE
PHALAKASANA

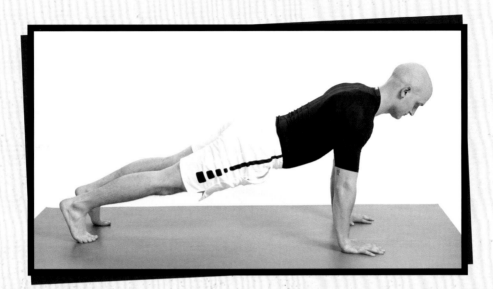

Plank pose is used widely in yoga as well as in the sports world. Although this pose looks like an insignificant transition move, it is a critical pose for assessing your body. This pose, like several in yoga, tends to go untaught, and teachers assume that the student is versed in the nuances of the pose. That is a mistake. Plank is a great teaching tool for the student.

Plank pose elongates the body and lengthens the neck. It is a neutral body position. It builds strength in the back, and it is a great pose for counteracting all the weakening the back undergoes each day. Building a strong back and abs at the same time is good for spinal support and for the development of better posture.

For athletes, this pose is particularly important for developing wrist integrity. Whether you play soccer where you are in danger of falling on your wrists, racket sports where power in the wrist is crucial, or on the offensive line in football where wrist strength will help determine how well you play and for how long, plank pose will help your performance in these and many other sports. Athletes should be able to open their wrists to a 90-degree angle to avoid injury and wear. Holding plank will accomplish that goal. Holding the body in the plank with knees off the floor challenges the athlete by using body weight to build strength while increasing flexibility.

BENEFITS

✓ Strengthens the arms, wrists, spine, quads, and abdominals

✓ Tones the core

CONTRAINDICATIONS

This pose is contraindicated for those with a history of carpal tunnel syndrome or degenerative low back problems. Note that even with a history of carpal tunnel syndrome, under the supervision of a highly qualified yoga teacher, plank pose can help with recovery from carpal tunnel syndrome. An athlete should be cleared for this pose by a medical professional before attempting it.

(continued)

HOW TO

1. Start in downward dog.

2. Lower the hips and bring your shoulders over your wrist joints. It is important to make sure the wrists are directly under the shoulders and the wrist forms a 90-degree angle.

3. The body should be in one line from the top of your head to your heels. You should not dip your hips or raise your hips. This is the same position as the top of a push-up.

4. Push back through your heels and forward through a neutral neck, out through the top of the head. Take a quick peek at your heels, and make sure that they are pointing directly up to the sky and that the feet are square.

5. At the same time, press firmly down through your whole hand, and keep the chest lifted. The hands should be totally engaged into the floor and flat. Spread the fingers, with even spacing between them. It is important not to press so firmly in this pose that you end up with a hyper-extended elbow.

6. Gently slide your shoulder blades down your back so your shoulders are out of your ears and your neck is elongated. Your head should be a natural extension of the spine.

7. If you experience slight pressure in the low back here, tuck the pelvis until the feeling dissipates. Legs are strong, straight, and engaged.

VARIATIONS

- Try plank pose on the forearms to open the shoulder joint (see variation 1). Here, instead of the wrists being under the shoulders, the athlete places the forearms on the floor with the elbows shoulder-width apart. The full expression of the pose is having the forearms parallel to each other, which will only happen if the shoulder joint is clean and open. Holding forearm plank, as you will quickly notice, is a great abdominal and shoulder strengthener.

- Try toe push-offs while in plank to give the athlete more power to push off and more strength in the feet and toes (see variation 2). In plank, push off the toes to bring more weight onto the upper body, and then return. This pose is reminiscent of the "on your marks" push-off action at the beginning of a race.

- Try wrist turns to further develop flexibility in the wrists (see variation 3). While holding plank, turn one hand around at a time until the fingers are pointing toward the toes. Hold for several breaths, returning one hand at a time to neutral position. It is important in wrist turns that you make sure the wrists remain under the shoulder and at 90 degrees. Watch how much heat you create in the body quickly by holding the wrist turn variation.

- Try elbow to knee to continue to challenge the wrists and shoulders while adding another level of intensity to abdominal training (see variation 4). In plank pose, draw your right knee to the right elbow and squeeze. Try both sides; also try bringing the right knee to the left elbow and the left knee to the forehead, among many other variations.

- Try opposite-arm opposite-leg reach to improve overall core strength and balance (see variation 5). In plank pose, lift the left arm and energetically extend it forward as though you were shaking hands with someone. At the same time, lift the right leg and press it toward the back of the room. This pose will improve overall core strength and balance.

VARIATION 1

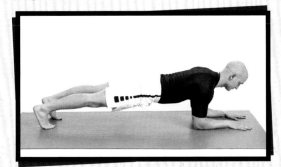

VARIATION 2

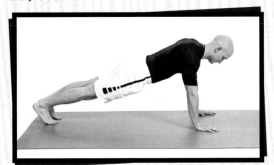

VARIATION 3

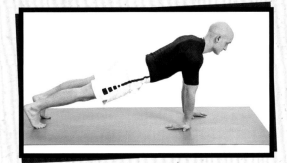

VARIATION 4

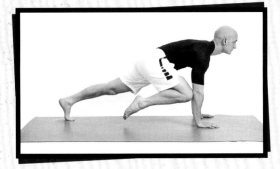

VARIATION 5

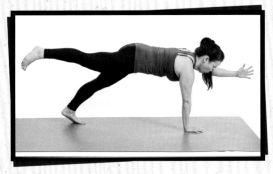

LOW PUSH-UP
CHATURANGA DANDASANA

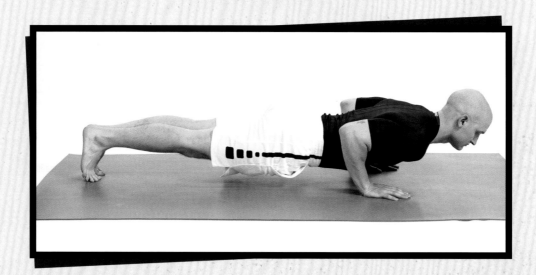

Most every workout you have ever done, whether it is based on yoga philosophy or not, has used the skill of low push-up. This is a great transition pose and overall strength builder. The power and control required to perform this pose properly is what makes it a great choice to add to most all Power Yoga for Sports routines.

For athletes, the beauty of this pose is that it offers the benefits of chest pressing motion without weights. Football linemen are familiar with this pose as part of their jobs, as are rowers who rely on tremendous push-pull power, but just about every athlete needs chest and anterior shoulder stability to perform better or to absorb a fall during play. You can use this pose as a transition in a routine or repetitively as a push-up exercise.

BENEFITS

✓ Strengthens the arms, chest, shoulders, and core

✓ Tones the abdominal organs

✓ Increases the flexibility of the shoulders

✓ Is a great pose of focus

CONTRAINDICATIONS

This pose is contraindicated for people who have had recent wrist surgery or are suffering from acute carpal tunnel syndrome.

HOW TO

1. Start in plank pose, tuck the tailbone under, and firm the shoulder blades to the back.

2. On an exhale, lower your torso and legs to the height of the elbows, when the elbows are in a 90-degree angle. Do not let your back sway.

3. Keep the space between the shoulder blades broad.

4. Don't let the elbows splay out to the sides; hold them close to the sides of the torso, and push them back toward your heels.

5. Keep the palms flat and the fingers spread.

6. Lift the heart; your head should look forward.

VARIATION

An extra challenge to chaturanga is to lower with one leg a few inches off the floor to further challenge the balance and strength of the upper body.

SIDE PLANK
VASISTHASANA

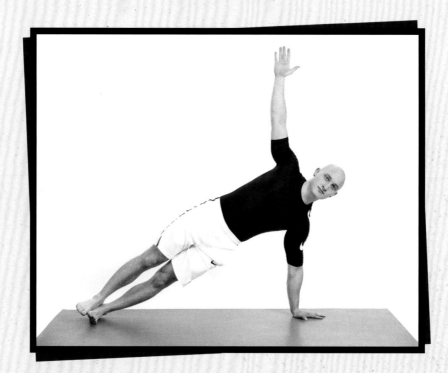

This pose is classified as a balancing pose. It demands full concentration as well as determination. Side plank is also the perfect pose for developing a strong, stable shoulder and wrist and for opening the chest and heart.

Any time your focus is on opening the chest, you are expanding the rib cage, which enables you to increase your lung capacity. This increases oxygenation to the body. This pose also helps you to strengthen the back and chest at the same time in order to achieve balance. In our overly forward-bending lives, we need to focus on the balance of strength and flexibility in the front and back to reduce the likelihood of injury to the spine. Since this is a balancing pose, it works our core, increasing strength through the midsection and reducing strain on the back.

For athletes, not only do I use this pose to increase abdominal strength (which is a concern for all athletes, from wrestlers to lacrosse players), I also use it to build a support system for the back muscles. Another reason to add this pose to the routine for athletes is to increase the strength, stability, and integrity of the wrist joint. Athletes who play tennis, golf, football, baseball, and other sports need to open the wrists and keep them flexible. Whether you are blocking a defender or swinging for a hole in one, rigid wrists increase the risk of sprains and carpal tunnel. The more open, strong, and flexible the wrist joint is, the more power you will gain in your sport. Also, in the event of a fall on the soccer field, a takedown in wrestling, or a powerful block as a goalkeeper, you want the wrists to be able to handle the force rather than break. Holding the side plank builds strength while stretching. Therefore, if you do fall on one hand during a game, your body is accustomed to taking the weight.

BENEFITS

✓ Strengthens the shoulder girdle, wrists, and elbow joints

✓ Increases abdominal strength

✓ Firms and tones the body

CONTRAINDICATIONS

This pose is contraindicated for those who have had recent abdominal, wrist, or shoulder surgery and for those who have serious eye problems or severe neck pain.

HOW TO

1. Begin in plank pose. Your shoulders should be directly above your wrists, creating a 90-degree angle; your body is in one line, without sagging in your hips or belly. Hold your legs strong and your core tight.

2. Drop your heels to the left, and slowly turn the body as you bring your right arm up to the sky.

3. Align your right arm to create a long line through your chest, down to your left wrist.

4. Open the chest.

5. Look up at your right hand. If you cannot, you will be able to in time; do the best you can.

6. Keep the legs and core strong throughout the hold. Maintain even, deep breaths, and elongate your body.

7. Hold for 5 to 10 breaths, then repeat on the other side.

VARIATIONS

- Try side plank mat touches to add strength to the obliques and shoulder joint (see variation 1). In side plank, take the top arm (right arm), and slowly lower it down and touch the outer left edge of your mat. Keep lifting the hips, then return to side plank.

- Try half side plank if your upper body is not strong enough to sustain plank (see variation 2). From plank, drop your right knee to the floor so the knee is directly under the hip. Bring the feet together, and lift your right arm up to the sky as you did in side plank. Once you become confident and strong and develop stable wrists, you will be able to execute this pose with the knee off the mat.

- Try extended-leg side plank as an advanced variation to challenge your core strength, balance, and shoulder stability (see variation 3). From side plank, lift the top leg off the lower leg and hold; if your right leg is on top, grab the right big toe with the right first two fingers and thumb of the right hand, and slowly extend the right leg toward the sky.

VARIATION 1

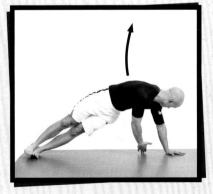

VARIATION 2

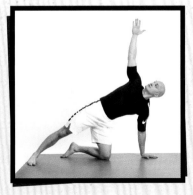

VARIATION 3

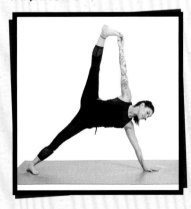

FOREARM SIDE PLANK
VASISTHASANA VARIATION

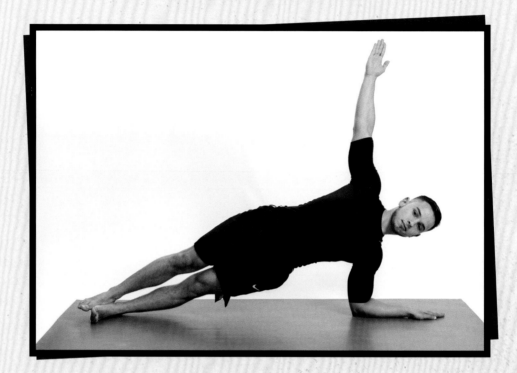

This is a good variation on extended-arm side plank. When you work from a bent elbow on your forearms, you face the truth of the shoulder's flexibility. You do not have the length of the arm and therefore more leverage to push into the shoulder joint.

This pose will steady the body and the mind. To hold your balance, focus your thinking and breathing. Holding your balance here is only possible if you engage the core and lift the kneecaps with the quadriceps muscles. It clarifies your awareness of the flexibility of the shoulders, the mobility in each shoulder, and how they differ. Holding this pose will start to engage and strengthen the smaller muscles of the shoulder joint rather than always focusing on the larger deltoid group.

Strong, supported shoulders are a must for athletes who use their arms a lot and depend on the shoulder for their success, like pitchers, tennis players, swimmers, and lacrosse players. The shoulder joint, like the hip joint, is a ball-and-socket joint. The main difference between them is that the shoulder joint is much less stable than the hip because it is much shallower. That is the reason why dislocated shoulders are more common than dislocated hips. That is also the reason it is so important to maintain strength and stability in the shoulder in all directions, not just in the front because that is the direction worked by chest and shoulder presses. This pose, along with downward dog, plank, and inverted table poses, creates strength and stability in multiple planes of motion.

BENEFITS

✓ Stretches shoulders and chest

✓ Creates balanced rotator cuff strength

✓ Increases abdominal strength

✓ Improves balance

CONTRAINDICATIONS

This pose is contraindicated for those who have had a recent shoulder dislocation or recent shoulder surgery.

HOW TO

1. Start on your hands and knees, lower down to the forearms, and set your elbows up directly under the shoulders.

2. Pivot the forearms so that they are as close to being parallel to each other as possible.

3. Straighten the legs out, and slowly drop the heels to the left.

4. Stack the feet, right foot on top of the left.

5. Raise the right arm straight up to the sky.

6. Try to create one long line from the right fingertips down the right arm, through the chest, and down through the left upper arm.

7. The left forearm and feet will eventually be in one line, like you are on a balance beam.

8. Hold for the desired length of time, 5 to 10 breaths.

VARIATIONS

• If you cannot stack your feet, keep the feet staggered (see variation 1).

• Try hip kisses to challenge the strength of the oblique muscles (see variation 2). While in forearm side plank, slowly lift and lower the hip that is closer to the floor.

VARIATION 1

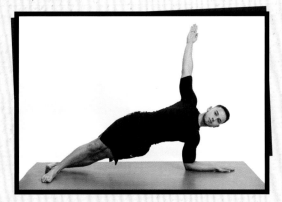

VARIATION 2

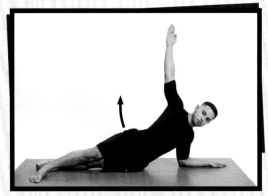

WRIST OPENERS

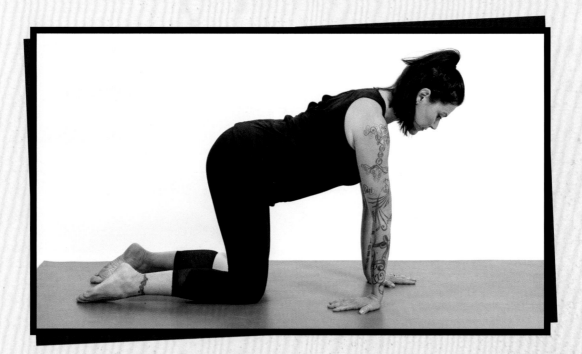

Everybody, whether you are a stay-at-home parent or a professional athlete, should consider adding wrist openers to their routine. If you have stiff wrists and fall, you might break a wrist and could also damage soft tissue. If your wrists are more flexible, you will better absorb the fall and perhaps walk away with only a strain and a little embarrassment. Take the time to open the wrists. If you work a lot at the computer or type a lot on your phone, you can develop carpal tunnel syndrome, and this stretch will help address that ailment as well.

For the athlete, wrist openers can stave off a more serious injury if you fall as a goalkeeper in soccer making a diving block, a receiver in football falling out of a play, or an outfielder in baseball motoring to make the catch. In addition to helping in a fall, more flexible wrists will give you more power if wrists are involved in your game like in pitching, throwing, or swinging a racket. Having more strength and flexibility in the wrist will improve the power equation in your Power Yoga for Sports program:

Strength + Flexibility = Power

BENEFITS

✓ Increases the mobility of the wrist joint

✓ Stretches the forearms and biceps

✓ Strengthens the chest and shoulders

✓ Warms the body

CONTRAINDICATIONS

This pose is contraindicated for those who have had recent wrist or biceps surgery or those who have a dislocated shoulder. If you have pins in your wrist, you should perform under the watchful eye of a trained professional.

HOW TO

1. Start on the knees in table pose.

2. Do one wrist at a time. Start by externally rotating your right arm so your fingers go from pointing to the 12 o'clock position through 1 o'clock, 2 o'clock, and 3 o'clock until they are at 6 o'clock.

3. Always start with the middle finger touching the kneecap. As you test the extent of your flexibility, you can slowly and carefully move your hand forward until one day the wrist joint is directly under the shoulder joint.

4. Push the floor away, and do not sink your shoulders into your ears; keep a long, extended neck. If you can place the wrist joint directly under the shoulder, you will slightly pull back the wrist joint and hold.

5. Since you are working smaller muscles, I recommend you do 30-second stretches two times on each side.

VARIATION

For the more seasoned yogi or athlete, these wrist openers can be done while in plank pose.

Prone Floor Pose

PUPPY POSE
UTTANA SHISHOSANA

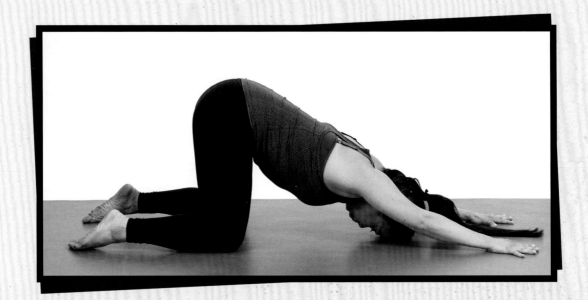

Puppy pose is, to me, the unsung hero of yoga stretches. It tends to be overpowered by its big brother pose, downward dog. When this pose is done properly, you can actually get a deeper stretch in the shoulders, lats, and chest and rest at the same time.

Many of us hold tension in the neck and shoulders without even knowing it. Stresses of the day, work, home life, and relationships easily get piled on the shoulders, causing stiffness, decreased blood flow in the head and neck, and just plain old pain. Puppy pose is a restorative hold that can bring your mind closer to the tightness in your shoulder girdle and neck. You can easily focus your mind and breathe here, liberating the neck and shoulders. When the neck holds less tension, breathing is easier, and the shoulders have more range of motion, therefore decreasing the likelihood of injury.

For the athlete, puppy pose offers a beautiful moment to release and relax the buildup of tension in the shoulders. This pose offers time to rest the head on the floor and focus on the tension being held. Once release begins, you can take advantage of the increased range of motion in the upper body. Athletes such as water polo players, volleyball superstars, racket sports competitors, and pitchers can all benefit from a five-minute hold here. When the neck is less tense, the shoulder can open to its full potential and lessen the load on the upper back, too. It is not a magic bullet; like all the rest of the poses in this book, it holds the potential to change your game when you apply it diligently.

BENEFITS

✓ Stretches the shoulder joint, chest, lats, and sides

✓ Opens the rib cage to increase depth of respiration

✓ Relieves tension on the neck

✓ Tractions the spine

✓ Improves mindfulness and stillness

CONTRAINDICATIONS

This pose is contraindicated for those who have had recent shoulder surgery or shoulder impingement.

HOW TO

1. Start on your hands and knees in table pose with the hip joints directly over your knees and the wrists directly under your shoulder joints.

2. While keeping your hips directly over the knees, start walking your hands out in front of you about 16 to 24 inches away from the starting position. The palms are flat, fingers spread, and hands are shoulder-width apart.

3. Feel as if you are gluing your hands down into the floor, arms straight, and start to slowly pull the hips back slightly. You will start to feel an itchy type of feeling in your stretch in the chest, shoulders, and side as you exaggerate each breath.

4. Rest your head on the floor.

5. Hold the pose and breathe until you start to feel the opening, release, and a bit more ease in the pose.

VARIATION

You can rest your head on a block if the forehead does not reach the floor.

Prone Floor Pose

DOWNWARD DOG
ADHO MUKHA SVANASANA

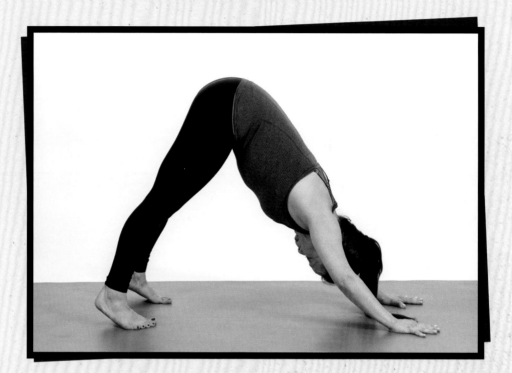

Most people have heard of the downward dog pose, whether they do yoga or not. As commonplace as it is, it is often assumed and not taught in the yoga studio, but it is not to be taken lightly. Downward dog has many functions; it can be used for assessment, transitions, resting, strengthening, inversions, and as an overall rejuvenator.

Downward dog elongates and lengthens the back. Think about how critical this is for someone who sits all day, hunched forward. As a matter of fact, most people—whether they are moms, brokers, drivers, or teachers—are in a constant forward bend and would benefit immensely by stretching and lengthening the back, shoulders, and front of the body. Downward dog is also a mild inversion (since the head is lower than the hips), and inversions are great for increasing blood flow to the brain and eyes and flushing the sinuses.

For athletes, this pose is vital for assessing their postural needs and imbalances. While in downward dog, tune in closely to the hamstrings, and notice if they differ in tightness; do the same with the shoulders and the hips. Athletes should check alignment daily, before something in the body gives way to injury. Downward dog can open the hamstrings for quickness and speed, stretch the shoulders for upper body mobility, and keep the wrists strong and supple for improving skills such as grip strength for baseball or pushing on the offensive line in football. This pose also keeps the lower back open and strong, complementing a strong core; this is key to agility in sports such as soccer, football, tennis, and golf. Finally, this pose will stretch the toes, calves, and arches. Open, flexible feet translate directly to speed for any sport that includes a run or sprint.

BENEFITS

✓ Stretches the shoulders and shoulder blade area, hands and wrists, low back, hamstrings, calves, and Achilles tendons

✓ Strengthens the entire back and shoulder girdle, easing back pains

✓ Elongates the cervical spine and neck, creating an opportunity to relax the head and to benefit from the traction

✓ Eases tension and headaches

✓ Expands the chest

✓ Deepens respiration

✓ Lessens anxiety and stimulates full-body circulation

✓ Stimulates the nervous system, which helps with memory and concentration

CONTRAINDICATIONS

This pose is contraindicated for those with a history of carpal tunnel syndrome; serious eye injury; sudden, sharp pains while performing the pose; and those in late stages of pregnancy.

HOW TO

1. Place the hands shoulder-width apart on the floor in front of you with the fingers spread wide and the middle finger pointing straight ahead. Engage or "plug" your entire hand fully into the floor at all times to avoid excess strain on your wrist joint, the line of which should be parallel to the front edge of your mat.

2. Your feet are hip-width apart and parallel to each other, meaning that your heel is directly behind your second toe. If you were to draw an imaginary line from the left middle toe down to the left heel, the left heel across to the right heel, the right heel up to the right second toe, and the right second toe over to the left second toe, this should create a perfect square. Look at your lower leg or shin area: from ankle to knee, you should see a perfect rectangle when in the proper position. Your lower leg should never look like a triangle with your knees knocking in toward each other; that creates a risk of tension on the inside of the knee.

3. Support yourself equally by your upper and lower body, not resting heavily in the legs. Always push the floor away and engage the shoulders and the upper body: elongate rather than sinking your neck into the shoulders and upper back. From a side view, you will see a nice V: no rounding in the back (especially the low back) and no arching of the back, either.

VARIATIONS

• If you have tight hamstrings, you can bend the knees.

• Try one-arm downward dog to increase the strength of the shoulder joint and increase focus (see variation 1). In downward dog, lift one arm, and place it at your low back.

• Try downward dog push-up to increase the strength in the shoulder joint and core and also stretch the chest and shoulders (see variation 2). In downward dog, bend the elbows until the top of your head touches the floor, and then straighten the elbows. This variation will increase the strength in the shoulder joint and core and will also stretch the chest and shoulders.

(continued)

- Try downward dog leg kicks to get the heart pumping and to strengthen the glutes while challenging the shoulder girdle and wrists (see variation 3). In downward dog, vigorously alternate kicking your legs to the sky, or repeatedly kick one leg at a time.

- Try dolphin pose to add an extra challenge to the flexibility of the shoulders. This pose is the same as downward dog except you are on the forearms instead of the hands. Your forearms should be parallel to reach other with the palms flat and completely grounded. Since you do not have the leverage of the entire arms' length, you will immediately notice the extent of the flexibility in the shoulder. You may need to soften the knees to accomplish a greater shoulder stretch.

- Try dolphin push-up to add more core strength, mental toughness, and a different angle of shoulder strength building (see variation 4). For this variation, keep the elbows shoulder-width apart and interlace the fingers, creating a triangle with the lower arms. You will exhale and dive the head and upper body forward until your face reaches beyond your hands and gently touches the floor and your chest is hovering over the floor; exhale and press back to dolphin pose.

VARIATION 1

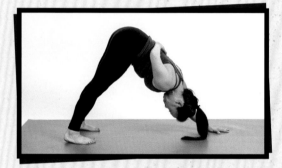

VARIATION 2

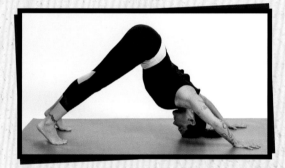

VARIATION 3

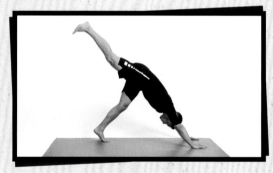

VARIATION 4

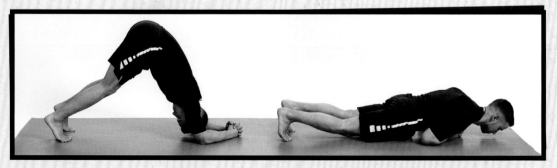

UPWARD DOG
URDHVA MUKHA SVANASANA

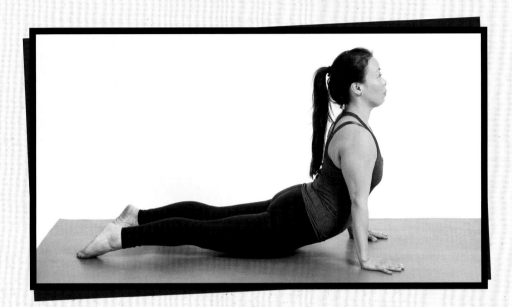

Aside from downward dog, upward dog is one of the most widely known and recognized yoga poses. Usually, upward dog is done during the Sun Salutation series. Upward dog has several functions, benefits, and therapeutic uses. It is the cousin to the cobra pose and is considered one of the easiest of the backbending poses. It is also considered a pose of assessment.

For the beginner, upward dog is just what the doctor ordered. Poses like this are critical for a healthy back. Backbending poses like upward dog counteract the problem of poor posture, which overstretches the back and weakens the abdominals. Upward dog allows our abdominal organs to function better, tones our arms and legs, and opens our hearts.

For the athlete, this pose works for many reasons. First, sports that require agility and speed often call for a supple, flexible spine. An open back is more efficient for making receiving plays on the football field, acrobatic plays in soccer, and strong swings in lacrosse. Second, upward dog stretches the quadriceps (front of the thigh) and the hip flexors (front of the hip). Balance between the front and back of the leg will keep the leg in harmony and lessen the risk of pulled hamstrings or quads. Third, upward dog develops strength and flexibility in the wrist, needed for powerful actions such as strong stick play in hockey or finesse shooting in basketball. Finally, the ability of this pose to open the rib cage and increase the breathing capacity is helpful for athletes in endurance sports. It may also help athletes who suffer from exercise-induced asthma by relieving tightness in the chest.

BENEFITS

✓ Strengthens the spine, arms, and wrists

✓ Firms the buttocks

✓ Stimulates the organs of the abdomen

✓ Improves posture by stretching the anterior spine and strengthening the posterior spine

✓ Stretches the chest, lungs, shoulders, and abdomen

✓ Helps to relieve depression, fatigue, and the pain of sciatica

✓ Opens chest space and increases lung capacity (may be therapeutic for those with asthma)

(continued)

CONTRAINDICATIONS

This pose is contraindicated for those with a history of carpal tunnel syndrome, those with serious back injury or disk issues, and those who are in the late stages of pregnancy.

HOW TO

1. Lie face-down on your mat. Feel the extension of the legs through the feet, which are about hip-width apart.

2. Bend your elbows, and place your palms flat on the floor with the fingers near the chest and spread wide, hands completely plugged into the floor. The elbows are at a 90-degree angle and close to your sides. The wrist joints are parallel to the front edge of the mat and at a 90-degree angle, also.

3. Press down through the tops of the feet and all 10 toes. Internally rotate the legs slightly (rolling the weight of the legs toward the pinky toes).

4. Press the palms down and gently lift your body off the floor. The only parts of your body touching the floor in upward dog are the tops of the feet and the palms of the hands.

5. Once your arms are fully extended, double-check that your wrist joint is still under your shoulder, stacking the wrist, elbow, and shoulder joints in one line. This positioning is critical and insures a safe, less stressed lower back. The most common mistake in upward dog is placing your hands too far in front of you or not stacking the joints of the arm, which can create tremendous low back pressure and pain.

6. Press down through your hands, and lift through the top of your head. Look straight ahead with a neutral neck to avoid compression on the neck and stiffening the throat. Lengthen the neck to avoid "the turtle head," where the head disappears into the neck.

7. Roll your shoulders back, pull the shoulder blades toward each other, and press your heart forward and up. Do not to let your elbows bow or hyperextend; the bends in the crooks of the elbows should face each other. To relieve pressure on the low back, press your tailbone down with a tucking action.

VARIATION

Try cobra push-ups to build shoulder and triceps strength and to add flexibility to the anterior space (see variation). In the upward dog position, repeatedly bend the elbows and lower your upper body down to the floor one vertebra at a time. Keep the palms flat and the fingers spread. On an inhalation, straighten the arms all the way.

VARIATION

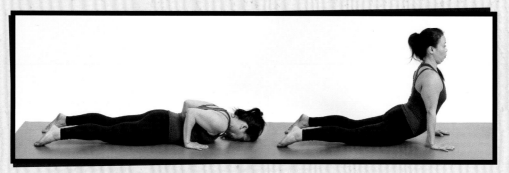

BOW POSE
DHANURASANA

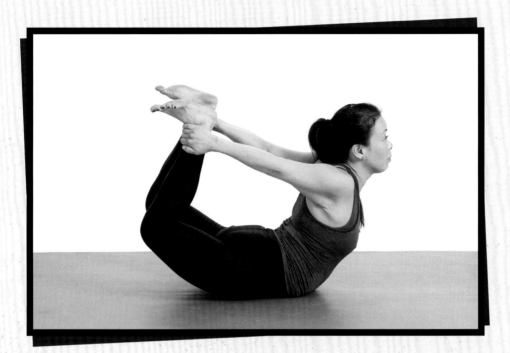

Bow is a therapeutic pose for those who often lean or bend forward throughout the day. The best way to undo a slouchy posture or long hours on the computer is by practicing bow pose.

Bow pose can alleviate constipation: the stretching of the anterior spine while in this gentle backbend creates a massage for the abdominal organs. It also eases tightness in the stomach and helps bring additional blood and oxygen to the area to aid in elimination. Regular practice of this pose will relieve lower back pain and will release tension and strain on the upper back and neck. I do not know anyone who would not benefit from some extra TLC for the back.

For athletes, this pose is a tremendous addition to their stretching routines. Athletes who play soccer, hockey, football, tennis, and wrestling all can appreciate the advantages of a flexible back. Athletic goal saves, powerful serve returns, and the compromising positions of wrestling all require great strength in the back. Most of these sports also encourage a spinal flexion position (forward bending). A hockey player constantly leans forward, for example, and the anticipatory ready position of a soccer player puts continuous stress on the spine. Being in this gentle back bend in bow pose is a welcome opener for the lungs and vertebrae. It also opens the hip flexors and psoas muscles. Greater spinal flexibility, better rotation, and less strain will improve agility and performance.

BENEFITS

✓ Strengthens the entire body, mostly the legs, back, and buttocks

✓ Improves digestion

✓ Helps people with respiratory ailments

✓ Relieves fatigue

✓ Decreases anxiety

✓ Stretches the whole anterior spine

✓ Improves posture

(continued)

CONTRAINDICATIONS

This pose is contraindicated for those who are pregnant or have had recent abdominal surgery and for those with high blood pressure, heart disease, and serious low back problems.

HOW TO

1. Lie on the floor face down. Extend and expand the body.

2. Bend both legs. Reach back, and try to grab onto your ankles or lower legs, thumbs facing down. For beginners, it is best to grasp the outer ankle. In time, you can externally rotate your shoulder and grab the leg on the inner ankle side, thumbs facing up.

3. Broaden your chest, and slide your shoulder blades toward each other, behind you and down your back. Relax your shoulders down and away from your ears. Lift the chest up by using the pure power of your legs to press back with your legs into your hands, arms straight and feet pressing up toward the ceiling.

4. Tilt the pelvis until you feel less strain in your lower back. Keep the chin tucked slightly to encourage a gradual backbend, finishing through the top of your head. Remember that your head is a natural extension of your spine. Keep your gaze neutral.

5. You can hold the pose as previously described while you breathe, or you can use this flowing option: On the inhalation, lift your upper body. On the exhalation, lift your lower body to initiate a gentle rocking motion with your breath. Press the chest and legs away from each other, "stringing the bow."

6. Gently let go, and release back into child's pose.

VARIATIONS

- If it's not possible for you to grab your ankles, you can wrap a strap around the legs and hold one side of the strap in each hand.

- Try side bow to open the side of the body and shoulders more (see variation). From bow pose, generate a little side-to-side momentum and roll completely over onto your right side, deepen the bow, and roll back to center, then over to the left side.

VARIATION

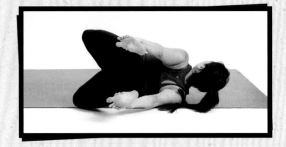

LOCUST
SALABHASANA

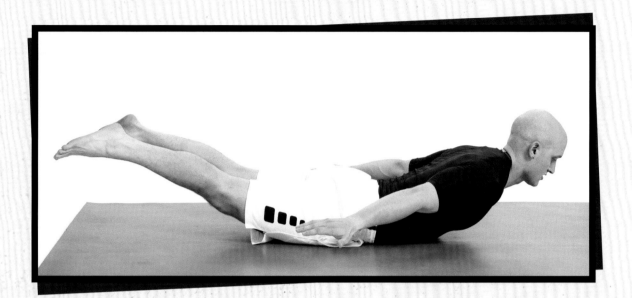

Locust pose is one of the best poses for developing posterior spine strength. Often we are slouched in our day-to-day lives, overstretching the back of the spine. This pose can be a challenge because unless you focus on it, your front spine is stronger than your back spine. If the posterior spine is untrained and unattended to, this will leave a great imbalance between the front and back of the body that will ultimately lead to injuries.

For the athlete, having balance in the spine is critical in addition to having strength in the back of the body. This pose is a good way to prepare for deeper back bends to further open the spine. I recommend that basketball players, volleyball players, outfielders in baseball and softball, goal-keepers, and lacrosse players add a lot of locusts to their routines because locust mimics the common moves they make during games. It will open the shoulders, increase the strength and flexibility of their reach, train the strength of the core, and help to protect the shoulder joint.

BENEFITS

✓ Increases back and shoulder strength

✓ Increases the flexibility of the core and shoulders

✓ Helps with constipation

✓ Helps with fatigue

✓ Decreases neck pain

CONTRAINDICATIONS

This pose is contraindicated for people who have had recent back or abdominal surgery and for women in the later stages of pregnancy.

(continued)

HOW TO

1. Lie on your stomach with the arms alongside your body.

2. Lengthen the legs, and on the exhale lift the upper and lower body, keeping the head in its natural alignment; do not overlift the chin.

3. On the inhale, lengthen the body; on the exhale, lift higher.

4. Keep the energy of the legs pressing back and the big toes toward each other.

5. You can extend the arms toward the front of the room, palms facing toward each other and upper arms alongside the head.

VARIATION

Try face-down snow angel to increase heart rate and respiration, to bring heat to the body, to increase back strength, and to improve the mobility of the shoulders (see variation). In locust pose, continuously make a snow-angel type of movement. Bring the arms to the front of the room and then down by your sides and the legs out wide and then close together, much like the action of a jumping jack. During this time, keep the upper body, arms, lower body, and legs off the floor.

VARIATION

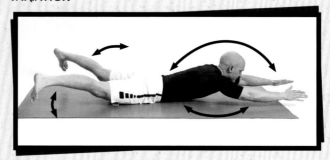

FACE-DOWN SHOULDER STRETCH
EKA BHUJA SWASTIKASANA I

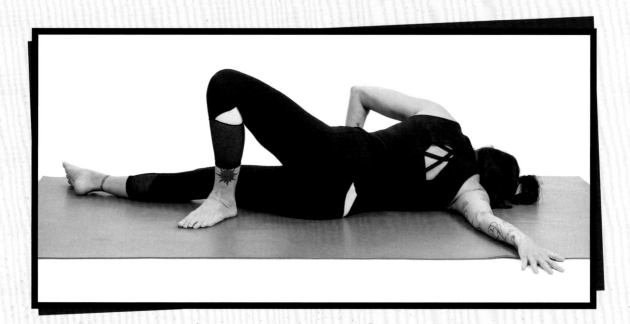

This pose is complicated and precise and should be done carefully without hands-on assistance from anybody, enabling you to breathe and go deep. This is a multifunctional pose to open many areas at the same time. It offers a stretch to the front of the shoulder, opens the chest and biceps, and at the same time provides a deep spinal twist to help improve posture. Some people, depending on their structure, may even feel a hip stretch. You need to take time to sink in here and feel the shoulder and spine open.

Athletes who need a large range of motion in the shoulder must increase strength and flexibility in all directions. This pose offers that multidirectional flexibility. Also, athletes, such as pitchers, whose elbow functions are critical to success will acquire deep opening by stretching the biceps. This is also a very safe pose because the floor does not allow hyperextension. I can see no better stretch for swimmers, fencers, softball and baseball pitchers, and even for defensive and offensive linemen who need shoulder flexibility to absorb the shock of big blocks and aggressive pushing.

BENEFITS

✓ Stretches the front shoulder, chest, and biceps

✓ Frees breathing

✓ Increases oxygenation

✓ Realigns the spine

✓ Increases flexibility of the neck

CONTRAINDICATIONS

This pose is contraindicated for those with unstable shoulders or for those who have had recent pectoral or shoulder surgery.

(continued)

Prone Floor Pose

HOW TO

1. Start lying face-down on the floor.

2. Straighten your right arm out to the side, palm facing the floor. See that your right middle finger is in line with your eyes so that the right arm is slightly higher than shoulder height.

3. Bend the left elbow, and place the left palm flat under the left shoulder, as though you were going to do a push-up.

4. Turn the head so you are resting on your right ear. Be sure to fully relax the head for the duration of the pose.

5. Bend the left knee; start to push into the left hand, rolling onto the right side of your body. Eventually, the left foot will be flat on the floor on the outside of the right leg, and the knee will be bent. Once you are very flexible here, both knees will be bent, both feet flat, and your butt will be flat on the floor.

6. With every exhalation, try to release the tension in the spine and right shoulder.

7. Use your left hand to support yourself in the pose, or gently press deeper into the pose.

8. Do not allow another person or outside force to push you deeper in this pose; let gravity intensify the pose.

9. Keep your right arm straight and your left palm flat on the floor.

10. Slowly roll back onto your stomach.

VARIATION

Try the 90-degree face-down shoulder stretch to open the shoulder joint at a slightly different angle (see variation). Follow the steps just as you do for the face-down shoulder stretch, except instead of having a straight arm, you will have the arm stretched at a 90-degree angle. Go into it slowly because you will probably not go as deep in this variation as you did in the straight-arm version.

VARIATION

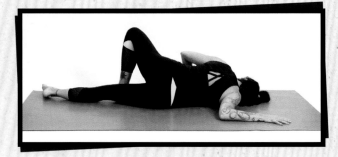

SPHINX
SALAMBA BHUJANGASANA

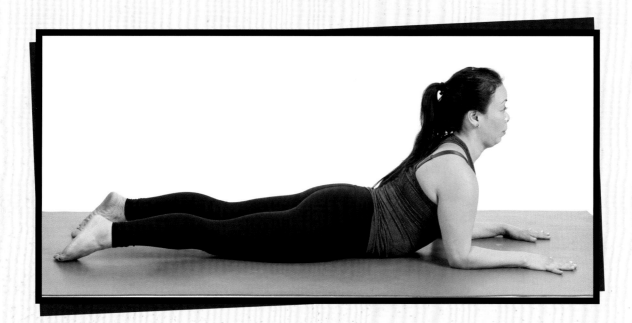

Sphinx, unlike plow, opens the front spine. It is also a great pose for those who suffer long hours at their desks or hunched over computers, playbooks, and phones. In these activities, you are probably shortening your anterior neck muscles and collapsing the chest. Being seated for long periods clamps your hip flexors in an engaged position, pressurizing the low back when you stand up. This is a relatively new ailment called tech neck and tech back. To prevent or alleviate it, you want to open your body in the opposite direction for optimum health. Holding this pose each day for one to three minutes will help immensely. This pose will open the front of the body from the top of the feet all the way through to the top of your head. Stress and pent-up feelings can make the shoulders tight, the chest constricted, and the posture less than stellar. Doing this pose will counter all that and will open the heart area, allowing for better breathing and freeing the upper body.

This pose is especially good for cyclists and others, like catchers, who spend long periods of time in deep-seated or squatting positions. They experience a shortening of the hip flexors and tightening in the low back. Sphinx pose will create balance in the hips, give you more ease of movement, and lengthen the quads. Wrestlers and others who are forced into awkward positions that compromise the spine and back should do this pose to help them absorb some of those forces and reduce potential back strains.

BENEFITS
✓ Opens up the chest cavity

✓ Strengthens the upper body

✓ Straightens and aligns the spine and internal organs for optimal functioning

✓ Stimulates the nervous system

(continued)

CONTRAINDICATIONS

This pose is contraindicated for those who have had low back fusions and recent abdominal or back surgery.

HOW TO

1. Start on your stomach and lift the upper body, placing the elbows directly under the shoulders, forearms parallel to each other, and palms flat with fingers spread.

2. Inhale and feel that you are creating length from the feet to the head, drawing the shoulders back toward each other and pressing the chest forward.

3. Don't let the head sink into the shoulders, but rather generate a proud chest and a lengthened neck posture.

4. Hold and breathe. When you feel more advanced, simply press into your hands and straighten the arms to increase the stretch.

5. To release: Exhale, and slowly lower the chest and head to the floor. Turn the head to one side; slide the arms alongside your body and rest.

CAT AND COW
MARJARYASANA AND BITILASANA

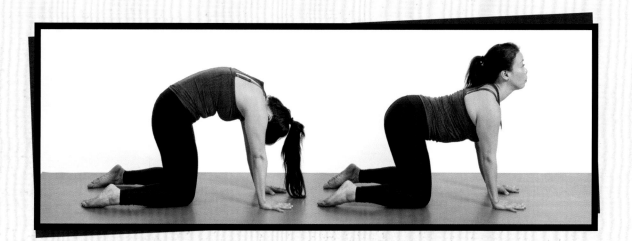

Cat and cow is a great transition pose and an easy way to warm up the spine and deepen your breathing. This pose is beneficial for increasing the suppleness of the spine. It allows you to get to the little spinal muscles; the larger spinal muscles; and the abdominals, neck, shoulders, and chest. Besides all those benefits, it just plain feels good. Cat and cow is a great way to pump the breath, refocus the mind, and get ready for deeper spinal work. It is another miraculous go-to yoga move for people who sit at desks for long hours or drive for many miles at a time. Doing this pose while seated on the edge of your bed before you even fully wake up in the morning will oxygenate the body and get you ready to face the day.

For the athlete, cat and cow movement is an enormously beneficial move: You cannot find a sport that does not need the cooperation of a flexible spine for more finesse and power. Incorporate this move as much as you can for every sport and position.

BENEFITS

✓ Assists with breathing

✓ Opens up the chest cavity, shoulders, and rotator cuff

✓ Creates a supple, flexible spine

✓ Frees tension in the neck

✓ Stimulates the thyroid gland

CONTRAINDICATIONS

This pose is contraindicated for those who have had recent neck or back surgery. Those who have had a back fusion should first perform the pose under supervision.

HOW TO

1. Start on your hands and knees, making sure your palms are flat, fingers spread, the wrists are directly under your shoulders, and the knees are directly under your hips.

2. Inhale into cat by arching your back and sucking the belly button up into the spine, pushing the floor away from you to feel it deep into the shoulders. At the same time, tuck your chin to your chest.

3. Exhale, and release the spine. Let the belly drop toward the floor into cow, creating a swayback as you lift the chin up to the sky.

THREAD THE NEEDLE
PARSVA BALASANA

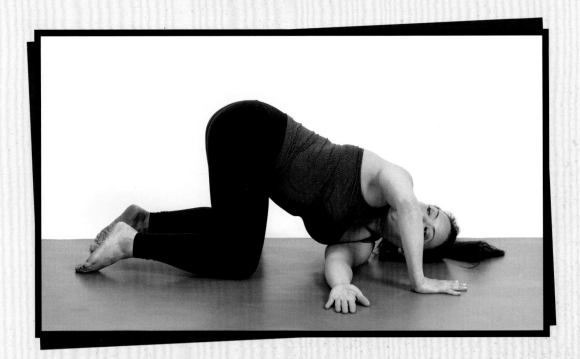

Threading the needle pose is the perfect way to sink in and stretch the side of the neck, shoulders, and traps and to get into a deep spinal twist. This is a chest-compressing posture to eliminate stagnant breath; it is important to focus on taking deep inhalations here to get the best lung cleanse.

For the athlete, this can be a calming pose. You get deeper on the exhalations and wring out the spine. I love this pose for wrestlers. It resembles a pose they often see themselves stuck in during a match. If your body is used to breathing in an awkward position and executing a certain pose, you will not become stressed when you face the same challenging pose in a match. The body has already been there, and the mind can remain calm.

BENEFITS

✓ Stretches the shoulders, traps, and neck

✓ Compresses the chest

✓ Calms the mind

✓ Detoxifies the body

✓ Increases neck and spine rotation

✓ Improves blood flow

CONTRAINDICATIONS

This pose is contraindicated for people with serious neck, shoulder, or back injuries.

HOW TO

1. Begin on your hands and knees in a neutral position with your palms flat, fingers spread. Your knees should be hip-width distance apart.

2. Walk your right hand forward one to two inches in front of your shoulder.

3. Turn your head toward your right hand as you slowly lower to the backside of your left arm onto your mat, palm facing up. Allow the left side of your head to rest on the floor.

4. Grab your left forearm with your right hand. The energy of the right hand should press the left forearm down and away from you. This action will make you want to twist the right side of your body open more and turn your chin to the right.

5. To release the pose, use your right palm, and push into the floor to come back to your hands and knees.

CHILD'S POSE
BALASANA

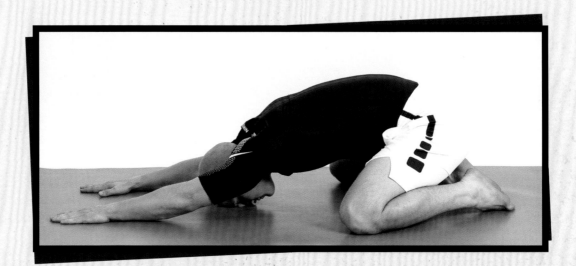

Often used as a respite for a yoga grind, child's pose is the option to turn to when you need a rest. Child's pose offers a range of benefits to consider.

Child's pose is a wonderful pose to practice when you are feeling overwhelmed, tired, or too challenged. It is also a comforting, protective pose to go to when you are feeling stressed. It eases low back tension and aids blood flow to the spine and brain. Child's pose is an easy place to stop and take breaths. You can get the benefit in the hips of a deep forward bend without the restraint of tight hamstrings. Stay here for anywhere from 1 minute to 10 minutes.

For the athlete, this pose offers other valuable benefits in addition to the de-stressing place. Athletes from long-distance runners to soccer players and golfers should visit this position to keep the ankles supple and flexible. It stretches the tops of the feet and shins, and regular practice can help to prevent painful shin splints. In addition, it increases flexibility in the knee joint. For sports such as hockey, a flexible knee joint is a huge advantage for avoiding injury and absorbing shock. Finally, child's pose opens the hips and eases the quads. Whether you play baseball and need great hip torque for power or you are a stop-and-go lacrosse player, many injuries can be avoided if the hips are open and strong.

BENEFITS

✓ Stretches the legs, including the ankles, thighs, hips, and knees

✓ Relieves stress and fatigue

✓ Calms the nervous system

✓ Releases back and neck tension

CONTRAINDICATIONS

This pose is contraindicated for those who have had recent knee or back surgery, those who have acute stomach problems, and those who are in late-stage pregnancy.

HOW TO

1. Start on your hands and knees.

2. Widen your knees to shoulder-width apart, big toes touching.

3. Slowly drop your hips back to rest on your heels.

4. Rest your forehead on the floor. You can either extend your arms straight out toward the front of the mat or place the backs of your hands near your feet to drape your arms on the floor alongside your body.

5. Focus your breath and intention, and rest your body with your full attention.

6. Continue to breathe and feel your spine lengthen, allowing the release of the low back.

VARIATION

If you have knee issues, roll up a towel, and place it behind the knee joint before you sit back on your heels.

PIGEON
KAPOTASANA

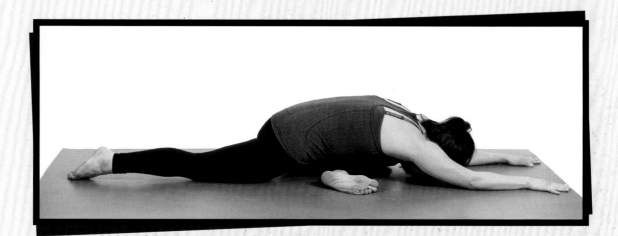

This is one pose just about everybody from professional athletes to office workers should include in their daily routines. It's a powerful hip opener as well as a significant pose to reduce the negative effects of stress on the body. I think it is the most valuable pose and should be considered an all star.

The hips are a storage depot for stress, trauma, fear, and anxiety. People suffering from any of those feelings should make a regular habit of stretching the hips. It is a primal reaction to store those feelings, creating unbelievable tightness and resistance in the hips. If you practice this pose regularly, you will realize how true this is: You may be able to gauge the type of week you are currently having by the tightness of your hips!

For the athlete, this pose is critical not only for stress relief but also to encourage speed and knee health. I don't know an athlete who is not interested in increasing speed and keeping the knees clear of injury. Open and strong hips equate with power; increased power is increased speed on the field of play. The greater the range of motion you have in the hip joint, the better your speed. Even more important is keeping the knees healthy, flexible, and strong. Any impact on the knee, whether from being hit, the chronic stress of running, or torque from sudden changes of direction, has to be absorbed in some way. If your hips are open, your whole body will be more accepting of the energy exchange. But if your hips are stiff and tight, the energy will go to the area that offers the least resistance, which is always the vulnerable, complex knee joint.

BENEFITS

✓ Opens the hip joint, hip flexors, chest, and shoulders

✓ Stretches the buttocks, anterior spine, gluteal muscles, and piriformis muscles, which is very helpful for sciatic problems

✓ Helps relieve low back pain and stiffness

✓ Increases depth of respiration

✓ Improves posture

CONTRAINDICATIONS

This pose is contraindicated for those who have had recent hip or knee surgery and for those who have severe sciatic aggravation; severe hip, knee, or low back pain; or any knee pain while in the pose.

HOW TO

1. Start on your hands and knees in tabletop position, with the hands under the shoulders and the knees under the hips.

2. Bring the left knee forward between the hands with the shin directly under the thigh into a modified pigeon pose.

3. Slide the right leg back as far as your hip flexor and quad will allow. Keep your hips square; do not list to the right or onto the left hip.

4. Slide your left thigh forward, from pointing straight ahead to having the knee point to one or two o'clock. Support your body by pressing down into the floor with your hands. Lengthen your torso.

5. On an exhalation, lower down to your forearms. Again, be sure your hips are square. With more practice, you will be able to bring your left foot and ankle closer to the front edge of your mat until your left shin is parallel to the front of your mat. As you sink into this pose, you should feel a deep stretch in your left glute or hip. Some people feel it radiate to their hamstring. You may also feel the stretch in the right hip flexor. If you feel knee pain here, be sure to only do this pose under careful supervision of a qualified yoga teacher. Blocks under the left glute can help eliminate the pressure on the knee.

6. Hold for the desired length of time, then switch sides.

VARIATIONS

- Try the quad variation of pigeon to intensify the stretch in the hip flexor and anterior space as it pressurizes the back (see variation 1). Leave the legs the same, tuck your tailbone, and lift and elongate the spine as close to perpendicular to the floor as you can. Slowly bend the back knee, and grab the foot or ankle with the same-side hand. Bring the heel as close to your glutes as possible, and hold for one minute. It is important to note that when you release this pose, do it slowly; do not spring out quickly because that is too shocking to the muscles.

- Try double pigeon for a very deep opening of the hip joint (see variation 2). From pigeon pose with the left leg forward, roll onto the left hip, and swing the back leg around to come to a seated position. In this variation, you will stack the right lower leg on top of the left lower leg; when you look at the inner edges of your legs, they should make a triangle shape. Sit up tall with the legs stacked. If this is enough of a stretch for the hips, stay there; if you need an additional challenge, fold forward from the hips until your head can rest on a block or on the floor. In time and with practice, you will stack the lower legs so that the right knee is directly over the left ankle and the right ankle is directly stacked onto the left knee. If you have knee pain here, sit on a block or come out of the pose.

(continued)

VARIATION 1

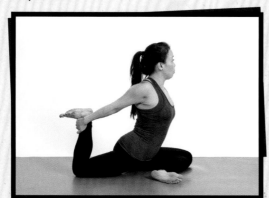

VARIATION 2

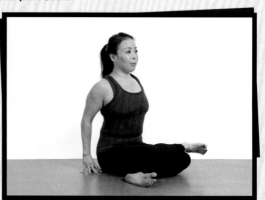

What are the two best poses for tight hamstrings?

Tight hamstrings are common; the only true remedy is a motivated athlete. Hamstrings have to be addressed every day for improvements to occur. Have your athlete try standing forward bend, standing forward bend against a wall, pigeon, and plow for five-minute holds every day.

WHEEL OF LIFE

SAMSARA

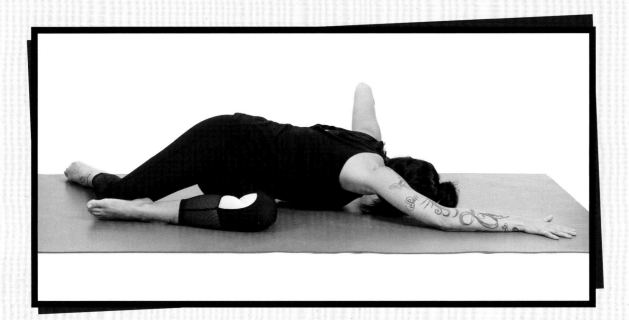

Perhaps the gold standard in full-body opening and spinal stretching is the wheel of life. My professional clients like to call it the wheel of death because it brings their awareness to areas of tightness and limitation.

The wheel of life is an extraordinary spinal alignment and spinal stretching pose. This pose wrings out the vertebrae from the tailbone all the way to the base of the skull. When you position yourself perfectly in this pose, you will sink in and detect the tight spots better than ever before. You should relax your weight fully into the floor or blocks and your head. Stress can cause the spine to tighten and can reduce blood flow and nerve impulses. This is a great hold to do to increase the rotation of the neck and align the cervical spine for optimum blood flow and oxygen to the brain.

For athletes who run and turn on a dime, constantly looking over their shoulders to defend, and for those who need their necks to rotate to the fullest for the widest field of view, this pose is critical. Many poses can target the rotation in the lower back and lumbar spine and perhaps even in the anterior shoulder and chest to help release the upper back, but this pose does it all, demanding attention as you breathe and fully surrender. This is one of the few poses that can help athletes to work on neck rotation. Wheel of life allows you to come to terms with stiffness as you sink in and try to place the chin easily over each shoulder. The more rotation you have, the better your "side view mirrors" are. Once you position your side view mirrors, you will be unstoppable, and nobody will come up from behind you to tackle or steal a ball. Imagine for a second what it would be like to drive for two to three hours with your side view mirrors folded down; it would be disconcerting, disabling, and blinding, leaving you at a huge disadvantage for sensing and responding to what is around you.

(continued)

BENEFITS

✓ Increases spinal flexibility and range of motion

✓ Stretches the neck, hips, and shoulders

✓ Increases oxygenation

✓ Realigns the spine

✓ Wrings out the organs

CONTRAINDICATIONS

This pose is contraindicated for those who have had spinal fusion or recent neck surgery and for those who have a weak and injured lower back.

HOW TO

1. Start in a seated position.

2. Put your weight on the left hip, and position the body so that the right knee is up against the bottom of the left foot.

3. Sit up nice and tall through the torso, and start to twist the body to the left.

4. Inhale as you lengthen the spine, and exhale to twist until you feel resistance and cannot twist anymore.

5. Start to lower the chest to the floor. Turn your head to the left, resting your right ear on the floor.

6. Place the palm of your left hand flat under your left shoulder as though you were going to do a push-up, and extend the right arm straight with the palm facing down.

7. Inhale as you press into the left hand, and exhale to spiral the right side of the chest closer and closer to the floor.

VARIATION

If it is too difficult to go all the way to the floor, place a block under the chest and right ear. If you cannot rest on your ear, put a block under your forehead until your neck flexibility improves.

FROG
MANDUKASANA

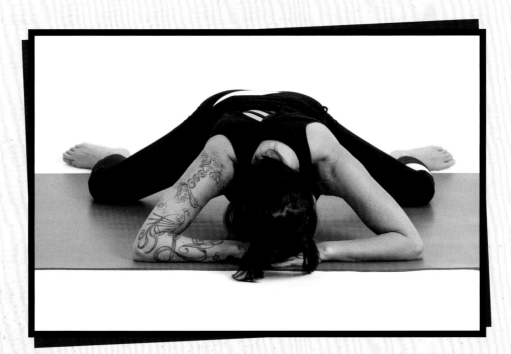

At first glance, frog is as awkward as the striking angles it displays. Frog pose is not as common as downward dog or warrior 1, but its benefits have made it a staple in my teaching repertoire.

Frog pose works well to hold for long periods of time and to perform a full breathing practice. Many people with poor posture and sedentary lifestyles end up with severe tightening in the hips. Even those of us with the best intentions and healthy routines can fall into the tight-hipped category. Frog gives you the opportunity to negotiate the opening of the hips. It also gives you the opportunity to tune into your hip tightness and discover whether you are tighter on one side. This helps you identify a potential problem that could result in injury before it actually happens. It's like rotating the tires on your car: If you drive for miles and miles and your car's alignment is off, you will eventually wear one tire bald, and it will blow. However, continually checking the tires and alignment enables you to avoid the blowout. The same holds true with your body. Knowledge is power. Frog is really a simple pose to execute; the yogic test comes by holding it and breathing.

For the athlete, frog should be a vital part of the routine. For hockey goalies, soccer players, and base runners, quick agility moves that can prove to be groin rippers will be a thing of the past when frog is a permanent part of stretching plans. As I mentioned before, giving the hips every opportunity to open and be loose in every direction has also been proven to reduce the risk of knee injury. Any quick torque or slick move will direct its energy to the point of least resistance, which is the vulnerable knee joint.

(continued)

BENEFITS

✓ Opens the hip joint

✓ Improves abduction

✓ Strengthens the low back while opening the hips

✓ Helps digestion

✓ Reduces knee strain

CONTRAINDICATIONS

This pose is contraindicated for those with inguinal hernia. Those who have knee or hip pain should perform it under supervision.

HOW TO

1. Begin in a tabletop pose on your hands and knees. Make sure your hips are directly over your knees and your lower legs are parallel to each other.

2. Lower down to your forearms and begin to slowly separate your knees as far as they can go. From a side view, your hip joint is in line with your knee joint, and your ankles are directly behind your knees. Your toes face out to the sides. Your knees, hips, and ankle joints will all be at 90-degree angles.

3. Lower down to a depth where you can feel a significant stretch and still breathe comfortably. Try to relax your shoulders out of your ears.

4. It is particularly comforting to hold this pose with blocks under your chest or pelvis. Once you release all your weight into the blocks, your groin will let go.

5. You can hold this pose for one minute, and you can work up to a mind-blowing 30 minutes for a mental toughness experience.

SUPPORTED FISH
SALAMBA MATSYASANA

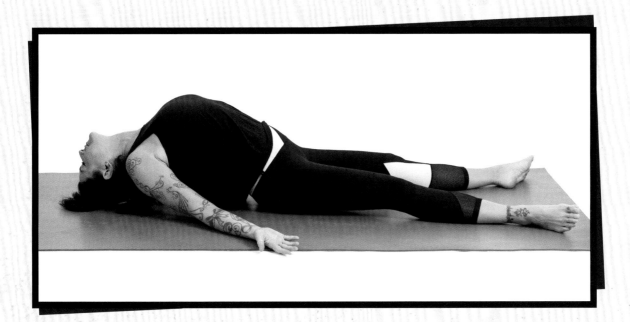

A pose that I recommend to everyone is supported fish. The middle back, the thoracic section, is the least mobile part of the spine due to the structure of the ribs. Opening this part of the spine is very freeing and contributes to the overall suppleness of the back.

Supported fish pose gives you the opportunity to traction the spine, surrender, and rest. It's the best pose for undoing the detrimental effects of tech neck and back pain. A person with beautiful and enviable posture probably also has great digestion, better organ function, and a healthier and more pain-free spine and probably looks great to boot. Supported fish pose helps to encourage good posture, counteracting the overstretched back and the tight or weak front and core muscles brought on by our forward-leaning everyday positions.

Athletes who depend on large rotational movements should consider holding this pose. The way to maximize spinal rotation is to lengthen the spine first. If you are hunched over and collapsed, your rotation is restricted. People who need flexion and extension in the spine, such as swimmers who perform the butterfly stroke, goalies, or strong servers in tennis, can use supported fish pose to increase extension in the spine. Athletes who need open, flexible anterior deltoid and chest muscles (such as pitchers, quarterbacks, and swimmers) should consider long holds here. In addition, holding this pose and being able to focus on diaphragmatic breathing can calm the body and mind.

BENEFITS

✓ Lengthens the spine

✓ Stretches the chest and front of shoulders

✓ Increases respiration and oxygenation of the body

✓ Improves posture

✓ Stimulates the thyroid

(continued)

CONTRAINDICATIONS

This pose is contraindicated for those with spinal fusions, serious neck issues, or vertigo and those who have had recent spinal or abdominal surgery.

HOW TO

1. Start in a seated position with your legs straight out in front of you and your feet about shoulder-width apart with the legs completely relaxed.

2. With the block in the side-up position behind you and centered on your spine, ground your hips, and slowly lie down over the block. Do not let your butt come off the floor. Let the arms relax on the floor, palms facing up.

3. The head touches the floor, and the eyes are closed.

4. As you inhale, emphasize lifting up through the belly button, over the block, and out through the top of the head like a rainbow.

5. As you exhale, envision the chest and heart center sinking down over the block through the front of each shoulder, down the arms, and out through the hands.

6. Hold and breathe for three to five minutes. To come out of the pose, very slowly roll onto your right side and into a fetal position. Stay here until you feel OK to sit up.

VARIATION

If your head does not reach the floor due to tightness or high stress levels, place another block under your head. Do not let your head just dangle without the support of a block.

VARIATION

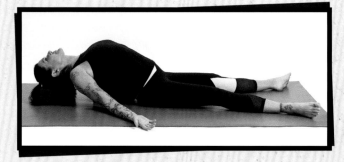

CORPSE
SAVASANA

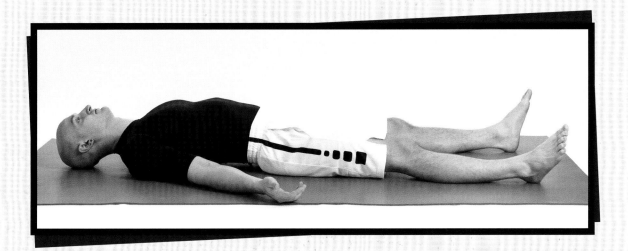

Corpse pose, otherwise known as final resting pose or savasana, may be the most anticipated pose of a yoga class. While it may seem as though you are preparing for a nap in corpse pose, you are relaxing in a pose that prepares your body for meditation, which is what the whole practice of yoga is preparing you for.

Performing savasana is an opportunity to leave the stress and trauma of life behind. Lying in a relaxation pose gives the body and mind time to decompress and come to terms with the rigors of the day. It allows you to train for deep breathing and to cleanse the body. This is the perfect chance to commit to a practice of meditation, which is vital to well-being.

For athletes, add these benefits to the opportunity to practice visualization during this pose. Visualization can be the missing puzzle piece that enables you to achieve the outcomes you desire. You envision details of the play, the game, the uniform, and the venue. Get as detailed as you can with your thoughts. Train your brain to think as though you already own the title, championship, or medal.

BENEFITS

✓ Calms and balances the body

✓ Relaxes the body to help ease blood pressure

✓ Encourages deep breaths

CONTRAINDICATIONS

This pose is contraindicated for those with low back herniation.

HOW TO

1. Lie on your back with the knees bent. Lift the hips off the floor as you lengthen the spine along the floor, then return the hips to the floor.

(continued)

2. Straighten your legs and let your feet fall out naturally to the sides. Slide the shoulders away from your ears and tuck the shoulder blades under you on the floor, creating space in the armpits and stretching your arms out long, palms facing up.

3. Let your head feel heavy on the floor.

4. Breathe naturally in and out through the nose, filling your throat, chest, and belly with every inhalation. Be sure to exhale fully.

5. Relax your eyes into their sockets, and focus your eyes on the inside of your forehead between your eyebrows. Feel a sense of stillness and calm, and continuously check your body for areas of tension. When you find tension, try to relax that area with each exhale. Stay in the pose for 5 to 30 minutes.

6. When finished, gradually wiggle your toes and fingers and bend your knees, bringing your feet flat. Roll to your right side, and curl into fetal position. Sit up when you feel ready.

VARIATIONS

- Try leg raises in corpse to increase abdominal strength (see variation 1). In corpse, place your hands palms down under your tailbone, engage the abdominals, and, with the legs together, lift and lower the legs.

- Try leg flutters in corpse to strengthen the abdominals and back (see variation 2). In the leg raise position, press the low back into the floor and alternately lift each leg 12 inches off the floor.

- Try banana pose to deeply open the sides of the body, shoulders, and hips (see variation 3). While lying in corpse pose, extend the arms over your head, and take the legs out wide; you should resemble an X. Cross your left ankle over the right ankle while keeping both hips flat on the floor, and gently press energy through your right heel. Inch your upper body to the right so your body resembles the shape of a banana, and grab your left forearm with your right hand. On every exhalation, lengthen the left side of the body. Keep both shoulders on the floor.

VARIATION 1

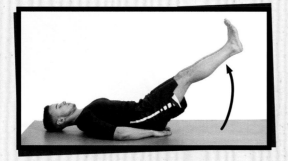

VARIATION 2

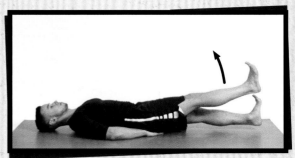

VARIATION 3

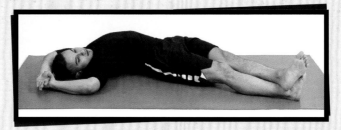

HIP FLEXOR OPENER

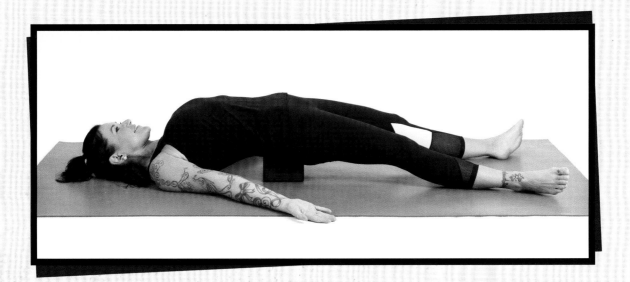

Low back issues, pain, and stiffness plague many people; this pose can be the game changer for all. The hip flexor opener stabilizes the pelvis, so the stretch targets the deep hip flexors with full surrender.

Most people find that they sit at their desks or in their cars for far too many hours per day. Sitting for lengthy amounts of time can tighten the hip flexors, which is why when you get up after a long day, it takes a moment or two to loosen. Tight hip flexors severely misalign the pelvis, pressurizing the low back and putting a lot of tension on the hamstrings. Tight hip flexors can cause alignment issues. That is why this pose is so exciting. This pose reduces the negative effects of sitting and also gives you time to fully surrender and relax.

Runners, cyclists, soccer players, rowers, and people in deep squat positions like catchers in baseball and softball are in danger of tightening the hip flexors and creating alignment issues. These athletes will especially benefit from this pose, especially when they hold it for three to five minutes.

BENEFITS

✓ Stretches the deep hip flexors

✓ Releases pressure on the low back

✓ Lengthens the hamstrings

✓ Releases the quads

✓ Induces relaxation

CONTRAINDICATIONS

This pose is contraindicated for those who have had recent low back surgery.

(continued)

HOW TO

1. Start by lying on your back with the knees bent and feet flat.

2. Lift your hips, and place a yoga block under the low back or tailbone area.

3. Slowly straighten the legs, and separate the feet about shoulder-width apart. Relax the legs completely, and let the arms relax on the floor, palms facing up. If there is any pressure on the low back, then you need to move the block toward your feet more.

4. As you get used to the pose or if you are taller, you can place two stacked yoga blocks under the low back.

VARIATION

Try half happy baby to increase the stretch in the hip flexors (see variation). Simply perform happy baby on each leg one at a time for two minutes.

VARIATION

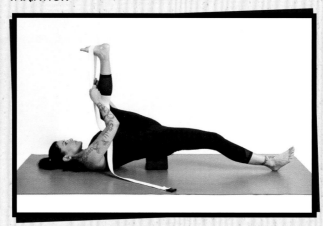

Psoas Health

The psoas, the major core muscle, is often overused by athletes during training. A tight psoas causes overworked quads, tight hamstrings, sciatic pain, groin difficulties, and pressure on the low back in addition to the following:

- Chronic low back pain
- Sciatica
- Intense menstrual cramping
- Hip socket tension
- Groin pain
- Chronic quadriceps strain

- Knee, neck, and ankle tension
- Bladder and digestive disturbances
- Structural imbalance
- Poor flexibility and strength in the core
- Lumbar joint immobility
- Organ dysfunction

For the athlete, if you find you have these issues regularly, look to the psoas for answers and healing. Most sports that involve running and jumping can exacerbate psoas injuries. Cyclists are very susceptible to psoas issues due to their position on the bike. When you do not allow full extension and when you ride for hours, the psoas shortens and potentially overstretches the back. Triathletes have difficulty because they are running and riding and therefore doubling their chances of issues. These athletes go from holding the psoas in a shortened position during the ride directly to running, which demands lengthening they may not possess.

Inversion

Inversions Q&A

How do inversions affect blood pressure?

You should check with your doctor about your case, but for people whose blood pressure is controlled by medication, our advice is to engage in exercise and other activities that a person with normal blood pressure would do. Therefore, it seems reasonable that you can safely introduce inversions if you do so gradually. Inversions temporarily reduce blood pressure, so theoretically, regular practice may enhance the treatment of your high blood pressure. If you have students whose blood pressure is not under control, you should hold off teaching them until you get an OK from their physicians.

When should I not teach inversions? Why?

Anyone who has high blood pressure, heart-related problems, eye issues (e.g., seeing floaters), neck problems, epilepsy, or previous stroke or sinus problems should never practice headstands or shoulder stands. Omit other mild inversions, or have them adjusted by the yoga teacher, unless they are cleared by a doctor.

Also, during any stage of pregnancy, yoga should be practiced in prenatal yoga classes specifically designed for that purpose or privately with a qualified pregnancy yoga teacher. If the athlete is pregnant and has been practicing all along, there should be no complications or restrictions. She should just be mindful that her center of gravity is changing daily, so inversions and balancing poses will be more difficult.

SHOULDER STAND
SARVANGASANA

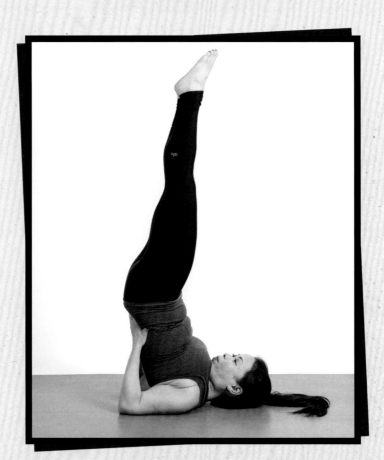

Shoulder stand is sometimes called the candle pose or queen pose. Shoulder stand translated from the Sanskrit name is "all limbed" or "whole body." Shoulder stand has many roles, including relaxation, inversion, gentle stretching, and revitalizing.

Shoulder stand opens and strengthens the upper shoulder girdle and stretches the back of the neck. Since it is an inversion pose and nourishes the brain, it offers a rich supply of blood and a flood of oxygen to the organs and glands of the upper body. Pressure is taken off the lower extremities, which can relieve pressure and swelling in the feet and legs caused by tough, long days at work and play. Getting extra blood flow to the brain, face, and head will give a tired mind and body the boost and glow you need to continue.

For the athlete, shoulder stand can be used for assessment. While you are holding the pose, you are in a perfect position to check your leg lengths and look for imbalances that may need adjusting. Being aware of differences in the length of your legs will help you to identify low back knots or tightness. Shoulder stand is also a great stretch for the neck. This is critical for high-contact sports such as hockey, wrestling, and football. Athletes in these sports often find themselves in twisted predicaments. If the neck is supple enough to enable the chin to touch the chest, then the risk of injury in a game situation is greatly reduced. The best part of shoulder stand for the athlete is the reverse lymph flow. It decreases the swelling of feet and legs and reduces the "heavy" postgame leg. I often have my athletes hold this pose for 10 or more minutes to help them get their quickness back. Beginners should always start with a 30-second to one-minute hold and work up to a longer time.

BENEFITS

✓ Helps with lymph drainage

✓ Promotes efficient thyroid gland function (The thyroid gland is responsible for managing your metabolism.)

✓ Promotes good circulation to the brain

✓ Stretches the neck, the upper back, and the entire spine

✓ Aids with constipation, indigestion, and asthma

✓ Increases blood flow to the brain, therefore reducing headaches and congestion

✓ Tones the legs and abdominals

CONTRAINDICATIONS

This pose is contraindicated for those with thyroid disease, high blood pressure, glaucoma, or a detached retina and those with any disorders or injuries to the neck or cervical spine.

HOW TO

1. Lie flat on the floor, with your arms alongside your body, palms facing down.

2. Exhale, and pull the knees into your chest.

3. Keep pressing down through your hands and arms as you bring your toes as close to the floor as possible behind your head. You should look as though you are in a seated forward bend, only upside down. It is important to position your arms under you and keep them shoulder-width apart, resting on your shoulder blades. Do this by interlacing your fingers together underneath you and wiggling the shoulders closer together under you.

4. Now bend your elbows, keep your upper arms (shoulder to elbow) on the floor shoulder-width apart, and place your hands on your low back. If you are new to this pose, bend your knees toward your forehead. If you can, lift the feet toward the sky as you straighten the legs.

5. As you advance in the pose, your hands will be closer to your shoulder blades, and your legs will be straighter, stretching your hamstrings (back of the thigh).

6. Positioning yourself deeply will create a 90-degree angle in your neck. While holding the pose, concentrate on your breath, and press down through your upper arms and up through your legs and feet. Gently squeeze your inner thighs together. Check out your leg lengths, and look for symmetry.

7. Check the rotation of your legs; notice the direction your knees and feet are pointing.

8. Adjust your feet so they are even and equal.

HALF HEADSTAND

SIRSHASANA

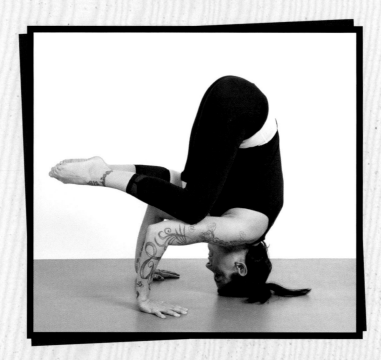

Half headstand is widely regarded as one of the most beneficial yoga postures for the body, mind, and spirit. It is understood to be one of the best stimulants for the brain and the spine as well as the cerebrospinal fluid. The pose's primary intention is to achieve the active reversal effect. This means toning the vital organs, stimulating the endocrine glands, and promoting the balanced and efficient functioning of our bodies. The secondary intention of headstand variations is to strengthen the neck, improve spinal integrity, and deepen respiratory rhythm. It's a crucial pose to add to your yoga practice.

Aside from its other benefits, half headstand is effective in relieving mild depression because it increases the level of blood, oxygen, and glucose going to the brain. This helps the brain create more dopamine and serotonin. Depressed people are deficient in both. This is one way to aid the body in producing higher levels naturally. The continued practice of half headstand can alter your brain chemistry. It is particularly effective in stimulating the pituitary gland, which releases endorphins and reduces the level of cortisol. Cortisol is a stress hormone.

For the athlete, half headstand has many major benefits to improve performance. This pose reverses the effects of gravity on the lungs and diaphragm, strengthening the diaphragm and assisting in more complete exhalation. The more efficient the breathing of a high-endurance athlete such as a track star or a tennis player, the better and longer quality play will be. Many athletes experience exercise-induced asthma, and when we assist the breathing mechanism, it increases the athlete's endurance. Another benefit of half headstand is that it teaches players to rest their bodies while in a state of activity. This translates nicely into finding calm and comfort in an uncomfortable situation, which is something familiar to all athletes. Finally, every inverted pose helps to drain the lymph glands. Many athletes find that after a hard day of competition or training, they have the "heavy leg" or "lead leg" feeling. Regular practice of inversions helps to increase lymph drainage.

BENEFITS

✓ Improves concentration, internal organ function, and circulation to the neck and brain

✓ Nourishes the skin of the face

✓ Calms the body and mind

✓ Relieves stress and tension

✓ Strengthens the shoulders, upper back muscles, and abdominals

✓ Relieves varicose veins

✓ Increases stamina

CONTRAINDICATIONS

This pose is contraindicated for those who have neck injuries, blood pressure extremes, ear and eye problems, back and shoulder injuries, certain heart diseases, stroke, hiatal hernia, or reflux.

HOW TO

1. Start by kneeling on the floor. You may want to practice close to a wall until you become confident and skilled.

2. On your hands and knees in table pose, be careful that your hands are shoulder-width apart with your palms flat. Rest your head on the floor.

3. Your head and two hands should make a perfect triangle, and your elbows and wrists should make a 90-degree angle.

4. Next, place your right knee on your right elbow. Stay here as long as needed, and switch sides, keeping your head in a straight line with the spine.

5. When you feel ready, place your right knee on your right elbow and the left knee on the left elbow at the same time. Hold and breathe.

6. On every exhalation, remember to lift your shoulders away from your ears and elongate your neck. Be sure to distribute the weight of your body equally on both hands and the top of your head.

7. Come out of the pose slowly, and lower into child's pose for several breaths.

WALL WALKS

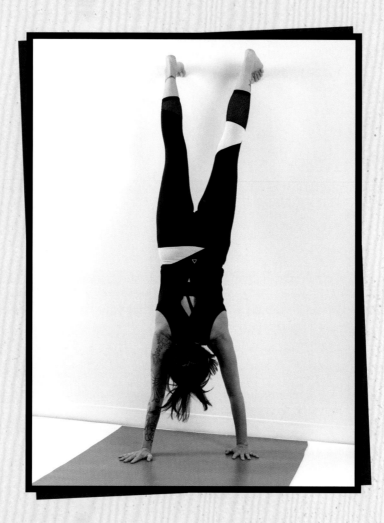

I fully believe in teaching wall walks to my athletes for the health and stability of the shoulder joint.
Typically, an athlete will focus on strengthening the shoulder joint with pull-ups, shoulder press-es, and chest pressing, but the shoulder joint is a ball-and-socket joint that is involved in many more movements than just pressing forward and over the head. You need to consider strength-ening the joint in every angle. Think of the positions on a clock. Wall walks is a functional strength move that will accomplish this for you. This movement will focus on wrist strength, too. This is especially important for athletes who need the hands and wrists to absorb their falls, like goal-keepers and wrestlers.

BENEFITS

✓ Strengthens the shoulder joint in all directions

✓ Stretches the chest and shoulder

✓ Increases abdominal and back strength

✓ Flushes the brain and sinuses

✓ Increases the strength and flexibility of wrists

CONTRAINDICATIONS

This pose is contraindicated for those who have had recent shoulder or wrist surgery.

HOW TO

1. Start in downward dog with your heels against a wall, set the hands flat, and push the floor away from you.

2. Bring one leg at a time onto the wall behind you. If you are a beginner, you will stay here, count to three, and return to downward dog.

3. Start to walk your hands toward the wall until you can bring your chest to the wall, take three breaths, and walk all the way back out.

4. Lower one leg at a time to the floor into plank pose, chaturanga, upward dog, and downward dog. That is one rep; in time and with practice, you will be able to do four sets of four reps.

Sport-Specific Sequences

8

This chapter will guide you through all you need to know to work successfully with athletes in specific sports and positions. Use it as a set of guidelines and as inspiration to add your own ideas. For each sport, I present a step-by-step way to incorporate yoga into your regime immediately. I have identified the most common injuries in each sport, by position where appropriate, and the top moves in each sport so you are not overwhelmed with options. Most important, I show you the top yoga pose or yoga move together with the actions of an actual player so you can see how similar the common moves and the yoga poses actually are. Finally, you will find a choreographed routine to incorporate until you are ready to start designing your own routines.

DESIGNING A POWER YOGA FOR SPORTS CLASS

There are many things to consider when designing Power Yoga for Sports classes. Here is a concise and comprehensive list. Do not overthink things, stay clear, and it will soon become second nature.

- What are the repetitive motions of the players in the sport?
- Look at videos and pictures; notice moves in the sport that resemble yoga poses.
- Be creative, and think of poses to keep muscles, joints, ligaments, and tendons open for the specific motions.
- What counter poses will work opposing muscles to retain symmetry, flexibility, and range of motion?
- Look at the needs of individual athletes (for example, I have a client with lordosis). What would be most effective for each person?
- What are the common injuries in each sport, and how can you help to prevent them?
- How can you predict what injuries could occur, based on repetitive movements you observe?
- Suggest abbreviated home routines to give to the athletes on their off days.

Is there a never-do pose or a never-do tip for teaching athletes?

Never force athletes into positions they are uncomfortable doing. Make sure they are not experiencing joint compression, be empathetic to their needs at all times, and stay focused on your teaching.

Things to Keep in Mind When Designing Your Session

When you are in a training session, you should already be well prepared, but consider what specific things will keep your athletes motivated and engaged. How can you help them to understand why yoga will help them excel?

- Think about what you are passionate about and how you want to communicate it through your teaching. If you are excited about what you are teaching, they will follow your lead and will realize how important the practice is to them.
- Understand why it is important to focus on the transitions as well as the poses themselves. Transitions between poses are important to keep the rhythm of the series and to save time. A routine that is not well thought out and is awkward to perform takes more time. When you work with athletes, it is likely you will only have a few precious moments to pack full of intelligent yoga.
- Write a sequence of 5 to 10 poses. This keeps the athlete moving and engaged.
- Create a warm-up sequence that you can use with athletes every session. It is familiar, it gets them centered, and it prepares them without immediately challenging them.
- Think about protecting the knee, foot, and leg placement at all times. The purpose of this yoga is always to protect the athlete, improve his game, and increase longevity, so form is crucial to success.
- Be clear and confident when adjusting your athletes. You should be deliberate when putting hands on, with a firm touch that will deepen or enhance the pose.
- Be mindful of where in the training cycle your athlete may be. This is important to providing the most effective training. Awareness of the training cycle means, for example, going slower after a game or going harder during the off-season. Every stage of the cycle presents opportunities for growth, so you must be absolutely clear where you are.
- Be aware of athletes' past or present injuries. Every time you work with a person or a group, ask about new injuries, or ask to be reminded of past injuries so that you continue to offer poses for growth, not setbacks.

Here are some additional features of effective Power Yoga for Sports classes:

- Motivated, willing athletes with a serious mindset to excel
- Warm-up poses, suggested by the typical warm-ups
- A series of poses appropriate to the sport and the position
- Breath work and reminders to incorporate breath peppered throughout the practice
- Long, deep holds relevant to the sport and the position at the end of the session
- A final resting pose (savasana) with guided meditation for recovery
- Constant reminders about why you chose a specific pose for the sport and how it will help the athletes

You must repeatedly remind athletes why you chose the poses you did so that they understand how your work is relevant to them. This is critical to their motivation, for without motivated athletes, you will be wasting your time.

Is it really important to teach different routines for each sport?

To make the best use of an athlete's time, it is the philosophy of PYFS that you cater each routine to the demands of the athlete by sport and position. This eliminates the fluff and focuses on specific needs for quicker gains.

How to Build Your Class

To create easy-to-follow, practical classes, follow the steps listed here. This chapter gives you a number of prebuilt classes for different sports and areas of the body. However, I want you to understand the process so that you can build your own effective classes.

1. Determine who the class is for and the sport, position, ailment, or body part to be addressed. Let's use tennis players as the example here. If you were building a series for tennis players, you would need to consider the following:

   ► Neck rotation, flexion, extension
   ► Shoulder flexibility and strength
   ► Chest openers
   ► Elbow safety
   ► Spinal rotation
   ► Hip strength
   ► Leg flexibility in all directions

2. Write down at least 10 poses that can be used to stretch the body. Using tennis players as the example, poses for stretching might include the following:

   ► Plow for neck flexion
   ► Wheel of life for neck rotation
   ► Face-down shoulder stretch for chest, shoulder, and elbow flexibility
   ► Face-up shoulder stretch for anterior shoulders
   ► Wrist openers for wrist flexibility
   ► Crescent lunge twist for spinal rotation
   ► Pigeon for hip flexibility
   ► Frog for groin health
   ► Hero's pose and hero's pose with toes tucked for the quads and feet
   ► Bow pose for the quads and hip flexors

3. Write down at least 10 poses that can be used to strengthen the body. Using tennis players as the example, poses for strengthening might include the following:

   ► Rock and rolls for spinal health
   ► Plank, low push-up, upward dog, and downward dog series for full-body strengthening
   ► Plank hold for core strength
   ► Inverted table to seated for the chest, shoulders, and arms
   ► Inverted plank to seated for the chest, shoulders, and arms
   ► Squat to standing to standing on the toes for leg strength

- ▶ Plank with opposite-arm opposite-leg reach series for glute strength and back strength
- ▶ Seated twists for spinal rotation and strength
- ▶ Half side squat for leg strength
- ▶ Eagle for overall strength and balance

4. Review the 20-plus poses you listed, and organize them in a way that flows easily. Using tennis players as the example and the poses listed previously, the flow for your class might look like this:

- ▶ Seated twists for two minutes
- ▶ Rock and rolls for two minutes
- ▶ Last roll into plow hold, then rock and roll to standing forward bend and hold
- ▶ Squat hold
- ▶ Squat to standing for two minutes
- ▶ Plank to low push-up to upward dog to downward dog 10 times
- ▶ Lower to the belly into face-down shoulder stretch on each side with bow hold in the middle during transition
- ▶ Downward dog to wrist turns—plank with opposite-arm opposite-leg reach—hero's toes tucked—untucked—frog
- ▶ Low push-up to upward dog to downward dog
- ▶ Step right foot forward into half side squat back and forth 10 times
- ▶ Standing forward bend
- ▶ Come to standing and into eagle
- ▶ Rock and roll 10 times to inverted table to inverted planks 10 times to downward dog
- ▶ Crescent lunge to twist to pigeon to wheel of life, then repeat on other side

Your Power Yoga Warm-Up

As mentioned in chapter 4, each yoga sequence in this chapter starts with a typical warm-up and takes the athlete through the poses needed to help her thrive in her sport and avoid injury. The typical warm-up is as follows:

POSE	PAGE	TIME
Easy cross-legged twist	103	2 min
Easy cross-legged pose with arm-ups	103	2 min
Seated cat and cow	173	2 min
Opposite arm opposite leg	122	2 min
Lying spinal twist (with block between thighs)	126	2 min
Reclining cobbler's pose	145	2 min
Diamond pose	146	2 min
Rock and roll	130	30 sec
Standing forward bend	54	30 sec

FOOTBALL

Football players are typically considered to be tough and to endure rigorous training to prepare their bodies for the often-jarring plays on the field. Football player types vary from the mindful, strategic position of quarterback to the solid, headstrong linemen to the elusive, acrobatic defensive backs and receivers. I have laid out several routines and examples to include all the different requirements of football players.

FOOTBALL: ALL POSITIONS

Regardless of their position, most football players need special attention on their backs and hips. You need to focus on their spinal rotation, flexion, and extension as well as strength. All positions rely on great strength, so it is important to keep the PYFS formula in mind and consistently work on their overall flexibility.

COMMON INJURIES IN FOOTBALL

Groin pulls and strains, hamstring pulls and strains, quadriceps strains, oblique strains, plantar fasciitis, Achilles tears and strains, shoulder subluxations and instability, neck strains

YOGA POSES CLOSELY RELATED TO MOVEMENTS IN FOOTBALL

Squat (pg. 79)

Most players need to explode from a still position, and squat prepares the hips and legs by increasing flexibility and strength.

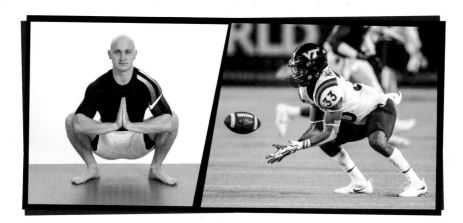

Goddess (pg. 72)

This pose is a deep groin opener that alleviates stress on the knee, open the hips, and develops stability.

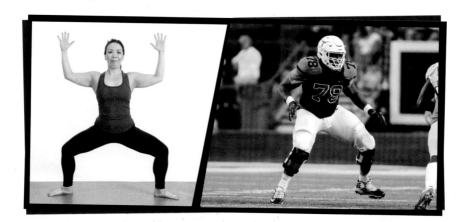

Extended Side Angle (pg. 66)

This pose opens the side of the body for better reach.

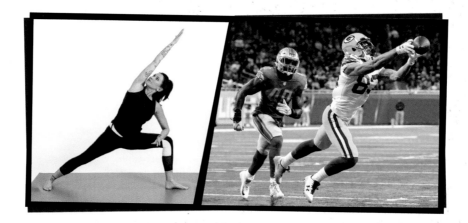

Straddle Forward Bend Twist (pg. 74)

This pose increases flexibility in the shoulder joint and chest and strengthens the core.

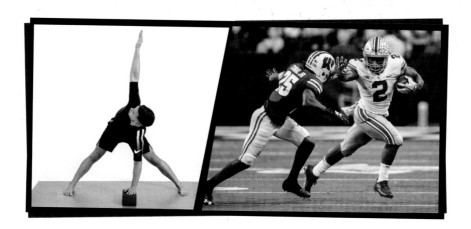

Face-Down Shoulder Stretch (pg. 169)

This pose lowers the risk of chest strain and shoulder injury, making players more resilient to a push or when making a block. It also enables them to better absorb a fall that is broken by the hands.

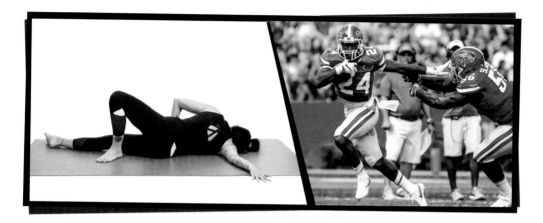

Lunge Twist (pg. 98)

This pose promotes powerful, flexible hip flexors, opens lats, and allows for deeper breathing.

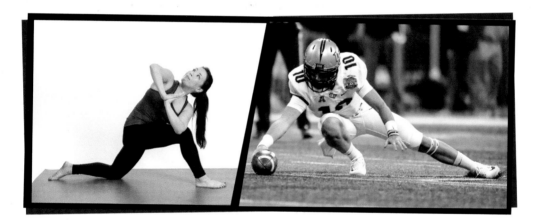

Crescent Lunge (pg. 69)

This pose mimics the running motion; elongates the spine for deeper rotation; and opens the feet, calves, and legs.

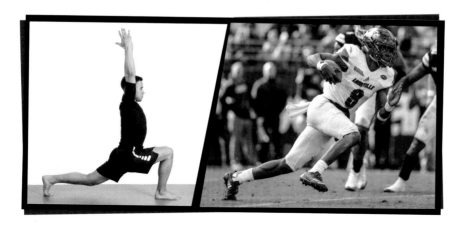

Half Hero's (pg. 114)

This pose stretches the quads, keeps knees supple, and opens the ankles and hamstrings.

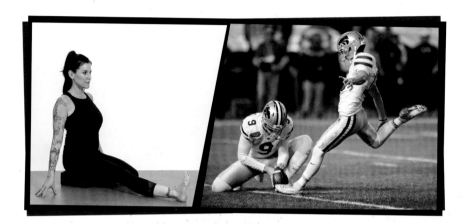

Warrior 2 (pg. 84)

This pose helps with running motion and power.

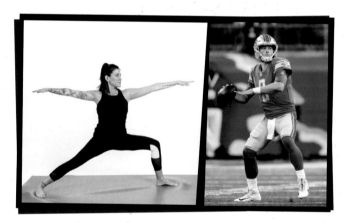

Revolving Triangle (pg. 63)

This pose opens the IT band for more supple knees and opens the hips.

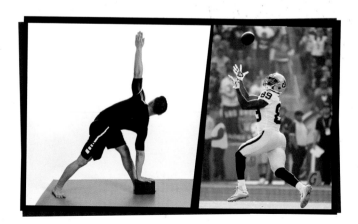

Tree Pose (pg. 90)

This pose encourages the strengthening of all the tiny muscles in the feet and lower legs, stabilizing the ankle joint and improving balance.

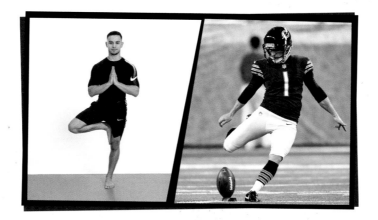

Low Push-Up (pg. 150)

This pose strengthens the chest and shoulder joints for better strength and stabilization of the joints and wrists. Plank holds are great for building push strength in addition to core stability.

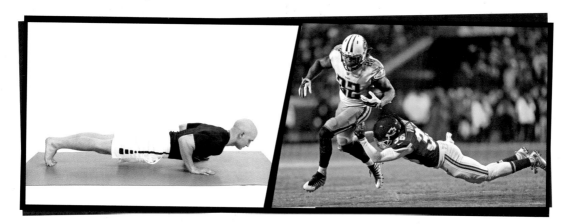

Chair (pg. 58)

This pose encourages the opening of the lats and ribs and at the same time strengthens the lower body .

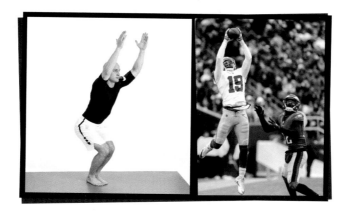

Warrior 3 (pg. 86)

This pose strengthens the smaller lower-leg muscles and helps develop ankle stability and balance.

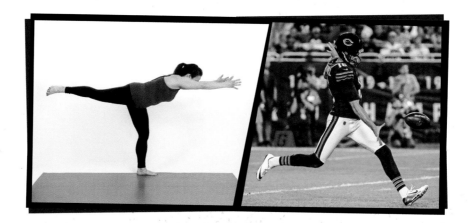

Opposite-Arm Opposite-Leg (pg. 122)

This movement helps develop range of motion and is especially great for punters and kickers.

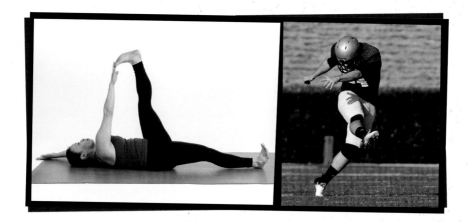

FOOTBALL: DEFENSIVE BACKS AND RECEIVERS

Players in these positions (and any other position where speed and agility are necessary) need great stamina, nimbleness, and strength. Strong, flexible legs are important because these players need to run at explosive speeds. Ankle integrity is critical to turning on a dime and making important plays. Abdominal and back strength is central to making a twisting catch and to being able to stay in bounds at the most crucial times, not to mention balanced shoulders and arms for the extraordinary reaching catches. Often overlooked is the need for stable wrists; it is very likely that players in these positions will fall during the play, and they need to be able to depend on their wrists to cushion their falls every time. If your wrists are tight and unforgiving, then you risk a break or a tear on a fall instead of getting up and getting ready for the next play.

COMMON INJURIES FOR DEFENSIVE BACKS AND RECEIVERS

Knee sprains, strains, and more; back problems, strains, and herniations; finger breaks; wrist and ankle strains, twists, and breaks; neck pain and stiffness

TOP FIVE YOGA POSES FOR DEFENSIVE BACKS AND RECEIVERS

The top five poses should be done several times a week as needed. Explore them and understand how they help you personally, and then you will use them best for recovery or before games to warm up.

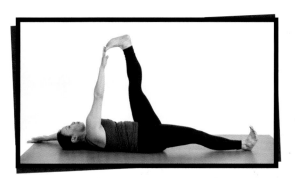

1. Opposite-Arm Opposite-Leg (pg. 122)

This movement is amazing for warming up the whole hip socket and shoulder socket before a game, as well as for syncing the breath with the movement and warming up the abs and trunk, which is critical for the quick, elusive moves you need on the field. Try it for two to four minutes.

2. Lunge Twist (pg. 98)

This pose increases strength in the legs and at the same time stretches the quadriceps and increases the rotation in the back. Watch a receiver and you will know how important it is to be able to twist to catch a less-than-perfect pass. Great execution of this pose also helps you to improve your balance, which can come in handy when landing from a leaping grab or when you need the presence of mind to keep your feet inbounds. Hold it for one to two minutes on each side.

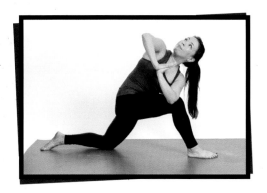

3. Elbow-to-Knee Plank (pg. 148)

Performing plank on its own will increase your abdominal and hip flexor strength, but adding the elbow-to-knee variation will deepen the abdominal crunch and strengthen the wrist joint. Having the best abdominal strength you can will support your back in all compromising positions on the field as well as develop your posture and oxygen intake. Do this for one to three minutes, alternating knees.

4. Face-Down Shoulder Stretch (pg. 169)

Doing this yoga pose gives you a deep opening in the anterior deltoid (front of the shoulder), stretching the biceps muscle, neck, and spine, all very important when turning on a dime to prevent or make a catch. Hold each side for three to five minutes.

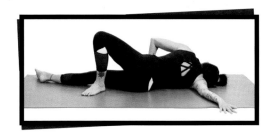

Football

5. Frog (pg. 183)

This pose is a long, deep hold. As soon as you are in the pose, you will begin to release the groin and inner thigh. The inner thighs need to be flexible to run, stop, and change direction without injury. This is another example of opening the hips in all directions to protect the knees from stresses and strains. Hold this pose for 5 to 15 minutes.

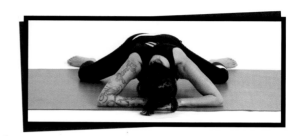

YOGA SEQUENCE FOR DEFENSIVE BACKS AND RECEIVERS

POSE	PAGE	TIME/REPS
Perform typical warm-up before you begin		
Rock and roll	130	1 min
Standing forward bend	54	1 min
Squat	79	1 min
Plank to forearm plank to plank	147, 148, 147	3 times, 10 sec each
Upward dog to downward dog and hold	163, 160	1 min
*Crescent lunge (right foot forward)	69	1 min
Lunge twist	98	1 min
Warrior 2 (hold)	84	1 min
Warrior 2 (bend and straighten right knee)	84	1 min
Warrior 1	82	1 min
Lower chest and belly to thigh, then return to warrior 1	82	3 times
Warrior 3	86	1 min
Stand up, hold knee to chest, and then into eagle pose (left leg over right)	76	1 min
Reach left leg back into crescent lunge	69	1 min
Return to eagle pose and back into crescent lunge 3 times		
Stand up and move into standing forward bend to low push-up to upward dog to downward dog	54, 150, 163, 160	1 time
Repeat on other side from * for 1-3 times each side; after last downward dog, continue with following poses		
Bow	165	1 min
Child's pose	176	30 sec
Bow	165	1 min
Child's pose	176	1 min
Face-down shoulder stretch	169	5 min each side
Frog	183	5 min
Hero's pose with toes tucked	115	2 min

FOOTBALL: OFFENSIVE AND DEFENSIVE LINEMEN, RUNNING BACKS, AND FULLBACKS

Players who excel in these types of positions (and any position that requires strength and stability) are powerful and explosive in the lower body. Their legs, hips, and feet need to be perfectly balanced in strength and flexibility to maximize their power. These athletes need flexible wrists to maintain a strong push without injury, and they need flexibility in the chest and anterior shoulder to absorb the push without damage to the shoulder joint.

COMMON INJURIES FOR OFFENSIVE AND DEFENSIVE LINEMEN, RUNNING BACKS, AND FULLBACKS

Pectoral tears and strains; wrist pain and injury; knee strains; plantar fasciitis; turf toe; Achilles tendonitis; and back pain, stiffness, and strain

TOP FIVE YOGA POSES FOR OFFENSIVE AND DEFENSIVE LINEMEN, RUNNING BACKS, AND FULLBACKS

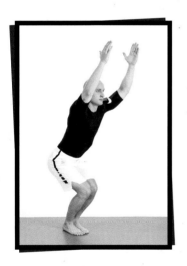

1. Chair (pg. 58)

Chair is a perfect pose to strengthen the back and quadriceps and to open the calves and Achilles tendons. Hold chair for 30 to 60 seconds at a time, and perform two to four reps.

2. Flat-Back Chair (pg. 59)

This flat-back variation of chair intensifies its ability to strengthen the back of a lineman. During games, the starting position of the player can be very forward and can put the spine in a flexed position. Flat-back chair pose offers relief to the back, increases the strength in the back of the spine, keeps the abs strong, and supports the back more completely. Do this variation between chair pose practices. Do it for 5 to 10 breaths.

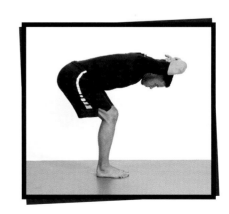

Football

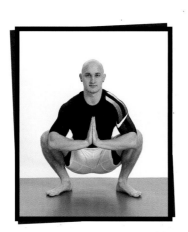

3. Squat (pg. 79)

Squat not only opens the hips very deeply, it also stretches and strengthens the calves, the Achilles tendons, and the lower legs, especially if you are patient and mentally tough enough to stay in the position for the maximum hold. Once players become seasoned in holding this squat, they can work on flattening the back and developing deeper hip, groin, and inner thigh elasticity. Hold for two to four minutes.

4. Plank (pg. 147)

Multiple benefits will arise from regular practice of this pose. You will undoubtedly increase abdominal strength, which will increase your stability. Also, it will increase the strength of the chest muscles and will stretch the wrist joints and the flexors and extensors of the forearm. When you consider the importance to linemen of having power in the wrists to push, block, and stop an opponent, you will understand that if the wrist joint is tight, your opponent will open it for you in an uncomfortable way, perhaps even damaging your wrists. This pose also comes in handy in the event you get knocked on your butt; your wrist will be able to take the weight of the fall with less risk of injury. Practice this one to three times for one minute each.

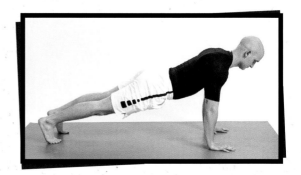

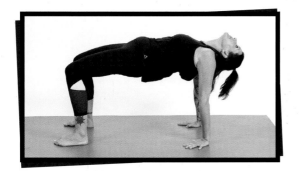

5. Inverted Table (pg. 139)

This pose loads you up with the same benefits as the forearm plank pose, but it will add a great shoulder and chest opener and quad stretch. At the same time, it will strengthen the back, chest, and shoulders. This can be a tough pose to accomplish for the bigger guys, but well worth the effort. Hold this for 30 to 60 seconds one to two times

YOGA SEQUENCE FOR OFFENSIVE AND DEFENSIVE LINEMEN, RUNNING BACKS, AND FULLBACKS

POSE	PAGE	TIME/REPS
Perform typical warm-up before you begin		
Rock and roll	130	1 min
Rock and roll to standing forward bend	130, 54	10 times; hold standing forward bend for 2 breaths, then repeat
Plow	132	1 min
Rock and roll to standing forward bend	130, 54	1 min
Squat	79	1 min
Squat turns	80	1 each way
Plank	147	1 min
Low push-up to plank	150, 147	3 times
Upward dog	163	1 min
Downward dog	160	1 min
Downward dog with leg kicks	160	1 min
*Half side squat (start with right knee bent)	96	4 times each side
Pyramid pose	64	30 sec
Revolving triangle	63	30 sec
Pyramid pose	64	30 sec
Triangle	61	30 sec
Return to pyramid pose and then back into triangle 5 times		
Standing forward bend to plank with wrist openers	54, 147, 156	3 times with 30 sec in each wrist position
Low push-up to upward dog to downward dog and hold	150, 163, 160	1 min
Repeat on other side from * for 1-3 times each side		
Jump to squat, jump back to plank and into downward dog and hold	79, 147, 160	1 min
Standing forward bend	54	1 min
Lower to toe balance	60	30 sec
Return to standing forward bend and then again into toe balance 10 times, holding each for 30 sec		
Happy baby	143	1 min

(continued)

Yoga Sequence for Offensive and Defensive Linemen, Running Backs, and Fullbacks *(continued)*

POSE	PAGE	TIME/REPS
Hip flexor opener	189	5 min
Frog	183	5 min
Lying spinal twist	126	3-5 min each side
Face-up shoulder stretch	134	2-4 min
Face-down shoulder stretch	169	2-4 min
Supported fish	185	5 min

SOCCER

Soccer players are known for their extraordinary stamina and aerobic ability that allow them to last in the grueling running game. They must have strong, flexible ankles and toes to be able to powerfully push off on the run and to kick effectively. Soccer's high, jumping header is a common movement that demands explosive power through the lower body. Agility is also needed to elude defenders. Strong, symmetrical legs; a flexible groin; and healthy knees are critical.

COMMON INJURIES IN SOCCER

Achilles tendon issues, back sprains and pain, hips issues, calf and foot pain, oblique strains, knee tears, groin and inner thigh pulls, wrist breaks and strains, plantar fasciitis, turf toe

YOGA POSES CLOSELY RELATED TO MOVEMENTS IN SOCCER

Lunge Twist (pg. 98)

Lunge twist and any lunge poses mimic the common moves on the field, preparing the body and back for lunging kicks. This pose also opens the ankle for more power, reducing the likelihood of plantar fascia problems. Deep opening of the spine increases range of motion and power to twist the core. These poses will open the player's legs and hips in all directions. They will also strengthen and stabilize the abdominals for better balance.

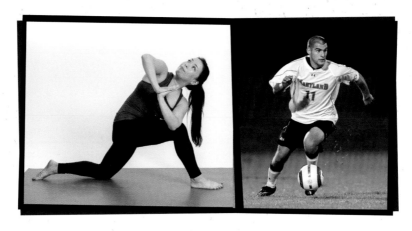

Wheel of Life (pg. 181)

This pose opens the lats and targets rotation in the spine and neck to give the player eyes in the back of his head.

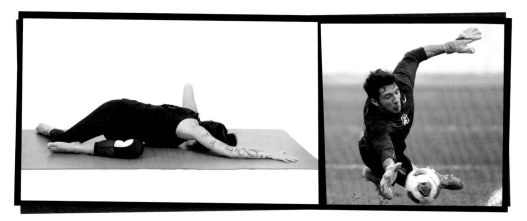

Reclining Big Toe Pose (pg. 124)

This pose is a great hamstring opener. It also increases flexibility in the inner thigh and groin.

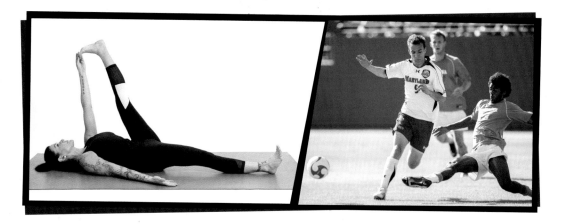

Warrior 3 (pg. 86)

This pose increases ankle stability. Standing balancing poses are added because they strengthen and stabilize the ankle joint.

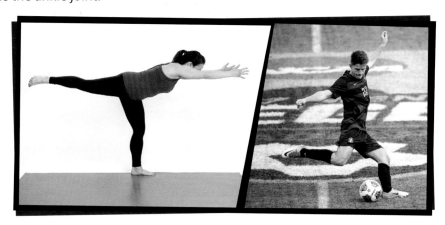

Revolving Triangle (pg. 63)

This pose targets IT bands, releases tension on knees and hips, and is the perfect preparation pose for the common twisting kick motion.

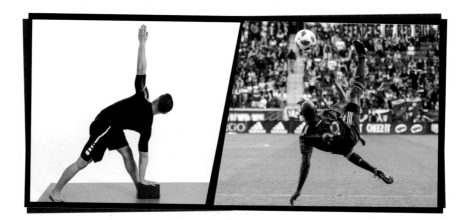

Hero's Pose (pg. 113)

This pose stretches the quads and shins and opens the ankle for more power to push off, and it helps to produce ease of movement.

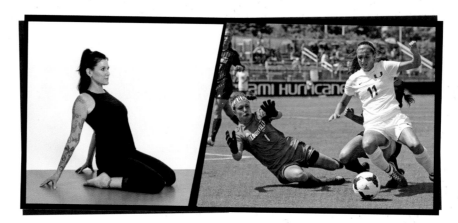

Low Push-Up (pg. 150)

This is a great pose, particularly for goalies who need strong wrists and forearms to avoid injury.

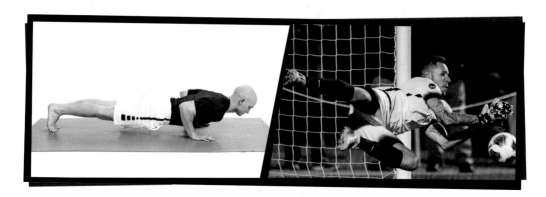

Face-Down Shoulder Stretch (pg. 169)

This pose is great for pec, bicep, and anterior deltoid flexibility and deep spinal rotation.

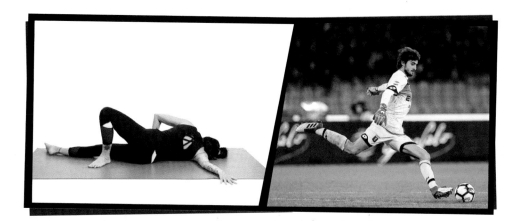

Wrist Openers (pg. 156)

Even though soccer players don't use their arms a lot, they tend to throw their bodies around a lot and fall. Wrist openers help the shoulders, arms, and wrists to absorb the falls.

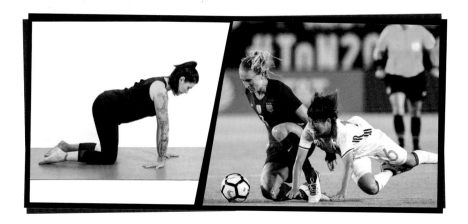

TOP FIVE YOGA POSES FOR SOCCER

1. Triangle (pg. 61)

Triangle pose is a great way for a soccer player to stretch the inner thigh and side of the body, which will help increase breath capacity while also increasing the strength and stability of the core. The revolving variation is important for opening up the ever-resistant IT band and the outer thigh muscles. Revolving triangle can increase the rotation in the spine, which is called upon continually during a soccer game. Do each pose for one to two minutes, two to three times each side.

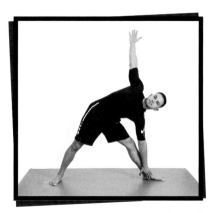

(continued)

Soccer

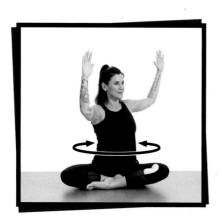

2. Easy Cross-Legged Twist (pg. 103)

This is a great way to warm up before your game. Sitting and twisting for one to four minutes increases the strength in your spine and improves spinal rotation. It will identify which side it is harder to rotate toward so that you can remove that asymmetry. A soccer player who displays tight rotation on one side is at risk of creating a blind side, and the ball will be taken from you on the blind side every time.

3. Squat (pg. 79)

Squat is a great way to get a deep stretch in the hips and groin to enable more range of motion. Also, this pose helps to elongate the Achilles tendon and calves, decreasing the strain on them.

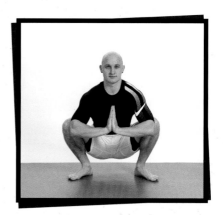

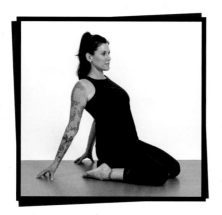

4. Hero's Pose (pg. 113)

Since soccer is one of the fastest-paced, most acrobatic sports, it is critical to keep the lower legs flexible, including the shins, the tops of the feet (extension), the calves, the Achilles tendons, the bottoms of the feet, and under the toes. Keeping all of these areas flexible and strong will preserve power for running, kicking, and movement on the field. Hold each type (toes tucked and toes untucked) for two minutes.

5. Pigeon (pg. 178)

Pigeon is a great way to keep the glutes and hips open. Doing this pose every day for several minutes on each side will maintain a flexible, supple hip. I cannot stress enough the importance of keeping the hips flexible to lessen the stress on the knees. Keeping the hips flexible in all directions reduces injury risks to the knee. Perform the pose on each side for three to five minutes.

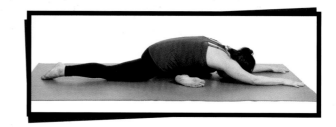

YOGA SEQUENCE FOR SOCCER

POSE	PAGE	TIME/REPS
Perform typical warm-up before you begin		
Rock and roll	130	1 min
Roll into standing forward bend and hold	54	1 min
Squat	79	1 min
Standing forward bend	54	1 min
Squat	79	1 min
Jump back to plank, then into low push-up to upward dog to downward dog	147, 150, 163, 160	1 time
*Bring right foot forward into warrior 1	82	30 sec
Warrior 2	84	30 sec
Reverse warrior	85	30 sec
Triangle	61	30 sec
Revolving triangle	63	30 sec
Repeat from warrior 1 to revolving triangle for a total of 5 times		
Standing split (left leg up)	88	30 sec
Tuck left knee behind right knee and lower as much as you can with right foot flat, return to standing split, lower, return to standing split, and lower	88	5 times
Step back on left foot, bring right leg over left for eagle pose	76	1 min
Grab right big toe with right hand and extend right leg out in front of you		1 min
Bring leg to right and hold		30 sec
Bring leg back to center, let go of toe, and keep leg as high as you can		10 sec
Bring leg down and sweep it through to warrior 3	86	1 min
Standing split (right leg up)	88	30 sec
Standing forward bend	54	30 sec
Squat	79	1 min
Repeat on other side from * for one to three times per side, and then go to floor		
Pigeon	178	3 min each side
Double pigeon	179	2 min each side
Frog	183	5 min
Hero's pose with toes tucked	115	2 min
Hero's pose	113	2 min
Lying spinal twist	126	3 min each side
Supported fish	185	3 min

Soccer

BASKETBALL

To succeed in basketball, athletes need strong legs for the intense running and aerobic game. Strong, flexible ankles are critical for turning on a dime and eluding defenders and for increasing vertical leaping ability while maintaining healthy, open knees. All players must display great agility, quick reactions, a supple spine, and a flexible groin.

COMMON INJURIES IN BASKETBALL

Low back problems, shoulder strains, oblique and abdominal strains, quad pulls, hamstring pulls, neck pain, tight chest, heavy legs, and knee strains

YOGA POSES CLOSELY RELATED TO MOVEMENTS IN BASKETBALL

Locust (pg. 167)

This pose trains athletic back extension that is needed for powerful dunks.

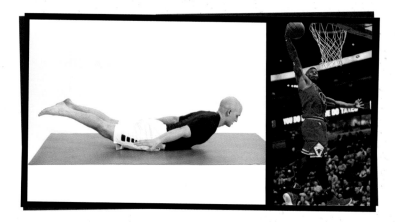

Crescent Lunge (pg. 69)

This pose trains the athlete to have great leg strength and flexibility; it also helps elongate the stride for faster drives down the court.

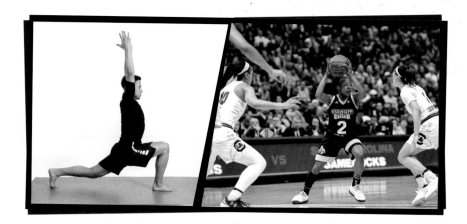

Straddle Forward Bend (pg. 75)

This pose allows for bigger strides and stable planting when preparing to make a shot.

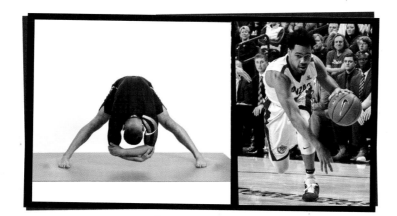

Extended Side Angle (pg. 66)

This pose helps with reach on defense and with shooting on offense.

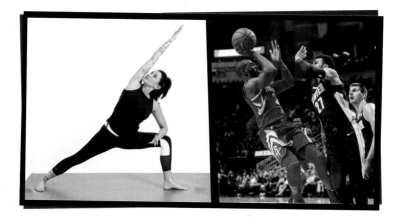

Standing Crescent (pg. 53)

This pose opens the side of the body and shoulders for a better reach.

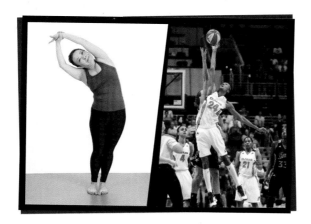

Wheel of Life (pg. 181)

This pose helps increase spinal rotation and arm reach as well as neck rotation for a better visual field.

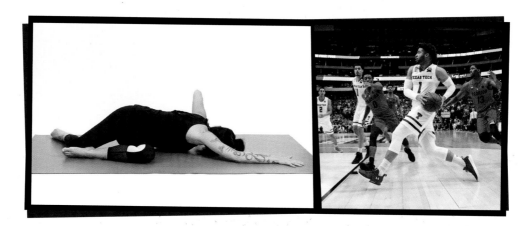

Revolving Triangle (pg. 63)

This pose helps build oblique strength, reducing injury risk and increasing strength, spinal rotation, and IT band flexibility.

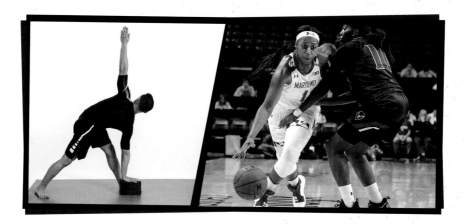

TOP FIVE YOGA POSES FOR BASKETBALL

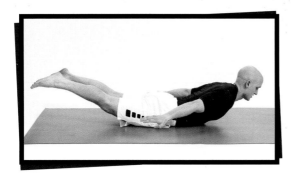

1. Locust (pg. 167)

Locust is a great option to strengthen the entire posterior spine. It actually simulates the look of getting air on the court before you stuff a basket. Locust is also great because it achieves back training on the floor, and the arm extension resembles blocking a shot at the hoop. Hold for 30 to 60 seconds for three to five reps.

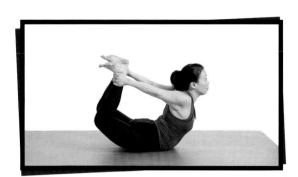

2. Bow (pg. 165)

Bow pose also stretches the anterior spine, building the flexibility of the back muscles. At the same time, bow promotes deep quad stretching and hip flexor flexibility. Both are important to the balance of leg flexibility and power. Open quads, hip flexors, and hamstrings allow overall balance in the legs. Hold 30 to 60 seconds for three to five reps.

3. Frog (pg. 183)

Basketball demands quick changes of direction. Keeping the groin open facilitates these quick moves and protects the vulnerable knee. If the groin can give a little, the knee stays safer. Hold this pose for 5 to 10 minutes.

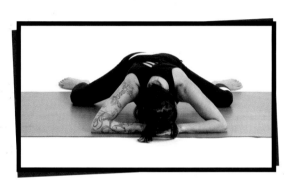

4. Hero's Pose (pg. 113)

Hero's pose (and hero's pose with toes tucked) allows continued opening in the quadriceps muscles but also keeps the knee flexible and gives it pliability in case of a jarring fall on the court. Hero's toes tucked allows you to open the Achilles tendon, calf, plantar fascia, and toes, all of which build more power to push off. The untucked version opens the shin and the top of the ankle for overall stability. Hold each type (toes tucked and untucked) for two minutes.

5. Warrior 1 (pg. 82)

This is a great pose for hoops players to strengthen the thigh and stabilize the knee and increase reach on defense; at the same time, it strengthens the back. Adding a twist in warrior 1 can enhance game form by increasing rotation of the spine to build your ability to twist out of compromising situations. Hold each side for 30 to 60 seconds three times on each side.

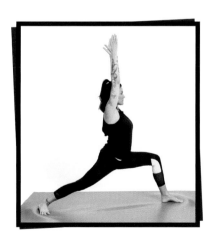

Basketball

YOGA SEQUENCE FOR BASKETBALL

POSE	PAGE	TIME/REPS
Perform typical warm-up before you begin		
Easy cross-legged pose with arm-ups	103	2 min
Rock and roll	130	1 min
Standing forward bend	54	1 min
Chair to standing forward bend and back to chair	58, 54, 58	10 sec each pose; 5 times
Chair to chair twist and back to chair	58, 60, 58	5 times each way
Plank	147	1 min
Plank with toe push-off	148	1 min
Plank with opposite-arm opposite-leg reach	147, 122	30 sec each side; 2 times
Low push-up to upward dog, then to downward dog and hold	150, 163, 160	1 min
*Step right foot forward outside of right hand to lizard and hold	71	1 min
Left hand stays down, twist right, and hold lizard twist	71	1 min
Bring right hand back down and place inside right foot to extended side angle	66	1 min
Repeat from * for 3 times each side		
Revolving triangle	63	30 sec
Triangle	61	30 sec
Repeat from revolving triangle for a total of 3 times and then lower to belly		
Locust (use arm variations)	167	30 sec
Face-down snow angel	168	1 min
Bow, side bow (right), bow, and side bow (left)	165, 166	10 sec; 3 times each side
Child's pose	176	1 min
Puppy pose	158	1 min
Sphinx	171	1 min
Repeat on other side from * for 1-3 times each side		
Face-down shoulder stretch	169	2 min each side
Happy baby	143	1 min
Heavy legs	140	2 min
Wheel of life	181	3 min each side
Frog	183	5 min

BASEBALL AND SOFTBALL

These sports demand quick reactions on the field, so you must be prepared to make diving and acrobatic moves instantly. The sport demands lunging, twisting, and constant focus. These sports are unusual because the athletes must be prepared to be in both offensive and defensive positions for each game. This type of demand develops mental fitness as well as physical fitness.

BASEBALL AND SOFTBALL: PITCHERS

A pitcher must demonstrate great poise and a calm demeanor on the mound. Pitchers also should have great reaction times for balls that are hit back at them to avoid injury, and they need bursts of high energy to deliver a fastball or to pick off a baserunner. It is crucial for a pitcher to have open, flexible, and strong hips, legs, and shoulders. Pitchers must have incredible balance and stability in their ankles. Most obvious is the need for stable elbows and strong wrists to deliver precision pitches. Pitchers need mental toughness and flexibility to stay calm during the toughest moments.

COMMON INJURIES FOR PITCHERS

Shoulder tears; shoulder instability; hip soreness; tired, heavy legs; neck strains and tightness; rotator cuff issues; elbow issues; back imbalance and strains; hamstring and groin injuries.

YOGA POSES CLOSELY RELATED TO MOVEMENTS IN PITCHING

Three-Legged Dog (pg. 94)

This pose is great for leg flexibility, ankle stability, and wrist and arm strength.

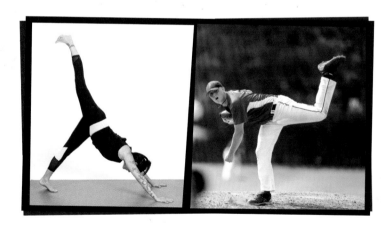

Warrior 1 (pg. 82)

This pose strengthens and stretches necessary areas for better pitching control.

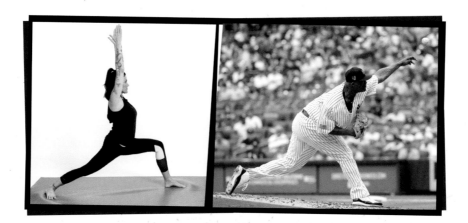

Warrior 2 (pg. 84)

This pose strengthens the legs, shoulders, and back.

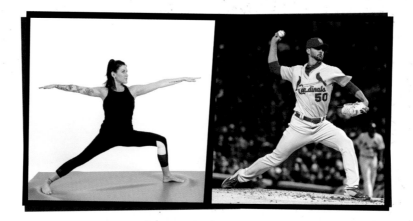

Warrior 3 (pg. 86)

This pose demonstrates the stability the ankle needs to balance on the pitcher's follow-through.

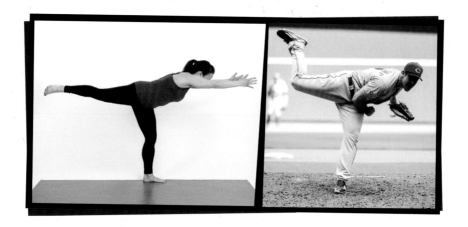

TOP FIVE YOGA POSES FOR PITCHERS

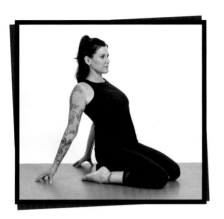

1. Hero's Pose (pg. 113)

This pose opens up the bottom of the pitcher's foot. It also gives more flexibility and power to his foot to push off. The more supple and flexible the toes are, the better the push-off, creating more force and speed in the pitch. Do each type (toes tucked and untucked) for two minutes.

2. Warrior 1 to Warrior 3 (pg. 82 and 86)

Going back and forth between these moves 5 to 10 times will develop the pitcher's balance. This creates strength and stability in the ankle. It will also create stronger quads and hamstrings, and it will develop deep glute strength to help the pitcher with hip force and power.

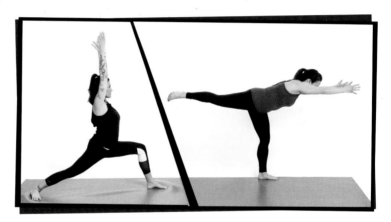

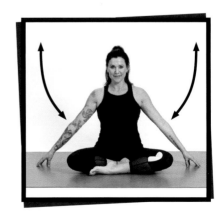

3. Warrior 2 (pg. 84)

Holding this pose for one to three minutes will not only help develop a strong knee joint from the support of the quad and hamstring, it will also help open the groin to prevent pulls and tweaks. In this pose, the practitioner focuses on tracking the knee over the toes to learn to protect the knee with proper form.

4. Easy Cross-Legged Pose with Arm-Ups (pg. 103)

This repetitive pose done from one to four minutes will help warm the shoulder joint and build functional strength in the vulnerable joint. It helps pitchers to start to sync their breath with their movement, preparing them for the mental rigors of game situations.

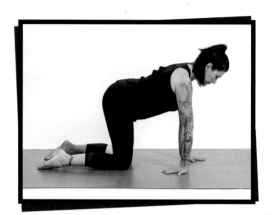

5. Wrist Openers (pg. 156)

This is a great one. Not only does this move strengthen and challenge the abdominals and legs, it opens the wrist joint to increase range of motion. Increasing the range of motion in the wrist will enable the pitcher to hold the ball more easily in all formations and will give the wrist snap. Finally, it will help relieve flexors and extensors in the forearm that could tighten up after a game or after the pitcher has gripped too hard. Do 30-second holds on each side three times.

YOGA SEQUENCE FOR PITCHERS

POSE	PAGE	TIME/REPS
Perform typical warm-up before you begin		
Rock and roll	130	1 min
*Standing forward bend	54	1 min
Standing backbend	53	1 min
Slide right leg back into crescent lunge	69	1 min
Right knee up and down in crescent lunge	69	10 times
Plank	147	30 sec
Side plank (right)	152	30 sec
Plank	147	30 sec
Low push-up to upward dog to downward dog	150, 163, 160	1 time
Knee-down crescent lunge (step right foot forward, left knee down)	71	1 min
Standing forward bend	54	1 min
Repeat on other side from * for 1-3 times each side; on last time through, end at downward dog		
**Bring right foot forward into warrior 1	82	1 min
Backstroke and front stroke with arms while in warrior 1	82	10 times each way
Plank to low push-up to upward dog to downward dog	147, 150, 163, 160	1 time
**Repeat on other side from ** **		
***Step right foot forward into warrior 2 to warrior 1 to warrior 3 and hold; touch left hand to floor, back to warrior 3, and again touch left hand to floor	84, 82, 86	10 sec per pose; 5 times

POSE	PAGE	TIME/REPS
Standing forward bend	54	1 min
Squat	79	1 min
Plank to low push-up to upward dog to downward dog	147, 150, 163, 160	1 time
Repeat on other side from ***		
Wrist openers	156	30 sec each position; 2 times
Elbow-to-knee plank	148	1 min
Lower to belly into bow	165	1 min
Face-down shoulder stretch (straight arm and 90 degree)	169	5 min each variation, each side
Pigeon	178	3-5 min each side
Frog	183	3-5 min

BASEBALL AND SOFTBALL: CATCHERS

Catchers are unique to the game. They have the only position that faces the entire field; therefore, they are very much in charge of directing play. They need strong, explosive legs and the ability to leap up from a squat and exert great torque to execute a precise throw. They need overall flexibility and strength and the ability to be mindful.

COMMON INJURIES FOR CATCHERS

Knee issues, low back strain and pain, shoulder problems

YOGA POSES CLOSELY RELATED TO MOVEMENTS IN CATCHING

Squat (pg. 79)

This pose mimics the needs of the catcher, strengthens and stretches legs and hips, and strengthens the back. Squat is a clear winner to prepare the knees, Achilles tendons, and ankles for nine innings in a squatting position.

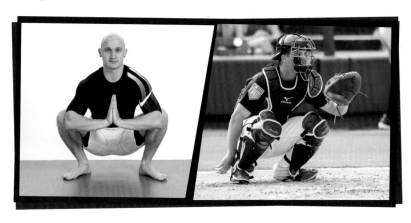

Baseball and Softball

Camel (pg. 117)

This pose prepares the body for blocking the ball by opening the quads and hip flexors and strengthening the ankles.

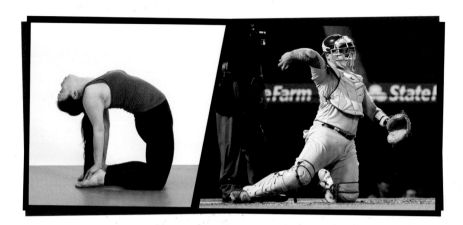

Warrior 2 (pg. 84)

This pose strengthens and stretches and mimics the moves the body performs when throwing to second base.

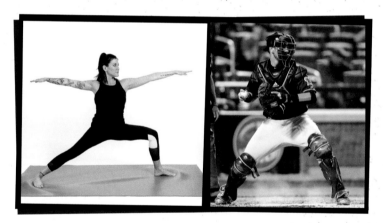

TOP FIVE YOGA POSES FOR CATCHERS

1. Squat (pg. 79)

Squat pose is the best way to open the hips and low back to prepare for long games behind the plate. It will also strengthen the back and take the load off the low back. Do this pose for one to three minutes.

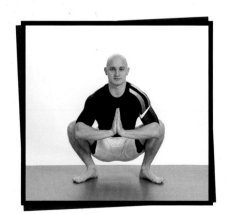

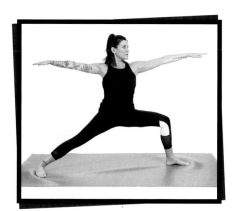

2. Warrior 2 (pg. 84)

This pose done on both sides is a way to strengthen and stretch the legs and inner thighs. It will tone the back and shoulders and strengthen the back all at the same time. Do this pose one to three minutes on each side.

3. Warrior 3 (pg. 86)

This pose helps to develop a strong ankle and strengthens the lower leg. When the catcher jumps up to make a throw to second base, she needs her lower body to be flexible enough to absorb the quick move. Do each side for one to three minutes.

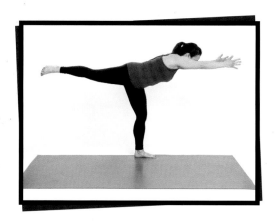

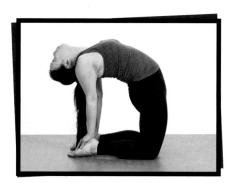

4. Camel Pose (pg. 117)

This is an essential pose to stretch a catcher's hip flexors. Holding the squat position during a game is a sure way to tighten the front hips and create pressure on the low back. Do this pose for relief. Hold it two to three times for one minute.

5. Bow Pose (pg. 165)

Bow is another great way to improve the strength of the hip flexors and to open the chest and anterior deltoids at the same time. For a catcher to have power in his throw, the front of his body must be pliable and supple. Do this pose for one minute three times.

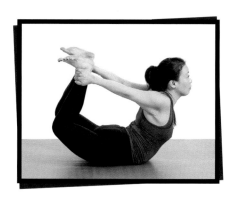

YOGA SEQUENCE FOR CATCHERS

POSE	PAGE	TIME/REPS
Perform typical warm-up before you begin		
Rock and roll	130	1 min
Standing forward bend	54	1 min
Standing backbend	53	30 sec
Standing forward bend to chair to standing forward bend	54, 58, 54	10 sec each; 3 times
Plank to low push-up to plank to low push-up	147, 150	1 time
Upward dog	163	1 min
Downward dog	160	1 min
*Bring right foot forward into half side squat	96	4 times each side
Warrior 1	82	1 min
Warrior 2	84	1 min
Windmill arms down to front of mat and lift left leg into standing split, then alternate legs for standing split kicks	88	1 min
Squat turn	80	1 time each way
Plank with wrist openers	147, 156	2 min; change wrist position every 30 sec
Plank with toe push-offs	148	1 min
Low push-up to plank to low push-up to plank	150, 147	1 time
Upward dog to downward dog	163, 160	1 min
Repeat on other side from * for 1-3 times each side		
Plank	147	30 sec
Bow pose to child's pose	165, 176	10 sec each, 10 times
Face-down shoulder stretch (straight arm and 90 degrees)	169	5 min each variation, each side
Child's pose	176	1 min
Hip flexor opener	189	5 min
Supported fish	185	5 min

BASEBALL AND SOFTBALL: FIELDERS

Infielders and outfielders should have a lot of flexibility to enable them to make diving plays that stretch the upper and lower body and ground-ball plays that require them to squat and get low. The hips should be open for these plays and to keep the knees safe.

COMMON INJURIES FOR FIELDERS

Leg muscle strains, low back pain, shoulder instability

YOGA POSES CLOSELY RELATED TO MOVEMENTS IN FIELDING

Extended-Leg Side Plank (pg. 153)

This pose lengthens the body and increases leg flexibility.

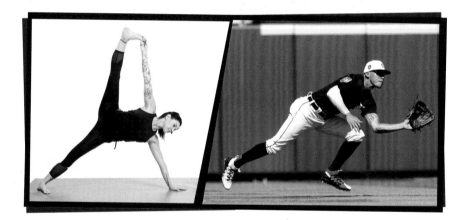

Split (pg. 71)

This pose mimics the needs of first basemen and increases flexibility.

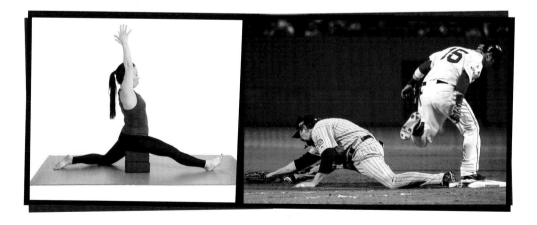

Crescent Lunge (pg. 69)

This pose opens the hip flexors and legs and preps the body for duties on the field.

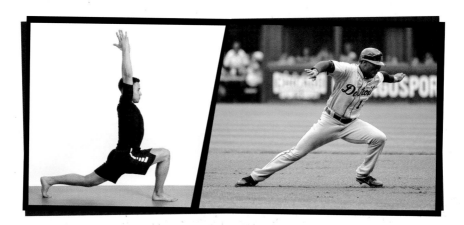

Wheel of Life (pg. 181)

This pose prepares the body for plays in all directions and increases spinal rotation, the ability to reach, and neck flexibility.

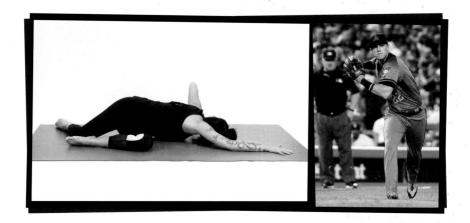

Locust (pg. 167)

This pose strengthens the back of the body and the spine for diving catches.

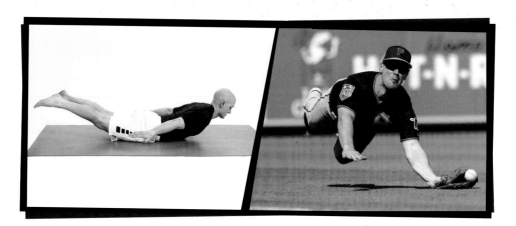

Squat (pg. 79)

This pose sets the athlete up for a perfect fielding position.

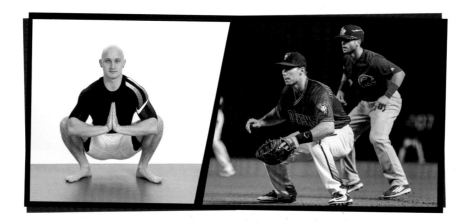

Warrior 2 (pg. 84)

This pose strengthens the upper body, increases strength and flexibility in the lower body, and develops a broad reach.

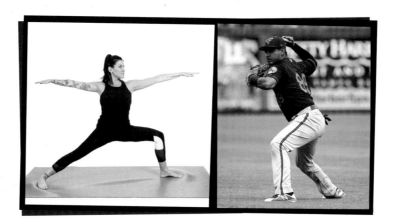

Chair (pg. 58)

This pose strengthens the legs and core and helps athletes maintain a ready position.

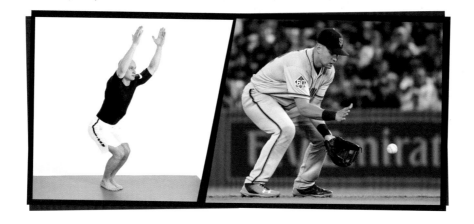

Lunge Twist (pg. 98)

This pose helps increase hip stability and spinal rotation for increased torque while batting.

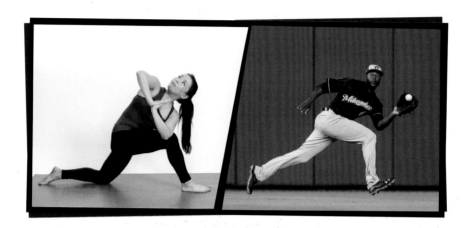

TOP FIVE YOGA POSES FOR FIELDERS

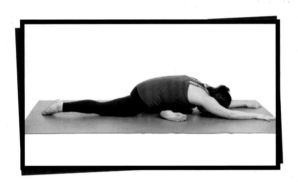

1. Pigeon (pg. 178)

It is important for players to keep their hips open in order to increase speed, agility, and torque and to lessen the potential stress on the knees. Pigeon pose opens deeply into the glutes and releases any pressure that could accumulate on the sciatic nerve. Do this pose five minutes on each side.

2. Frog (pg. 183)

Frog enables a player to open the hips and at the same time to stretch the inner thigh and groin, which is an area of injury for a lot of baseball players. You should hold this pose for 2 to 20 minutes.

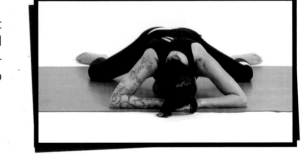

3. Standing Forward Bend Against a Wall (pg. 56)

As an alternative to seated forward bend, which is often done incorrectly, this pose enables gravity to take over while you fold in half facing the wall and stabilize your feet on the floor while leaning against the wall. This enables you to get deeper faster with the hamstrings, a resistant set of muscles. Learn to hold this pose for one to three minutes; you will find your mental toughness and focus challenged here.

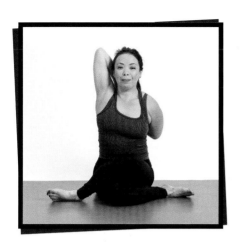

4. Cow Face Pose (pg. 119)

Baseball players need strong, open, stable shoulders. This stretch focuses on the anterior deltoid (front of the shoulder), which is often the tightest part of the intricate shoulder, and the rotator cuff. You can add plank pose held for a minute to increase the stability of the shallow, vulnerable shoulder joint. Do this pose three minutes on each side.

5. Easy Cross-Legged Twist (pg. 103)

This is a great movement for a softball player to increase the rotation in her spine on the nondominant side. Equalizing flexibility helps maintain a more symmetrical body, which is more stable. Having a strong, deep rotation will help with torque. This exercise also helps build strength in the back and to sync the breath with the movement. All athletes can benefit from increased breath capacity to remain calm in the most stressful situations. Continue fluid twisting for two minutes.

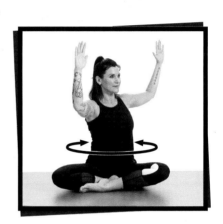

YOGA SEQUENCE FOR FIELDERS

POSE	PAGE	TIME/REPS
Perform typical warm-up before you begin		
Rock and roll to standing forward bend and hold	130, 54	1 min
Plank to low push-up to upward dog to downward dog and hold	147, 150, 163, 160	1 min
Bring right foot forward into warrior 1	82	30 sec
Straighten right leg and turn left into straddle forward bend	75	1 min
Stand up and flap arms vigorously		1 min
Windmill arms to front and into plank to low push-up to upward dog to downward dog	147, 150, 163, 160	1 time
Repeat on other side from * for 1-3 times each side; on last downward dog, hold for 1 min		
Step right foot forward outside right hand into lizard	71	1 min each side
Squat	79	1 min
Squat turns	80	1 time each way

(continued)

Yoga Sequence for Fielders *(continued)*

POSE	PAGE	TIME/REPS
Standing forward bend	54	1 min
Stand up into mountain pose to standing crescent	52, 53	1 min each side
Standing forward bend to plank to low push-up to upward dog to downward dog	54, 147, 150, 163, 160	1 time
**Step right foot forward into warrior 2	84	30 sec
Extended side angle (right)	66	30 sec
Warrior 1	82	30 sec
Crescent lunge	69	30 sec
Step forward into tree pose	90	30 sec
Repeat from ** for a total of 5 times, and on last tree pose, hold for 1 min		
Squat	79	1 min
Repeat on other side from ** for 1-3 times each side		
Pigeon	178	3-5 min each side
Hero's pose	113	2 min
Hero's pose with toes tucked	115	2 min
Cow face pose	119	2 min each side
Frog	183	5 min

HOCKEY

Hockey players of all positions need incredible balance; ankle strength and stability; sound Achilles tendons; strong legs; flexible spines; open necks; clear vision; strong, open wrists and forearms; and supple hips. Hockey also demands players make deep twisting plays to save and redirect the puck and develop speed with intense eye focus.

COMMON INJURIES IN HOCKEY

Back pain and problems; knee tears and strains; groin pulls; wrist injuries; elbow tendonitis; ankle trauma; tight hips; strained forearm muscles; asymmetrical back strains

YOGA POSES CLOSELY RELATED TO MOVEMENTS IN HOCKEY

Frog (pg. 183)

This pose prepares the groin for goal saves.

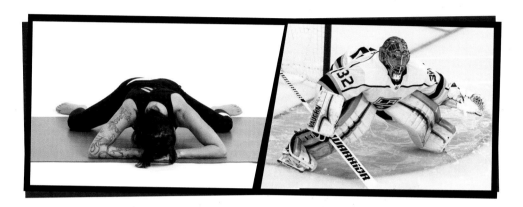

Lunge Twist (pg. 98)

This pose is great for building leg strength and encouraging spinal rotation.

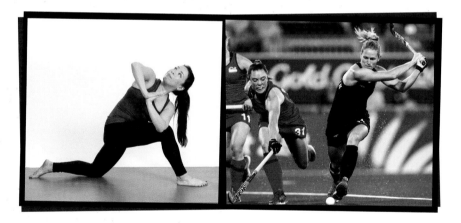

Eagle Pose (pg. 76)

This pose helps with balance and ankle stability.

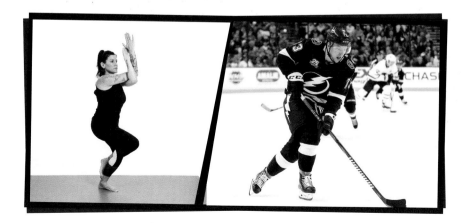

Boat Pose (pg. 111)

This pose is great for abdominal strength.

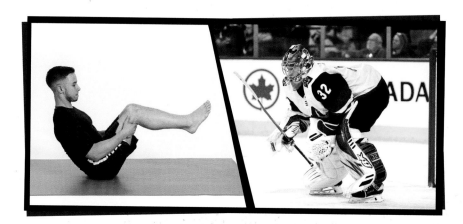

Half Side Squat (pg. 96)

This pose opens the groin and increases balance and leg strength.

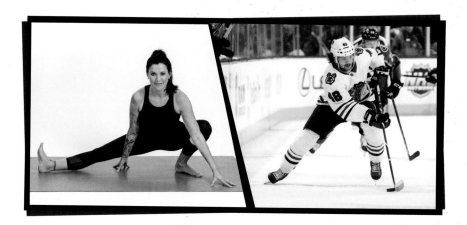

TOP FIVE YOGA POSES FOR HOCKEY

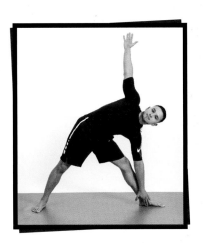

1. Triangle (pg. 61)

Triangle is a great pose for hockey players because the sport puts a high demand on the thighs and legs. Triangle opens the legs but also strengthens the back and obliques so a player has greater power to change direction on the fly. Hold this pose one minute on each side.

Hockey

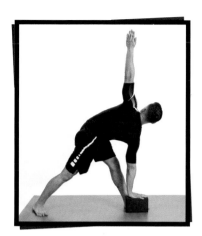

2. Revolving Triangle (pg. 63)

Revolving triangle has the same benefits as triangle except that it adds flexibility to the IT bands. The more open they are, the less the strain on the knees and back, especially during powerful twisting or rotating moves on the ice. Hold this pose one minute on each side.

3. Lunge Twist (pg. 98)

This pose gives you more time to work to increase spinal rotation, which is critical to hockey. Strong and deep rotation enhances the player's ability to respond to the direction of the play. Hold this pose for one minute on each side.

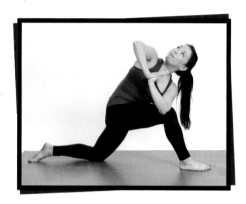

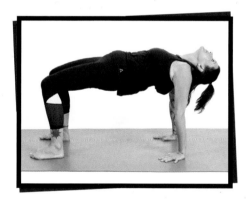

4. Inverted Table (pg. 139)

Inverted table is beneficial for two reasons: First, it opens hip flexors, which reduces strain on the low back by stabilizing and releasing the pelvis; second, it opens the wrist joints and forearms, giving players better control of the hockey stick and improving the wrists' ability to absorb shock during falls on the ice. It also opens the chest for increased power in the slap shot. A tight chest has limited range of motion. Do this pose 10 times, holding for 10 seconds.

5. Frog (pg. 183)

Frog is the perfect pose for long hours on the ice. Skating places constant demands on the inner thighs. The frog pose before or after a game for five minutes is awesome for releasing the tension and increasing the stride.

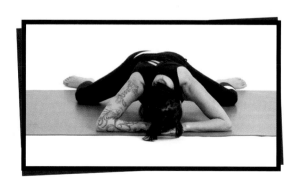

YOGA SEQUENCE FOR HOCKEY

POSE	PAGE	TIME/REPS
Perform typical warm-up before you begin		
Rock and roll	130	1 min
Rock and roll to squat pike and hold; after last pike, try to go to standing position from pike (advanced)	81	3 times each side
Standing forward bend	54	1 min
Plank to low push-up to upward dog to downward dog	147, 150, 163, 160	1 time
*Step right foot forward into pyramid pose (bend and straighten the knee)	64	1 min
Triangle to revolving triangle to triangle	61, 63, 61	30 sec each; 3 times
Windmill the arms into standing forward bend and hold	54	1 min
Squat (arms overhead)	79	1 min
Squat to standing on toes	79	10 times
Standing forward bend	54	1 min
Plank to low push-up to upward dog to downward dog	147, 150, 163, 160	1 time
Step right foot forward into crescent lunge	69	30 sec
Lunge twist	98	30 sec
Come to seated position and into inverted table	139	15 times
Inverted plank	138	15 times
Roll over onto hands and knees and into plank to low push-up to upward dog to downward dog and immediately press into plank	147, 150, 163, 160, 147	1 time
Repeat on other side from * for 1-3 times each side		
Pigeon (quad variation)	178	3 min each
Frog	183	5 min
Lying spinal twist	126	3 min each side
Face-up shoulder stretch	134	3 min each side
Supported fish	185	5 min
Hip flexor opener	189	5 min

LACROSSE

Lacrosse players need strong legs and great endurance. In addition, strong, flexible wrists and forearms will help with stick handling precision; flexible spines, open necks, and agility will promote quickness and accuracy on the field.

COMMON INJURIES IN LACROSSE

Wrist problems, back tightness and pain, shoulder tears, knee problems, groin pulls, hip tightness, neck issues

YOGA POSES CLOSELY RELATED TO MOVEMENTS IN LACROSSE

Locust (pg. 167)

This pose helps improve an athlete's reach for more incredible plays defending the goal or for scoring points.

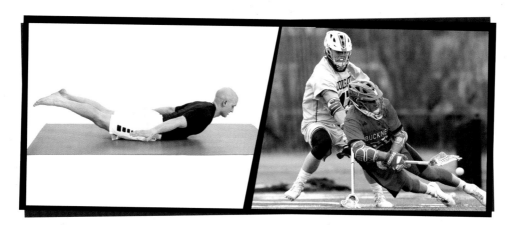

Crescent Lunge (pg. 69)

This pose strengthens the legs and prepares the groin for long strides and speed.

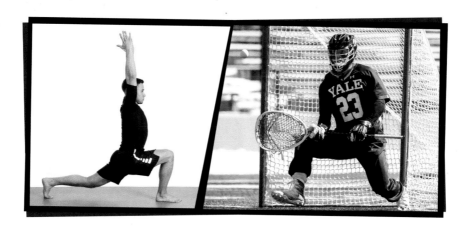

Lunge Twist (pg. 98)

This pose helps develop power and torque for changing direction on the field, attempting to score, and defending the goal.

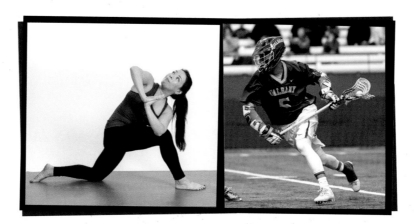

Goddess Pose (pg. 72)

This pose increases leg and hip flexibility and helps protect the knees.

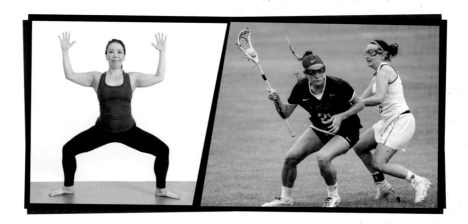

TOP FIVE YOGA POSES FOR LACROSSE

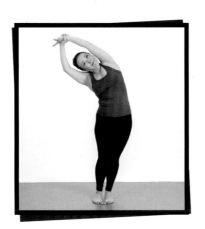

1. Standing Crescent (pg. 53)

This pose increases strength in the obliques and lateral movement in the spine, simulating the wild strength moves on the field of play. It also opens shoulders in a fully extended posture much like you do in the game. Do each side for one minute.

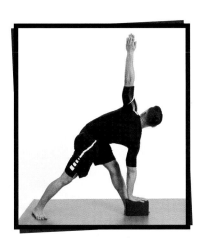

2. Revolving Triangle (pg. 63)

Opening the IT band is important in lacrosse because the legs get very tight with miles of running on the field per game. The more open they are, the better the protection of the knee, giving it a little more leeway for twists and turns. Do each side for one minute.

3. Warrior 1 (pg. 82)

Warrior 1 is another way to strengthen and increase flexibility of the legs as well as the back while the arms are extended over the head. Longer holds in this position truly prepare the player for short spurts of needed strength on the field. Do each side for one minute.

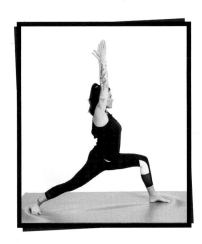

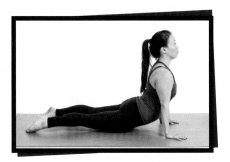

4. Upward Dog (pg. 163)

Upward dog while doing wrist openers is also beneficial for the lacrosse player; it brings the back into full extension, and it opens and stretches the wrists and forearms for better stick control. This pose also opens the chest to counterbalance the repetitive motion of being forward and running while contracting the chest in front of you to hold the stick. Do this pose for one minute.

5. Child's Pose (pg. 176)

This pose is a delight for the lacrosse player to ease the low back from miles of pounding from running on the field. It is also a mild back stretch and hip release. Hold this pose for two minutes.

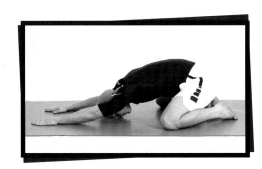

YOGA SEQUENCE FOR LACROSSE

POSE	PAGE	TIME/REPS
Perform typical warm-up before you begin		
Easy cross-legged pose with arm-ups	103	1 min
Rock and roll	130	1 min
Standing forward bend	54	1 min
Straddle forward bend to goddess	75, 72	30 sec each; 5 times
Straddle forward bend twist to right	74	30 sec
Place right arm behind back and make small shoulder rolls on right side		30 sec
Straddle forward bend twist to left	74	30 sec
Place left arm behind back and make small shoulder rolls on left side		30 sec
Windmill arms and step to front of mat into plank to low push-up to upward dog to downward dog	147, 150, 163, 160	1 time
*Step right foot forward with left knee down into crescent lunge	69	30 sec
Remain in crescent lunge and lift knee up and down	69	10 times
Remain in crescent lunge and twist to right	69	30 sec
Crescent lunge to warrior 3	69, 86	10 sec each; 5 times
Plank to low push-up to upward dog to downward dog	147, 150, 163, 160	1 time
Plank with wrist openers	147, 156	30 sec each wrist position; 2 min
Downward dog	160	1 min
Repeat on other side from * for 1-3 times each side		
Lower to belly into locust (use arm variations)	167	1 min
Bow pose	165	1 min
Face-down shoulder stretch	169	3 min each side
Wheel of life	181	3 min each side

VOLLEYBALL

Volleyball players need great agility to make lunging plays; an open groin to absorb shock; strong, flexible ankles for power to push off; and great range of motion in the shoulder joints. In addition, volleyball players' wrists must be open enough to be able to absorb the shock of constant falls.

COMMON INJURIES IN VOLLEYBALL

Ankle injuries, knee issues, wrist problems, back strains, neck issues, shoulder problems

YOGA POSES CLOSELY RELATED TO MOVEMENTS IN VOLLEYBALL

Standing Crescent (pg. 53)

This pose opens the side of the body for better reach and better defensive plays on the court.

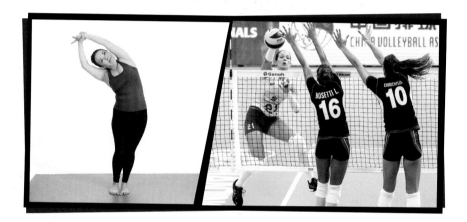

Locust (pg. 167)

This pose stretches the shoulders and opens the back, enabling players to make extraordinary saves.

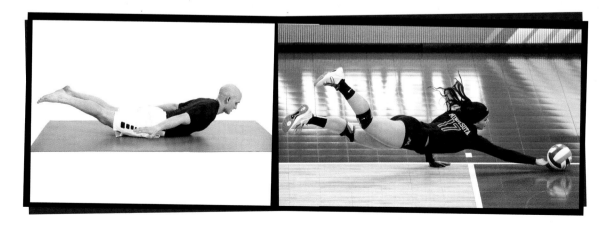

Volleyball

Crescent Lunge (pg. 69)

This pose helps build strong legs and flexible hip flexors, making the player more explosive and powerful.

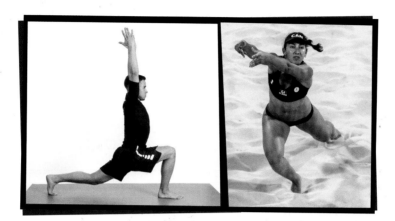

Half Side Squat (pg. 96)

This pose opens a different angle in the hips that players often face.

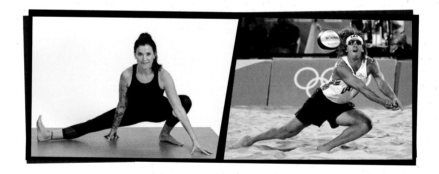

TOP FIVE YOGA POSES FOR VOLLEYBALL

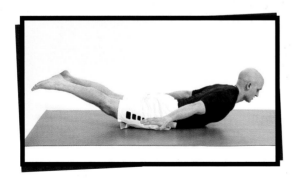

1. Locust (pg. 167)

Locust pose is a perfect choice to increase back extension and back strength. This pose also stretches the abdominal wall and chest for increased depth of breath. Hold this pose for 30 seconds five times.

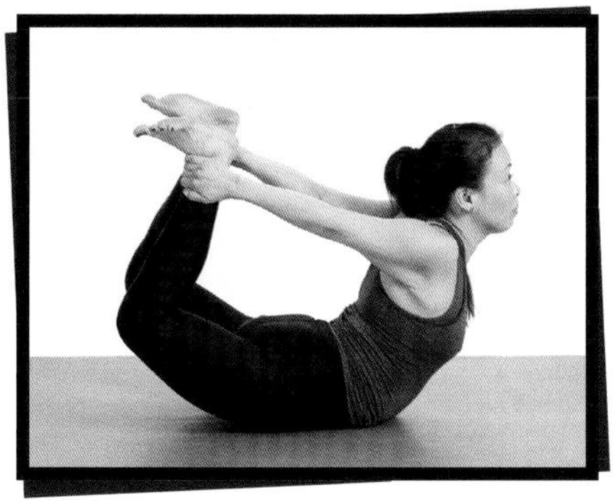

2. Bow Pose (pg. 165)

Bow pose builds on the benefits of locust, and it adds the element of a quad stretch and deeper back extension. Hold this pose for one minute three times.

3. Half Side Squat (pg. 96)

Half side squat protects the integrity of the knee joint, opens the hips, and strengthens the back at the same time. At first, this pose is difficult when done alone, not in a game situation, but in time the execution becomes much easier and deeper. Do this pose for 30 seconds on each side four times.

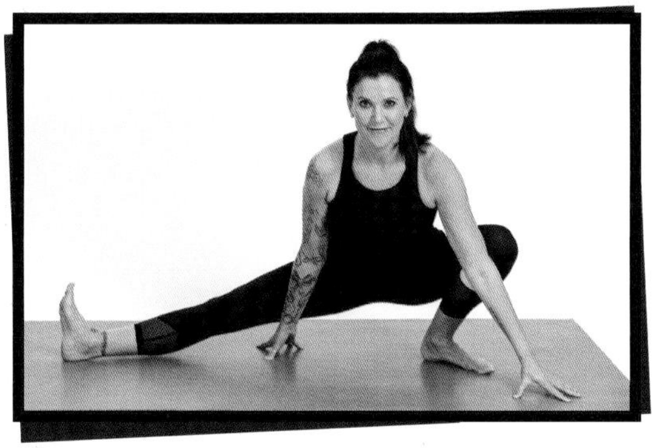

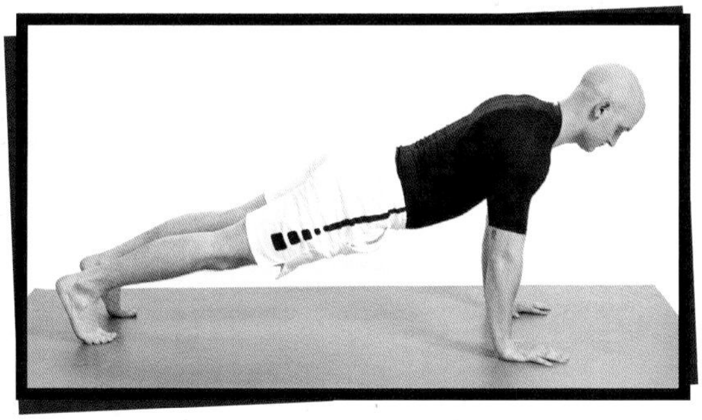

4. Plank (pg. 147)

Plank pose stretches the wrists and strengthens the abdominals. It forces athletes to focus on their breathing to stay determined and focused. Hold this pose for one minute.

5. Downward Dog (pg. 160)

Downward dog eases the stress on the back; it deeply opens the chest, shoulders, and hamstrings. In this pose, you can pedal the feet out and increase the flexibility of the Achilles tendons, calves, and toes for more power to make lunging saves. Hold downward dog for one minute.

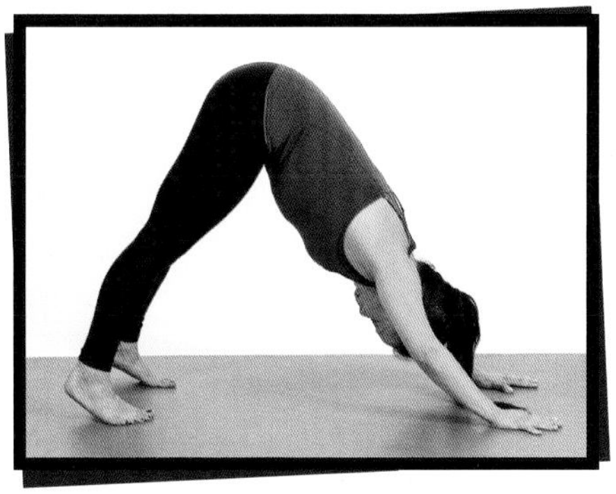

YOGA SEQUENCE FOR VOLLEYBALL

POSE	PAGE	TIME/REPS
Perform typical warm-up before you begin		
*Three-legged dog (right leg up)	94	10 sec
Pyramid pose (right foot forward)	64	1 min
Turn left into half side squat	96	4 times each side
Crescent lunge	69	1 min
Lunge twist	98	1 min
Crescent lunge to warrior 3 to lunge	69, 86, 147	5 times
Plank with wrist openers to low push-up to upward dog to downward dog	147, 156, 150, 163, 160	1 time
Squat	79	1 min
Standing forward bend	54	1 min
Repeat on other side from * for 1-3 times each side		
Lower to belly into locust	167	5 times; 30 sec each
Child's pose	176	1 min
Puppy pose	158	1 min
Pigeon	178	5 min each side
Wheel of life	181	3 min each side
Child's pose	176	10 breaths
Supported fish	185	5 min

WRESTLING

All wrestlers will benefit from having symmetrical back strength; flexible hips to protect their knees; and flexible spines in flexion, extension, and rotation. They must have strong, flexible necks to avoid awkward torqueing and twisting injuries. In addition, open wrists and strong grips, incredible overall strength and stamina, and tremendous mental toughness will help any wrestler prevail in the most challenging moments.

COMMON INJURIES IN WRESTLING

Neck pulls, back strains, knee tears, ankle injuries, shoulder and hamstring strains

YOGA POSES CLOSELY RELATED TO MOVEMENTS IN WRESTLING

Hero's Pose (pg. 113)

This pose prepares the ankles and quads for a match, enabling wrestlers to push out of awkward contortions and avoid being on their backs.

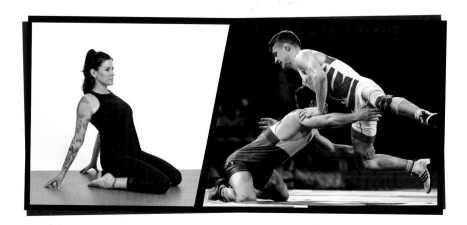

Bridge (pg. 136)

This pose is reminiscent of positions in which wrestlers may find themselves, and it opens the hip flexors and back.

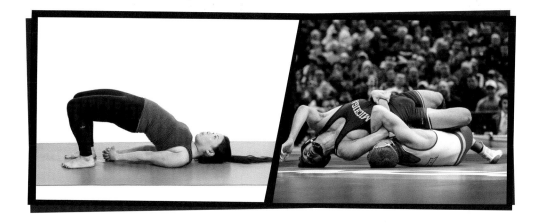

Straddle Forward Bend Twist (pg. 74)

This pose promotes overall leg flexibility and shoulder range. Wrestlers need profound shoulder flexibility. During a match, the opponent is trying to put you in a compromising position to win, and you must be able to endure the twists without damage to your shoulder.

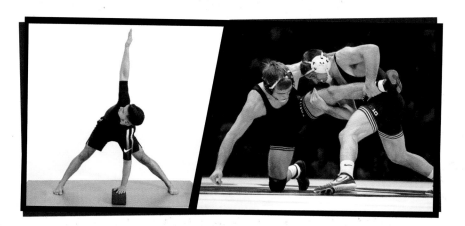

Hero's Pose with Toes Tucked (pg. 115)

This pose is good for foot and leg strength, flexibility, and power to push off.

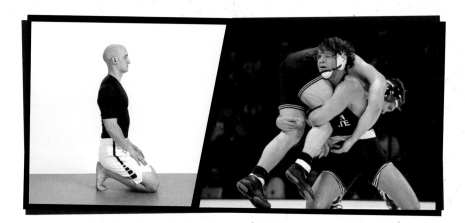

TOP FIVE POSES FOR WRESTLING

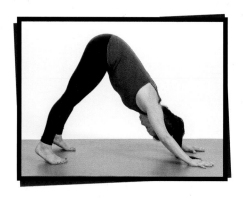

1. Downward Dog (pg. 160)

Wrestlers obviously need overall flexibility; otherwise, your opponent will stretch you beyond your limits. Downward dog stretches the chest, shoulder, and hamstrings and builds strength in the arms and shoulders for critical moves of strength and precision. Hold downward dog for one to two minutes.

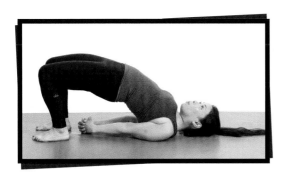

2. Bridge (pg. 136)

Bridge is a great pose to open the back of the neck. Wrestlers can often find themselves in positions that compromise neck safety. Bridge also allows you to open the shoulders and chest and stretch the anterior spine. Do this pose for one minute three times.

3. Inverted Plank (pg.138)

A more advanced pose, but a marriage made in heaven for wrestlers. Being able to open the anterior spine to the fullest while also bearing weight on the wrists, arms, and shoulders prepares the wrestler to escape compromising situations with less effort. Hold for 10 to 15 breaths.

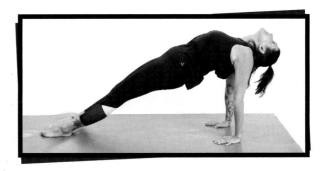

4. Warrior 3 (pg. 86)

While a wrestler would not mimic this pose in a match, it is important for building strength, stability, and flexibility in the ankles and deep glutes while training for balance. Strong legs, quads, and flexible ankles with power to push are critical to come out of the referee's position and escape so you can come to standing and get neutral. Hold each side for one minute.

5. Face-Down Shoulder Stretch (pg. 169)

This pose should be every wrestler's go-to long, deep hold. It opens the chest, shoulders, and biceps for better range of motion and therefore enables wrestlers to endure whatever position opponents put them in. This pose is also great for increasing spinal rotation so you can roll out of sticky situations and avoid the pin. Hold each side for three to four minutes.

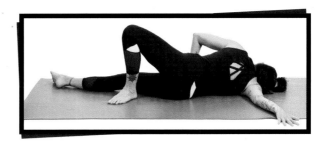

YOGA SEQUENCE FOR WRESTLERS

POSE	PAGE	TIME/REPS
Perform typical warm-up before you begin		
Rock and roll	130	1 min
Standing forward bend	54	1 min
Squat	79	1 min
Plank to low push-up to upward dog to downward dog	147, 150, 163, 160	1 time
From downward dog, jump through to seated position and into plow	132	1 min
Backward roll into downward dog	160	5 times
*Step right foot forward into half side squat	96	Hold 30 sec; 4 times each side
Crescent lunge	69	30 sec
Lunge twist	98	30 sec
Unwind to crescent lunge and step into warrior 3	69, 86	30 sec
Go to standing and bring knee to chest		30 sec
Warrior 3	86	30 sec
Crescent lunge to warrior 3	69, 86	5 times, 10 sec each
Stand up and extend leg		1 min
Warrior 3	86	30 sec
Crescent lunge	69	30 sec
Lizard	71	30 sec
Squat	79	1 min
Squat (turn 360 degrees)	79	1 time each way
Standing forward bend	54	1 min
Plank to upward dog to downward dog	147, 163, 160	Repeat for 1 min
Repeat on other side from * for 1-3 times each side		
Frog	183	5 min
Hero's pose with toes tucked	115	2 min
Hero's pose	113	2 min
Happy baby	143	1 min
Heavy legs	140	3 min
Plow	132	2 min
Shoulder stand	192	2 min
Half headstand	194	1 min

GOLF

Golfers require great hand grip and open forearms, symmetrical back muscles, and back strength. They also need open hips and deep spinal rotation for powerful torque. Finally, they need flexible necks, clear eyes, a calm mind, and calm breathing to deal with high-pressure situations.

COMMON INJURIES IN GOLF

Back problems, imbalance issues, tight hips and wrists, neck strain, mental challenges

YOGA POSES CLOSELY RELATED TO MOVEMENTS IN GOLF

Lunge Twist (pg. 98)

This pose improves overall balance and stability and increases spinal rotation, which will give the golfer more power.

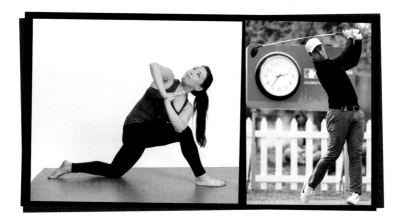

Lizard (pg. 71)

This pose clearly mimics the needs of the focused golfer, with its deep twisting action and rotation of the neck to track the rolling ball's potential path.

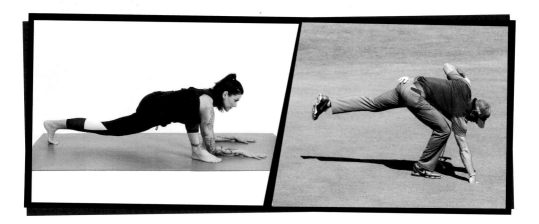

Squat (pg. 79)

This pose opens the groin and inner thigh to help release pressure on the knees and free up the spine for better rotation.

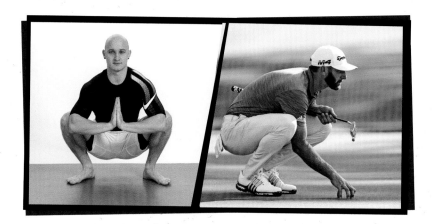

TOP FIVE POSES FOR GOLF

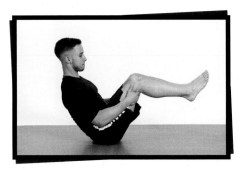

1. Pigeon (pg. 178)

It is very important for a golfer to have clear, open hips to rotate and drive the ball. It is important to always open both sides, not to surrender to the massive imbalance that golf creates. Pigeon is preferred to get a deep hip stretch and opposite quad flexibility. Do this pose for five minutes on each side.

2. Hero's Pose with Toes Tucked (pg. 115)

Picture the finished pose of driving the ball, up on that back toe. Hero's pose with toes tucked supports great finesse at the finish. Do this pose for two minutes.

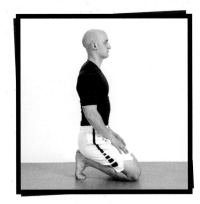

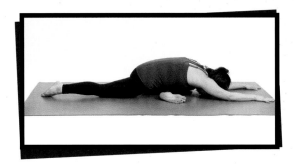

3. Boat Pose (pg. 111)

This pose not only strengthens a golfer's core but also increases back strength and improves posture for better breathing in critical pressure spots. Do this pose for one minute three times.

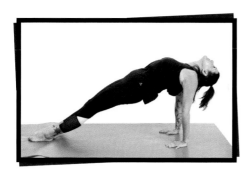

4. Inverted Plank (pg. 138)

This pose is a nice complement to golf. This pose opens the chest and anterior shoulder for better posture and increased spinal rotation. It strengthens the arms, opens the wrists to decrease wrist strain, and increases grip strength. It also adds a little power to the legs. Do this pose for one minute three times.

5. Lunge Twist (pg. 98)

This pose increases power and strength in the legs and at the same time enables the golfer to increase spinal twist for more power on the tee. Do this pose for one minute on each side.

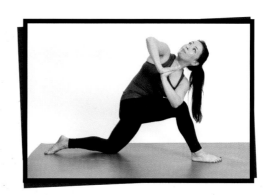

Golf

YOGA SEQUENCE FOR GOLF

POSE	PAGE	TIME/REPS
Perform typical warm-up before you begin		
Rock and roll	130	1 min
Standing forward bend	54	1 min
Standing mountain pose	52	5 breaths
Standing crescent (left and right) to standing backbend	53	1 min each; 3 times
Fold forward into plank to low push-up to upward dog	147, 150, 163	Repeat for 1 min
Downward dog	160	1 min
*While in downward dog, take right arm under you to grab outside of left leg and twist		1 min
Downward dog	160	1 min
Three-legged dog (alternate leg kicks)	94	2 min
As a continuous motion, go into standing split (right leg up) then tuck right knee behind left knee and lower as low as you can with left foot flat before extending back to standing split	88	1 min
Come to seated and into cow face pose with left leg on top	119	3 min
Cat and cow	173	1 min

(continued)

Yoga Sequence for Golf *(continued)*

POSE	PAGE	TIME/REPS
Puppy pose	158	1 min
Thread the needle	174	1 min each way; 2 times
Downward dog	160	1 min
Repeat on other side from * for 1-3 times each side		
Standing forward bend	54	1 min
Toe balance	60	1 min
Toe balance to standing	60	10 times
Squat	79	2 min
Rock and roll	130	1 min
Bridge	136	1 min
Happy baby	143	1 min
Heavy legs	140	3 min
Hip flexor opener	189	2-4 min
Supported fish	185	3-5 min

RACKET SPORTS

The racket athlete needs to display great agility, ankle strength and stability, and superior spinal rotation for powerful serves and returns. In addition, a quick mind favors success on the court. Your ability to maintain a strong grip, strong forearms, open wrists for power, and lightness on your feet will ultimately increase your success and longevity in the sport.

COMMON INJURIES IN RACKET SPORTS

Achilles tendonitis; wrist strains, sprains, and breaks; ankle instability; tightness in the legs; back problems; lack of rotation in the spine and neck; knee problems; groin pulls; hamstring injuries; knee injuries; elbow issues

YOGA POSES CLOSELY RELATED TO MOVEMENTS IN RACKET SPORTS

Camel (pg. 117)

This pose opens the hip flexors and increases back extension to decrease shoulder strain.

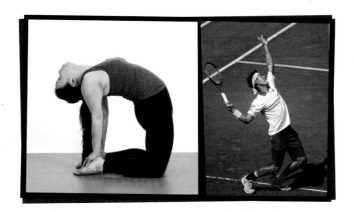

Wheel of Life (pg. 181)

This pose prepares the spine for great torque, increases power, and stretches the side of the body and neck for better reach and ability to track the ball.

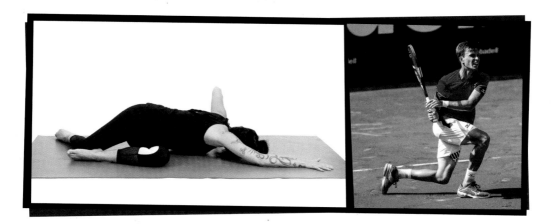

Warrior 2 (pg. 84)

This pose prepares the legs for a strong, powerful stride. Also, warrior 2 develops the wide wing-span needed for great returns.

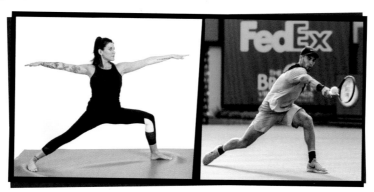

Lunge Twist (pg. 98)

This pose is great for balance, flexibility, and overall strength, enabling a player to reach for a return and recover in time for the next play.

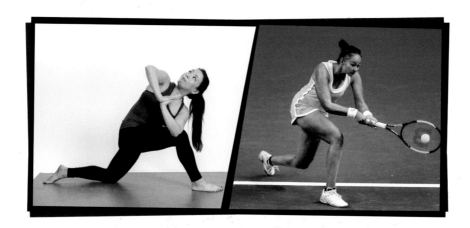

TOP FIVE YOGA POSES FOR RACKET SPORTS

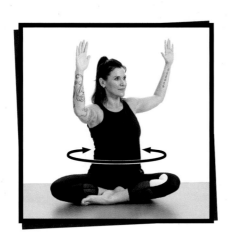

1. Seated Spinal Twist (pg. 128)

This is the best yoga pose to do for warming up your spine and synchronizing your breath with your movement. It is important to do this before the match, because racket sports require great range of motion in the spine in all directions, especially rotation. It gives you a good opportunity to see which side may be restricted for you on any given day and then to open your body accordingly. Do this movement for one to three minutes.

2. Easy Cross-Legged Pose with Arm-Ups (pg. 103)

This, too, is a great pregame warm-up. Arm-ups will completely warm up the shoulder joint. This is important for any racket sport to decrease injury, increase flexibility, and therefore increase power on the court. Do this for two minutes.

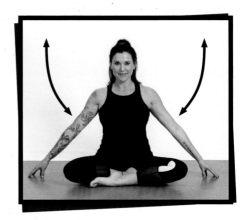

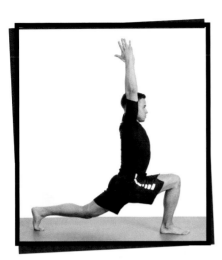

3. Crescent Lunge (pg. 69)

Lunges are imperative for racket sports because a lunge position is a common movement in the sport. There is not a minute when the athlete is not lunging. This makes it very important to keep your body open and receptive to this position so you do not pull muscles or get extremely sore afterward. This pose opens the hip flexors, quadriceps, ankles, and calves as well as stretches the torso. The forward rock variations open the bottoms of the feet, the bottoms of the toes, and the Achilles tendons and calves, giving you greater power to push off and increase quickness. Do this pose one minute on each side.

4. Supported Fish (pg. 185)

This is a great passive stretch to increase back extension and power. Do this pose for five minutes.

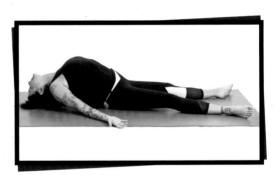

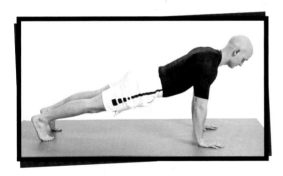

5. Plank (pg. 147)

This pose simultaneously strengthens the core and the legs, stretches the ankles and plantar fascia, and opens the wrists. Increasing wrist integrity is important for power and for protecting the wrist from injury if you fall. Do this pose twice for one minute each time.

YOGA SEQUENCE FOR RACKET SPORTS

POSE	PAGE	TIME/REPS
Perform typical warm-up before you begin		
Easy cross-legged pose with arm-ups	103	2 min
Rock and roll	130	1 min
Standing forward bend	54	1 min
Chair to standing forward bend and back to chair	58, 54, 58	10 sec each pose; 5 times
Chair twist (right and left)	60	10 sec each pose; 5 times
Standing crescent	53	1 min each side
Standing backbend	53	1 min
Standing forward bend	54	1 min
Plank to side plank to plank	147, 152, 147	10 sec per pose; 5 times each side
Lower to belly into cobra push-ups	164	2 min
Puppy pose	158	30 sec
Camel	117	30 sec
Forearm plank to forearm side plank	148, 154	10 sec each pose; 5 times each side
Dolphin	162	1 min
Dolphin push-ups	162	1 min
Puppy pose	158	30 sec
Downward dog to upward dog (toes tucked)	160, 163	1 min
Child's pose	176	30 sec
Repeat 1-3 times		
Hero's pose	113	2 min
Hero's pose with toes tucked	115	2 min
Seated forward bend	108	4 min
Seated straddle forward bend	109	4 min
Lying spinal twist	126	3 min each side
Face-up shoulder stretch	134	3 min each side
Supported fish	185	5 min

SKIING

Skiers need great endurance, superior breath work, and control to conquer often-unfavorable weather conditions. Critical to a skier's success is achieving great knee stability, strong and supple hips, a strong back, and a strong core. The maneuvers that skiers make demand constant fluctuations to conform to unstable surfaces. A next-level skier must also focus on mental toughness and breath to conquer the most intimidating runs.

COMMON INJURIES FOR SKIERS

ACL and knee problems, low back strain and tightness, quad pulls, tight hamstrings and hips, ankle and Achilles injuries, foot cramping, neck tightness

YOGA POSES CLOSELY RELATED TO MOVEMENTS IN SKIING

Chair Twist (pg. 60)

This pose mimics the common positions in skiing and helps prepare your legs and back to make subtle lateral moves.

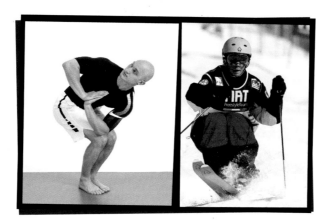

Chair (pg. 58)

This pose mimics the needs of a skier and enhances leg strength and spinal flexibility.

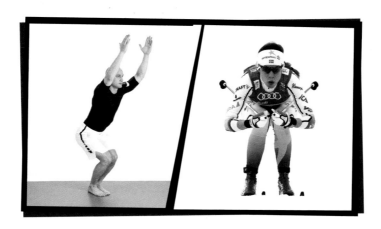

Warrior 2 (pg. 84)

This pose is great for leg strength and core stability, two important factors in a skier's success.

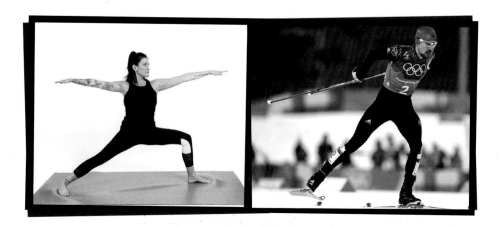

Half Side Squat (pg. 96)

This pose is great for leg and inner-thigh flexibility, and it helps protect the knee.

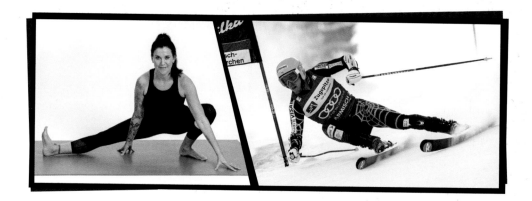

TOP FIVE YOGA POSES FOR SKIING

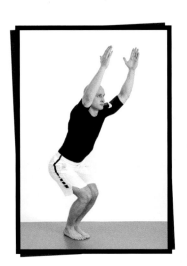

1. Chair (pg. 58)

This pose (and chair twist) simulates the skiing position, strengthening the legs and back as well as the inner thighs. It also applies a challenging stretch to the Achilles tendon. Adding a twist gives a skier a much-needed release of built-up tension in the back. Hold for one minute.

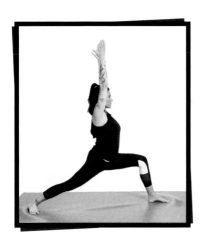

2. Warrior 1 (pg. 82)

This pose builds overall leg strength and flexibility while adding core strength. Warrior 1 is a great pose to hold for a minute to challenge the skier to build stamina as well.

3. Triangle (pg. 61)

Skiers need flexible legs, and triangle is a nice way to open the groin and the inner thigh and at the same time to build strength. Hold this pose on each side for one minute.

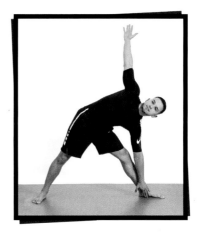

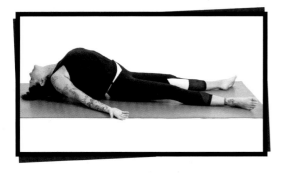

4. Supported Fish (pg. 185)

Most of the time, the forward motion of the skier can cause tension to build in the back. Supported fish is phenomenal for counterbalancing this motion. It also opens the chest and anterior spine as well as the front of the shoulder and neck. It is also a great way to release and open the hip flexor muscles. These muscles are constantly contracted while skiing, and they are often overworked and abused. Hold this pose for five minutes.

5. Plank with Wrist Openers (pg. 147, 156)

A multitasking pose for skiers, plank not only builds crucial core strength, it also builds strong arms and breeds nice, open wrists and forearms for a more relaxed grip on the ski poles. Adding wrist turns steps the stretching up a notch and commands the abs to work harder. Do this pose for two minutes, turning the wrists one at a time every 30 seconds.

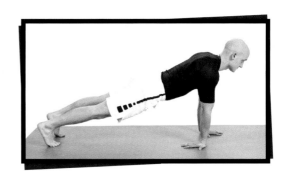

YOGA SEQUENCE FOR SKIING

POSE	PAGE	TIME/REPS
Perform typical warm-up before you begin		
Rock and roll	130	1 min
Cat and cow	173	1 min
Standing forward bend to chair and back to standing forward bend	54, 58, 54	10 sec each pose; 5 times
Chair to chair twist (left and right) and back to chair	58, 60, 58	10 sec each pose; 3 times
Standing forward bend	54	1 min
Standing split (alternate leg kicks)	88	1 min
Jump back to plank	147	30 sec
Low push-up to upward dog to downward dog	150, 163, 160	5 times
Lower to knees to seated position and into boat pose	111	1 min
Boat (progression 3)	111	1 min
Inverted plank to seated, inverted plank to seated	138	Repeat for 1 min
Hero's pose	113	2 min
*Pigeon (right leg)	178	5 min
Seated spinal twist	128	1 min
One-leg seated forward bend	109	3 min
Double pigeon	179	3 min
Cow face pose	119	3 min
Repeat on other side from * and repeat full routine one to three times		

SWIMMING

Swimmers need great range of motion in the shoulders, exaggerated symmetry to stay in their lanes effortlessly, flexible ankles to propel them forward, power in the legs, great neck rotations, and superior breath control.

COMMON INJURIES IN SWIMMING

Shoulder problems, back tightness, abdominal strains, neck tightness, chest and back strain

YOGA POSES CLOSELY RELATED TO MOVEMENTS IN SWIMMING

Wheel of Life (pg. 181)

This pose opens the spine, chest, shoulder, and neck for effortless strokes.

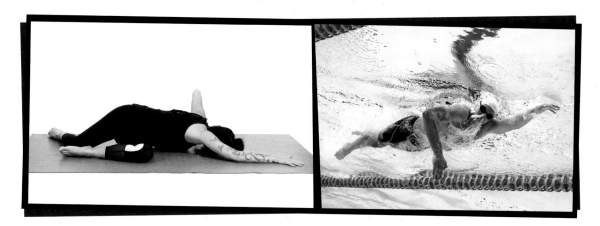

Face-Down Shoulder Stretch (pg. 169)

This pose prepares the shoulder joint and chest for great overall range of motion.

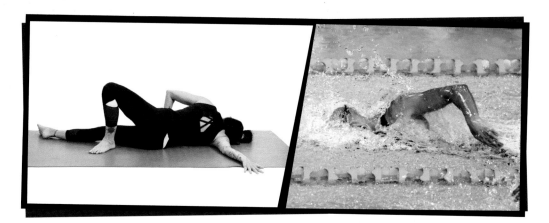

Swimming

Inverted Plank (pg. 138)

This pose opens the chest and shoulders for better range of motion and the wrists for more power.

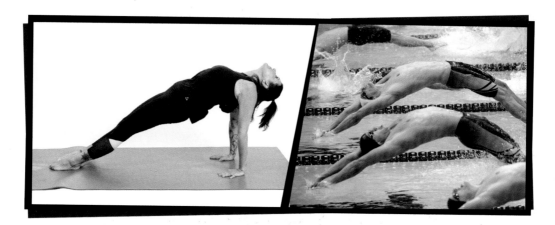

Extended Side Angle (pg. 66)

This pose is great for flexibility in the sides of the body and shoulders and helps strengthen the legs.

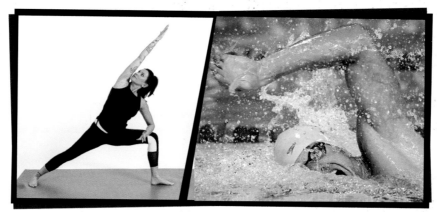

Standing Forward Bend (pg. 54)

This pose is great for leg flexibility to increase kicking power.

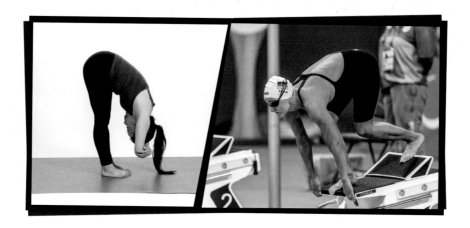

TOP FIVE YOGA POSES FOR SWIMMING

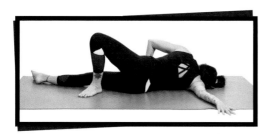

1. Face-Down Shoulder Stretch (pg. 169)

This pose enhances the range of motion not only in the shoulders but also in the chest. This will increase power against the water's resistance. Do this pose for five minutes on each side.

2. Supported Fish (pg. 185)

This pose counterbalances the forward contraction of the chest in strokes like the breaststroke and the freestyle. This pose opens the back, neck, spine, and chest. Supported fish also helps increase lung capacity, which is of great concern for swimming. Hold this pose for five minutes.

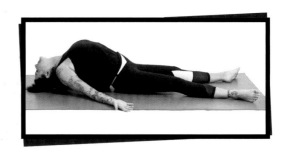

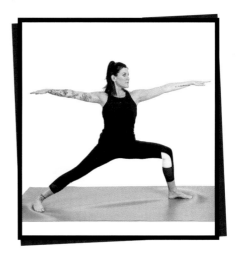

3. Pigeon (pg. 178)

Although range of motion in the lower body is not a critical focus in swimming, the power of the legs can make or break a champion. Opening hips and quads will maximize the power needed against the resistance of the water. Do this pose for two minutes on each side.

4. Warrior 2 with Arm Circles (pg. 84)

Holding warrior 2 opens the groin and inner thighs and strengthens the legs and hips; lowering into a right angle variation and circling the arms simulates the motions used in swimming, prepping the shoulders for a great race. Do this variation for two minutes on each side.

Swimming

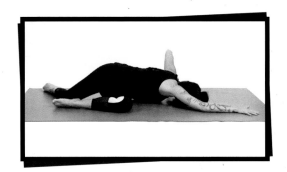

5. Wheel of Life (pg. 181)

This pose is a great way to open the spine all the way up to the neck while being fully supported by the floor and able to sink in. This pose is unique in that it enables you to stretch the neck and achieve full rotation, chin over shoulder. This will facilitate turning the head to the side to inhale in the crawl stroke. Not many poses allow you to open the neck without effort as this pose does. It opens the spine, which can help reduce the effort needed to make flip turns off the pool wall. Do this for four minutes on each side.

YOGA SEQUENCE FOR SWIMMING

POSE	PAGE	TIME/REPS
Perform typical warm-up before you begin		
Easy cross-legged pose with arm-ups	103	2 min
Hold arms directly out front of shoulders with hard flex in wrists		1 min
Repeat easy cross-legged pose with arm-ups and wrist flex for total of 3 times		
Cat and cow	173	2 min
Rock and roll	130	1 min
Standing forward bend	54	1 min
Remain in standing forward bend and interlace fingers, resting them at base of skull for neck traction		1 min
Remain in standing forward bend and interlace fingers at low back, bringing arms up		1 min
Lower to plank with wrist openers	147, 156	Change wrist position every 30 sec for 2 min
Low push-up to upward dog to downward dog	150, 163, 160	1 time
*Step right foot forward into warrior 1	82	30 sec
Remain in warrior 1 and circle arms (backstroke and front stroke)	82	1 min each way
Warrior 2	84	30 sec
Reverse warrior	85	30 sec
Warrior 2	84	30 sec
Remain in warrior 2 and interlace fingers behind neck, moving elbows together and out	84	1 min
Extended side angle	66	1 min
Front stroke left arm in extended side angle	66	1 min

POSE	PAGE	TIME/REPS
Backstroke left arm in extended side angle	66	1 min
Plank to low push-up to upward dog to downward dog	147, 150, 163, 160	1 time
Hero's pose with toes tucked	115	2 min
Hero's pose	113	2 min
Repeat on other side from * for 1-3 times each side		
Easy cross-legged pose with cow face arms	102, 119	2 min each side
Face-down shoulder stretch (arm straight and 90 degrees)	169	3 min each pose, each side
Face-up shoulder stretch	134	3 min each side
Puppy pose	158	1 min
Child's pose	176	1 min
Wheel of life	181	4 min each side

RUNNING

Runners need incredible discipline and mind control, better-than-average breath control, open and flexible hamstrings, supple quads and hip flexors, flexible ankles and feet with open toes, and back extension to protect posture.

COMMON INJURIES IN RUNNING

Pulled hamstrings, strained quads, torn Achilles tendons, shoulder tightness and fatigue, plantar fasciitis, low back problems and strains

YOGA POSES CLOSELY RELATED TO MOVEMENTS IN RUNNING

Hero's Pose with Toes Tucked (pg. 115)

This pose relieves many foot issues associated with running, such as cramps, plantar fascia issues, and Achilles tendon aches. This pose also enables increased power to push off.

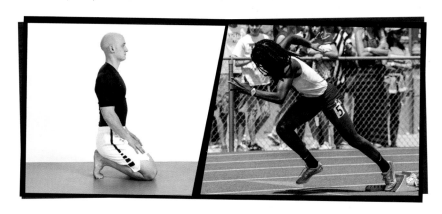

Crescent Lunge (pg. 69)

This pose opens the stride and strengthens the legs. Crescent lunge also strengthens the back and stretches the hip flexors.

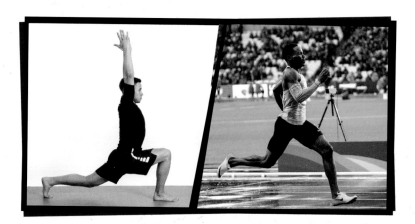

TOP FIVE YOGA POSES FOR RUNNING

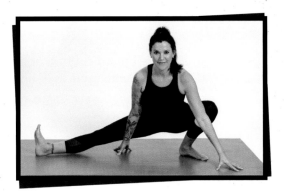

1. Half Side Squat (pg. 96)

Runners should get in the habit of doing this pose to open the inner thigh and groin deeply; it will also stretch the Achilles tendons, calves, and deep hips. This is important for healthy long-term running before and after taking to the street. Do each side for 30 seconds three times.

2. Standing Forward Bend Against a Wall (pg. 56)

Most people will perform standing forward bend seated. It has been my experience that this is frustrating to athletes, and they make little progress over years of trying because they are doing it wrong and overstretching their backs. Stretching the hamstrings is very important to runners; folding over and leaning your back against the wall to open the hamstrings is very deep, and you will get results faster when you do this regularly and for a three- to five-minute hold.

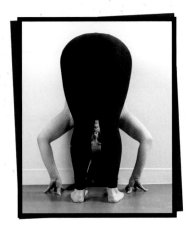

3. Hero's Pose (pg. 113)

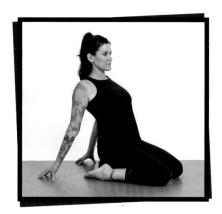

Hero's pose (toes tucked and untucked) keeps a nice flexion in the knees while also stretching the quadriceps. By keeping the toes untucked first and holding for two to three minutes, you are stretching deep into the shin, which is otherwise hard to access, and you are opening the top of the foot to increase range of motion in the ankle for greater quickness and power to push off. Doing the toes-tucked version opens the Achilles tendon and plantar fascia (bottom of the foot, arch area) as well as the bottoms of the toes; the combined effect of this is to increase the ankle's range of motion and to make for smoother and easier running. Do each version for two minutes.

4. Pigeon with Quad Variation (pg. 179)

Pigeon pose is a beloved position for runners because it releases the hips and glutes and relieves sciatic pain. Bending the back leg to add a quad stretch to the position opens the quads and deep hip flexors to enhance range of motion. All of this together will also help to alleviate stress on the back. Any time you keep the hips open and supple, you minimize stress and strain on the knees. Hold for five minutes on each side.

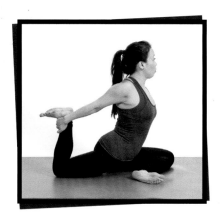

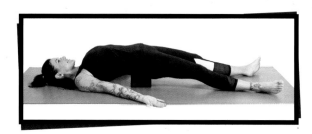

5. Hip Flexor Opener (pg. 189)

This stretch releases the deepest hip flexors to increase the range of motion in the hips and to minimize strain and excess pull on the low back and hamstrings that can plague runners every day. Hold this pose for five minutes.

YOGA SEQUENCE FOR RUNNING

POSE	PAGE	TIME/REPS
Perform typical warm-up before you begin		
Rock and roll	130	1 min
Standing forward bend	54	1 min
Squat	79	1 min
Standing forward bend	54	1 min
Squat	79	1 min

(continued)

Yoga Sequence for Running *(continued)*

POSE	PAGE	TIME/REPS
Lower to plank	147	1 min
Low push-up to upward dog to downward dog	150, 163, 160	1 min
In downward dog, raise high on toes and lower heels	160	10 times
*Step right foot forward into warrior 1	82	30 sec
Warrior 2	84	30 sec
Triangle	61	30 sec
Pyramid pose	64	30 sec
Turn left into straddle forward bend to halfway up with flat back	75	5 times
Stand up and windmill arms forward and lower into plank pose 147		
Lower into plank to side plank (right) to side plank (left)	147, 152	30 sec each pose; repeat 3 times
Plank to low push-up to upward dog to downward dog	147, 150, 163, 160	1 min
Repeat on other side from * for 1-3 times each side		
**Step right foot forward into warrior 2	84	30 sec
Triangle to pyramid pose	61, 64	30 sec each pose; 3 times
Right angle pose	67	30 sec
Half moon	68	30 sec
Standing split with right foot down and left leg up	88	30 sec
Standing forward bend	54	30 sec
Plank to side plank (heels to right; left arm and leg up)	147, 152	30 sec each pose; 1 time
Remain in side plank, bend left knee and place it in front of right knee while pushing down in foot and lifting hips for IT band stretch	152	30 sec
Plank to low push-up to upward dog to downward dog	147, 150, 163, 160	1 time
Repeat on other side from **		
Seated forward bend	54	4 min
Seated straddle forward bend	109	4 min
Seated spinal twist to cow face pose	128, 119	2 min each pose, each way
Seated cat and cow	173	1 min
Puppy pose	158	1 min
Pigeon with quad variation (left)	179	2 min each pose
Wheel of life (left)	181	3 min
Pigeon with quad variation (right)	179	2 min each pose
Wheel of life (right)	181	3 min
Hero's pose with toes tucked	115	2 min
Frog	183	5 min

CYCLING

Cyclists have great imbalances in the anterior and posterior spine. They need to improve back extension; open hip flexors; develop strong, flexible ankles; and have open chests for maximum lung capacity. They also need great aerobic ability, a strong core, and great focus to track their routes in the longest of races.

COMMON INJURIES IN CYCLING

Wrist injury, forearm tightness, hip flexor strain, low back pain, shoulder and chest problems

YOGA POSES CLOSELY RELATED TO MOVEMENTS IN CYCLING

Eagle Pose (pg. 76)

This pose is great for overall flexibility because of the intricacy of executing the pose, and it improves balance by challenging the body on one leg.

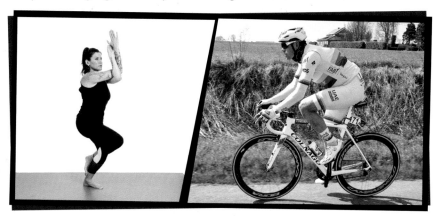

Chair (pg. 58)

This pose is great for leg strength and back strength. Cyclists hold their backs in compromising positions for long periods of time, so back strength is important.

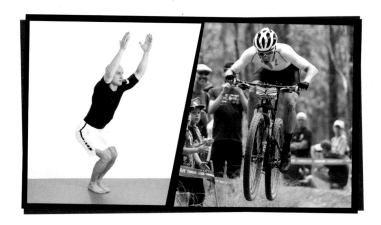

Pyramid (pg. 64)

This pose is great for leg and hamstring flexibility to improve cyclists' power on grueling rides, especially with power demands on hill work.

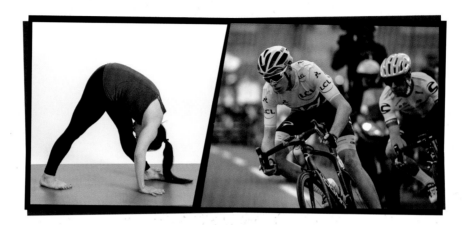

Standing Forward Bend (pg. 54)

This pose is great for leg flexibility and neck traction. Caring for the neck is often overlooked; cyclists put great demands on their extended necks, so they need to pay equal attention to flexibility, strength, and rotation.

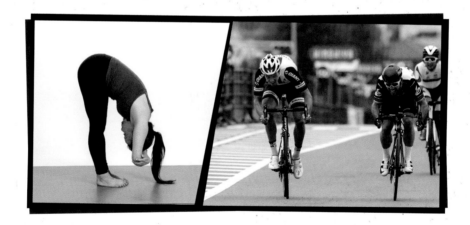

TOP FIVE YOGA POSES FOR CYCLISTS

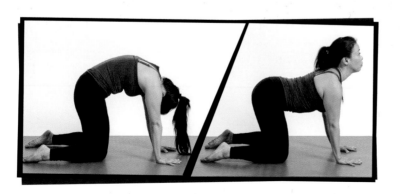

1. Cat and Cow (pg. 173)

This yoga move opens the spine, the ribs, the lungs, and the neck and truly warms you up from the inside out. The posture you hold on the bike will overstretch the back and weaken the abdominals, but this move evens you out and gets the breath going like no other. You will instantly counteract the slumped posture. Do this pose for two minutes.

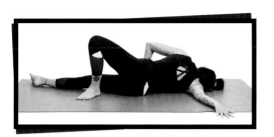

2. Face-Down Shoulder Stretch (pg. 169)

This stretch opens the anterior deltoid, or front of the shoulder, so you do not destroy your posture when you are off the bike. Hold this pose for two to three minutes on each side and watch the chest release and relax.

3. Bow Pose (pg. 165)

Bow pose is important for opening the hip flexors and quads. It also does double duty because it opens the anterior spine, which tightens up from bike riding, and it stretches the chest as well. If you had to pick one to do every day, it would be this one. Hold for 10 breaths four times.

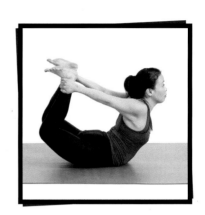

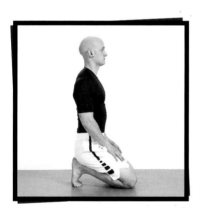

4. Hero's Pose with Toes Tucked (pg. 115)

Hero's pose with toes tucked will help elongate the Achilles tendons, stretch the bottoms of the feet and toes, and stretch the calves, too. It may not be enjoyable at first, but with time and attention, you will understand its importance. Do the same pose with the toes untucked to open the shins and the tops of the ankles. This will produce an overall open, supple, flexible, powerful ankle. Hold each variation for two minutes.

5. Heavy Legs Pose (pg. 140)

This may become your favorite pose if you ever have long training days that leave you sluggish and exhausted with legs that feel like cement. Doing this pose before or after a ride will lighten the legs back up and quicken your pace again. An added bonus is that your hamstrings get a light stretch, too. Hold it for two minutes.

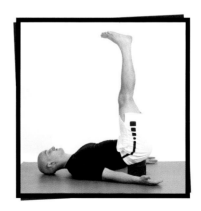

Cycling

YOGA SEQUENCE FOR CYCLING

POSE	PAGE	TIME/REPS
Perform typical warm-up before you begin		
Easy cross-legged pose with arm-ups	103	2 min
Rock and roll	130	1 min
Standing forward bend	54	1 min
Plank with wrist openers	147, 156	30 sec each wrist position; 2 min
Low push-up to upward dog to downward dog	150, 163, 160	1 min
*Step right foot forward into crescent lunge	69	1 min
Remain in crescent lunge and interlace fingers behind low back and dive forward so right ear is next to inner right lower leg	69	1 min
Remain in crescent lunge and stand upright with fingers still interlaced behind low back, then lower back down	69	5 times
Turn left into standing straddle with fingers still interlaced behind low back		1 min
From standing straddle, stand up, and then lower back down, keeping fingers interlaced behind low back		3 times
Step to front of mat into chair and then standing forward bend, keeping fingers interlaced behind low back	58	3 times
Release arms and lower into standing forward bend	54	1 min
Plank to low push-up and then to belly	147, 150	1 time
Bow pose to side bow	165, 166	30 sec each pose; 3 times
Downward dog and jump into squat	160, 79	1 min
Squat to standing	79	10 times
Repeat on other side from * for 1-3 times each side		
Standing forward bend	54	30 sec
Rock and roll	130	30 sec
Plow	132	2 min
Shoulder stand	192	2 min
Pigeon	178	3 min
Double pigeon	179	3 min
Face-down shoulder stretch	169	3 min
Repeat on other side from pigeon		
Hero's pose with toes tucked	115	2 min
Hero's pose	113	2 min
Hip flexor opener	189	4 min
Supported fish	185	4 min

MIXED MARTIAL ARTS

Mixed martial arts (MMA) fighters need to have quick bursts of energy, very flexible legs and hips, and strong and supple ankles. They also need to have full range of motion in the shoulder joints and neck and equal strength on both sides.

COMMON INJURIES IN MMA

Hamstring pulls, hip issues, back strains, neck injuries, shoulder instability

YOGA POSES CLOSELY RELATED TO MOVEMENTS IN MMA

Warrior 2 (pg. 84)

This pose helps with lunging and stretching movements to create powerful kicks during competition.

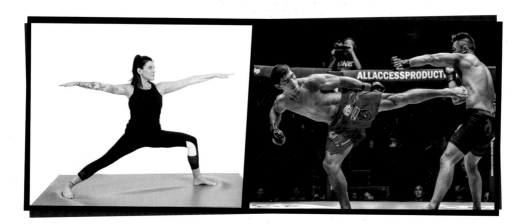

Camel (pg. 117)

This pose prepares the back for overextension, which is a common movement when trying to avoid a punch or kick or absorbing a landed punch or kick.

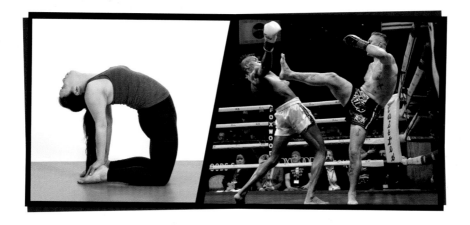

Bridge (pg. 136)

This pose prepares the back for overextension and kick avoidance. In addition, the back needs to be flexible in all directions to execute dancelike moves around the ring.

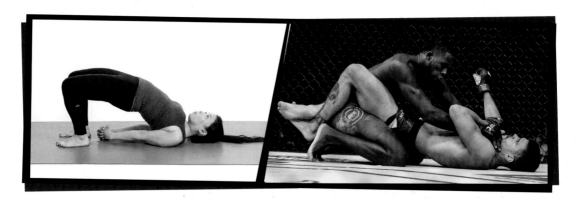

Reclining Big Toe Pose (pg. 124)

This pose opens the hamstrings to prepare for powerful kicks.

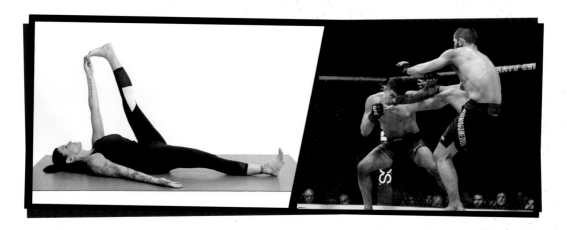

Pigeon (pg. 178)

This pose opens the glutes and hips for graceful kicking.

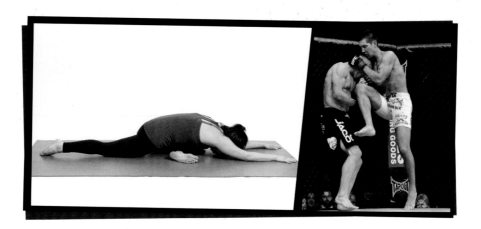

TOP FIVE POSES FOR MMA

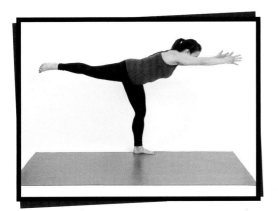

1. Warrior 3 (pg. 86)

This pose prepares the ankles to provide great stability and support. In addition, it strengthens and stretches the legs for better range of motion and power to kick. Hold this pose for one minute on each side.

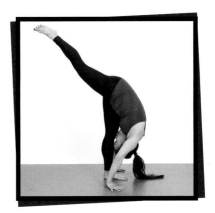

2. Standing Split (pg. 88)

This pose opens the hips and hamstrings; adding a repeated kicking motion will build power in the glutes. Hold on each side for one minute.

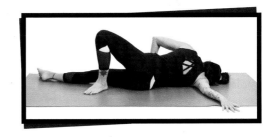

3. Half Side Squat (pg. 96)

This pose stretches the groin and inner thigh to reduce strain on the inner knee while at the same time strengthening the back and abdominals. Do each side for 30 seconds four times.

4. Face-Down Shoulder Stretch (pg. 169)

Face-down shoulder stretch increases the flexibility and range of motion in the chest and anterior shoulders, which will add power to punches and absorb impact with less injury. It will also increase spinal rotation to create an effortless spin kick move. Hold each side for five minutes.

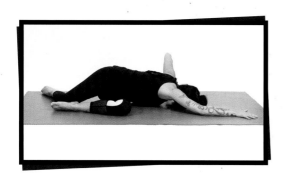

5. Wheel of Life (pg. 181)

This pose opens the lats and increases reach, deepens spinal twisting to increase lunging capacity and power, and opens the neck to be able to broaden your view. Hold on each side for five minutes.

YOGA SEQUENCE FOR MMA

POSE	PAGE	TIME/REPS
Perform typical warm-up before you begin		
Rock and roll	130	1 min
Standing forward bend	54	1 min
Squat	79	1 min
Standing forward bend to plank to low push-up to upward dog to downward dog	54, 147, 150, 163, 160	1 time
*Step right foot forward into crescent lunge	69	1 min
Remain in crescent lunge, lower left knee to the floor, then return	69	10 times
Warrior 1 to warrior 2 to warrior 3	82, 84, 86	1 min each pose
King dancer to standing extended leg	92	30 sec each pose; 3 times
Standing split kicks (left leg)	88	1 min
Standing forward bend	54	1 min
Plank to low push-up to upward dog to downward dog	147, 150, 163, 160	1 time
Repeat from * on the other side		
Standing forward bend	54	1 min
Squat	79	1 min
Half side squat	96	Alternate sides 4 times
Frog	183	1 min
Downward dog	160	1 min
Face-down shoulder stretch	169	3 min each side
Face-up shoulder stretch	134	2 min each side
Diaphragmatic breathing		2 min

9

Ready-to-Use Yoga Sequences

The yoga sequences provided here are meant to inspire you as a Power Yoga for Sports teacher. You can use them as written, or you can take parts of different routines and combine them. The suggested times to hold the poses and the number of reps should be adjusted as appropriate. The number one rule is that the routine should be created for the athlete you are working with; it should not be guided simply by what is easy to remember or by what you personally like to do.

Should I memorize a routine before I teach it?

First, I am adamant that my teachers never use a cheat sheet because it diminishes your credibility and you will lose your athletes' trust. Second, you should have an idea to whom you are directing your teachings before you go in so you are most effective. However, you do not always have this information ahead of time. Being a PYFS teacher who is well-studied in yoga, the needs of athletes, and, most of all, the game they play and the demands it puts on their body is ideal.

Your Typical Warm-Up

As discussed in chapter 4, it is important to get your athletes used to warming up before going deep into their yoga poses. The following warm-up will prepare the muscles and joints for yoga and will give you insight into your athletes' imbalances, so you can design a better class for the day. Many of the typical warm-up postures can double as assessment poses, which will make your class very efficient.

(continued)

Your Typical Warm-Up *(continued)*

POSE		TIME
Easy cross-legged twist with goalpost arms		2 min
Opposite arm opposite leg reach		2 min
Knees into chest and roll ankles		1 min
Lying spinal twist with block between knees		2 min
Reclining cobbler's pose with feet close to body		2 min
Reclining cobbler's pose with feet away from body		2 min

ARM AND SHOULDER YOGA SEQUENCES

While the following sequences develop strength and flexibility in the arms and shoulders, know that the entire body, mind, and breath are in cohesive union throughout. Strong, flexible arms help support the vulnerable shoulder joint, protect the back and neck, and enhance strong arm movements.

ARMS AND SHOULDERS SEQUENCE 1

POSE	PAGE	TIME/REPS
Perform typical warm-up before you begin		
Low push-up to upward dog to downward dog	150, 163, 160	1 time
*Step right foot forward and bring left knee down into crescent lunge	69	1 min
Crescent lunge twist with goalpost arms	71	1 min
Remain in crescent lunge, bring arms straight up, then to heart center and into crescent lunge twist	69, 71	1 min
Remain in crescent lunge, bring arms back up, and backstroke both arms in big circles	69	1 min
Remain in crescent lunge, interlace fingers behind low back, and slide hands down back of left thigh	69	30 sec

POSE	PAGE	TIME/REPS
Remain in crescent lunge, keep fingers interlaced behind low back, and dive forward so right ear is near right ankle, bringing interlaced arms up to sky	69	30 sec
Remain in crescent lunge, come back up, release and bring arms up and then to heart center and twist right	69	1 min
Repeat from * for total of 3 times		
Remain in crescent lunge and bring chest and belly to right thigh, reaching hands to front of room	69	3 breaths
From crescent lunge, move into warrior 3	86	1 min
Standing split (left leg up)	88	30 sec
Return to warrior 3	86	1 min
Return to crescent lunge and repeat from * for total of 3 times each side		
Warrior 3 into standing split with right leg forward and left leg up	86	1 min
Lift left leg up into handstand		As long as possible
Standing forward bend	54	1 min
Squat	79	1 min
Squat to standing	79	10 times
Bring left foot up into tree	90	30 sec
Bring left foot into half lotus tree	91	30 sec
Half lotus tree in single-leg chair	58	30 sec
Release and lower into low push-up to upward dog to downward dog	150, 163, 160	1 time
Bring left foot forward into crescent lunge and repeat from beginning on other side for 2-4 times		
Cow face pose	119	3 min each side
Face-down shoulder stretch	169	3 min each side
Banana pose	188	2 min each way

ARMS AND SHOULDERS SEQUENCE 2

POSE	PAGE	TIME/REPS
Perform typical warm-up before you begin		
Roll into downward dog	160	1 min
Step right foot forward into crescent lunge with arms up	69	30 sec
Remain in crescent lunge and straighten legs while bringing arms down	69	30 sec
Lower back into crescent lunge and bring arms straight out to sides	69	30 sec

(continued)

Arms and Shoulders Sequence 2 *(continued)*

POSE	PAGE	TIME/REPS
Lower into low push-up and then onto belly into cobra push-up	150, 164	30 sec
Downward dog	160	1 min
Repeat sequence from beginning on other side		
*Step right foot forward into warrior 1	82	1 min
Warrior 1 with cow face arms (left arm up)	82, 119	30 sec
Warrior 2 with cow face arms	84, 119	30 sec
Warrior 1 with cow face arms	82, 119	30 sec
Warrior 2 with cow face arms	84, 119	30 sec
Square feet and fold into straddle forward bend with cow face arms	75	1 min
Lift halfway up to flat back with cow face arms	119	30 sec
Fold back down into straddle forward bend with happy cow arms	75	30 sec
Lift halfway up to flat back with cow face arms	119	30 sec
Stand up, release arms, and windmill them to front of mat, lower to plank to low push-up	147, 150	1 time
Cobra push-up	164	30 sec
Downward dog	160	1 min
Child's pose	176	1 min
Repeat on other side from *		
Plank	147	30 sec
Forearm plank	148	30 sec
Plank	147	30 sec
Forearm plank	148	30 sec
Plank	147	30 sec
Side plank (right)	152	30 sec
Plank	147	30 sec
Side plank (left)	152	30 sec
Forearm plank	148	30 sec
Dolphin	162	30 sec
Dolphin push-ups	162	30 sec
Face-down shoulder stretch	169	3 min each side
Roll over onto back and into lying spinal twist	126	3 min each side
Face-up shoulder stretch	134	3 min each side
Corpse	187	30 sec

ARMS AND SHOULDERS SEQUENCE 3

POSE	PAGE	TIME/REPS
Perform typical warm-up before you begin		
Easy cross-legged pose with arm-ups	103	2 min
Rock and roll	130	30 sec
**Standing forward bend	54	1 min
Squat	79	1 min
Standing forward bend	54	1 min
Squat	79	1 min
Roll up to standing and into eagle pose (right leg over left) with arms out like you're holding a tightrope and pulse	76	1 min
Eagle	76	1 min
Unwrap right leg into warrior 1, keeping arms in eagle	82, 76	1 min
Remain in warrior 1 and fold forward, bringing ear to knee and keeping arms in eagle	82, 76	30 sec
Remain in warrior 1, and lift up into backbend and fold back down, keeping arms in eagle	82, 76	3 times
Unwind arms into warrior 1	82	30 sec
Square feet into straddling forward bend with fingers interlaced behind low back	74	1 min
Stand up into warrior 1, keeping fingers interlaced behind low back	82	1 min
*Remain in warrior 1, and slide hands down back of right leg	82	30 sec
Remain in warrior 1, bend forward, bringing arms up and over	82	30 sec
Repeat from * for total of 3 times; after last time, stand up into warrior 1 and bring hands down to floor and press back to plank	82	
Chaturanga (low plank) to upward dog to downward dog	150, 163, 160	3 times
Jump forward into standing forward bend	54	1 min
Roll up and into standing backbend	53	30 sec
**Repeat on the other side from **		

ARMS AND SHOULDERS SEQUENCE 4

POSE	PAGE	TIME/REPS
Perform typical warm-up before you begin		
Rock and roll	130	30 sec
Standing forward bend	54	30 sec
Plank to low push-up to upward dog to downward dog	147, 150, 163, 160	30 sec

(continued)

Arms and Shoulders Sequence 4 *(continued)*

POSE	PAGE	TIME/REPS
Upward dog to downward dog	163, 160	21 times
Jump forward into standing forward bend	54	30 sec
Standing crescent	53	30 sec each side; 3 times
Come to center and fold into standing forward bend	54	30 sec
Rock and roll	130	30 sec
Standing forward bend	54	30 sec
Chair to standing forward bend	58, 54	30 sec each; 3 times
Return to chair and interlace fingers behind back	58	30 sec
Release arms and fold into standing forward bend	54	30 sec
Rock and roll	130	30 sec
Stand up into chair and then into chair twist	58, 60	30 sec each; 3 times
Rock and rol	130	30 sec
Face-up shoulder stretch	134	3 min each side
Rock and roll	130	30 sec
Standing forward bend	54	30 sec
Chair twist	60	30 sec each side; 3 times
Rock and roll	130	30 sec
Downward dog	160	2 min
One-arm downward dog	161	30 sec each; 2 times
Step forward into standing forward bend	54	30 sec
Chair twist	60	30 sec each side; 3 times
Rock and roll	130	30 sec
Plank to forearm plank	147, 148	30 sec each; 4 times
Plank with wrist openers	147, 156	30 sec each wrist position; 3 times
Downward dog	160	2 min
Step forward into standing forward bend	54	1 min
Chair with fingers interlaced behind low back	58	1 min
Chair fold into standing forward bend with fingers interlaced behind low back	58, 54	30 sec
Repeat chair and chair and fold for total of 3 times		
Rock and roll	130	30 sec
Plow	132	2 min
Roll out slowly and into rock and roll	130	30 sec
Standing forward bend	54	30 sec

POSE	PAGE	TIME/REPS
Rock and roll	130	30 sec
Come onto hands and knees into cat and cow	173	5 breaths each; 5 times
Repeat from beginning for 1-3 times		
Wheel of life	181	5 min each side

ARMS AND SHOULDERS SEQUENCE 5

POSE	PAGE	TIME/REPS
Perform typical warm-up before you begin		
Rock and roll	130	15 times
Stand up into standing backbend	53	30 sec
Standing forward bend	54	30 sec
*Remain in standing forward bend, interlace fingers behind lower back, and bring arms up and over	54	30 sec
Release arms into chair	58	30 sec
Standing forward bend	54	3 breaths
Low push-up to upward dog to downward dog	150, 163, 160	30 sec
Standing forward bend	54	30 sec
Repeat from beginning for total of 3 times		
Bring hands to floor, and step right leg back into crescent lunge	69	30 sec
Remain in crescent lunge and twist left	69	30 sec
Remain in crescent lunge, and return hands to floor inside left leg	69	30 sec
Plank to low push-up to upward dog to downward dog	147, 150, 163, 160	1 time
Step right leg forward into crescent lunge	69	30 sec
Remain in crescent lunge and twist right	69	30 sec
Bring hands to floor and step forward into standing forward bend	54	30 sec
Repeat from * 1-3 times; after last time, go to standing mountain pose	**52**	
Jump back to plank and into downward dog	147, 160	1 min
**Step right foot forward outside of right hand		30 sec
Lower to plank, then step left foot forward outside of left hand	147	30 sec
Repeat step with right foot, plank, and step with left foot for total of 3 times		
Step right foot forward outside of right hand and reach right arm to twist open		30 sec
Bring right arm behind back and roll right shoulder forward and backward		30 sec
Circle right arm around to floor inside of right foot and open to right angle	67	30 sec

(continued)

Arms and Shoulders Sequence 5 *(continued)*

POSE	PAGE	TIME/REPS
Bring left arm behind back, tuck left arm in on right thigh, and roll left shoulder (forward and backward)		30 sec each way; 3 times
Lower into plank	147	30 sec
Downward dog	160	30 sec
Repeat on other side from ** and hold last downward dog for 1 min		
***Step right foot forward between hands and pivot left into straddle forward bend	74	1 min
Roll to standing, bringing arms behind the back where opposite hand touches opposite elbow and into standing backbend	53	30 sec
Fold forward into standing forward bend, keeping arms behind back	54	30 sec
Lift halfway up to flat back		30 sec
Forward fold to halfway lift		3 times
Stand up and release arms to sky into standing backbend	53	30 sec
Fold halfway down into flat back with arms still extended		30 sec
Lower into standing forward bend	54	30 sec
Forward fold to halfway lift		3 times
From standing forward bend, let left arm hang down and twist to the right with right arm up to the sky	54	30 sec
Bring right arm behind back, tuck right arm in on left thigh and roll right shoulder (forward and backward)		30 sec each way
Release arm and repeat on other side from *		
Stand at front of mat into standing forward bend with cow face arms (right arm up)	54, 119	1 min
Stand up, bringing arms to sky, then to cow face arms (left arm up) and folding into standing forward bend	119, 54	1 min
Repeat from beginning for 2-4 times		

ABDOMINAL YOGA SEQUENCES

Sequences that focus on the abdominals build overall strength, balance, and stability as well as strong abdominal muscles. Athletes who would benefit from these sequences are those who need to propel their bodies in awkward positions, those who must change direction on a dime even when their momentum takes them in a different direction, and those who need spine-protecting cores of steel, such as MMA fighters and wrestlers.

ABDOMINALS SEQUENCE 1

POSE	PAGE	TIME/REPS
Perform typical warm-up before you begin		
Rock and roll	130	1 min

POSE	PAGE	TIME/REPS
Low push-up to upward dog to downward dog	150, 163, 160	1 min
***Step right foot forward into crescent lunge	69	1 min
Half side squat	96	4 times each side
Crescent lunge	69	30 sec
*Crescent lunge twist to right	71	1 min
Remain in crescent lunge twist to right and circle right arm clockwise	71	30 sec
Place right hand inside of right foot into right angle	67	1 min
Remain in right angle and circle left arm clockwise	67	30 sec
Repeat from * for total of 3 times		
Bring both hands down into lizard	71	1 min
Plank	147	1 min
Forearm plank	148	1 min
Plank	147	30 sec
Forearm plank	148	30 sec
**Drop heels to left into forearm side plank	154	1 min
Forearm side plank with hip kisses	155	30 sec
Forearm plank	148	30 sec
Repeat from ** for total of 3 times		
Dolphin	162	1 min
Dolphin push-ups	162	1 min
Downward dog	160	1 min
Repeat on other side from * then repeat from beginning for 1-3 times; after last downward dog, lower into plank**		
****From plank, drop heels (left and right)	147	3 times each way
Side plank (right)	152	30 sec
Remain in side plank and touch left elbow to left knee	152	10 times
Lower to plank and into downward dog	147, 160	30 sec
Squat	79	1 min
Standing forward bend	54	1 min
Lower into plank to low push-up to upward dog to downward dog	147, 150, 163, 160	1 min
Repeat on other side from ** 1-3 times (you can do extra round on each side, doing all planks on forearms)**		
Sphinx	171	3 min
Puppy pose	158	2 min
Bridge	136	30 sec; 3 times
Hip flexor opener	189	3 min
Supported fish	185	5 min

ABDOMINALS SEQUENCE 2

POSE	PAGE	TIME/REPS
Perform typical warm-up before you begin		
Rock and roll, and after the last roll, go into standing forward bend	130, 54	1 min
Stand up into chair	58	30 sec
Chair twist (right)	60	30 sec
Chair	58	30 sec
Chair twist (left)	60	30 sec
Chair	58	30 sec
Repeat from first chair for total of 4 times		
Standing forward bend	54	1 min
Plank	147	1 min
Forearm plank	148	1 min
Forearm side plank (right)	154	1 min
Forearm side plank with hip kiss	155	30 sec
Forearm plank	148	30 sec
Side plank (left)	152	1 min
Side plank with hip kiss	155	30 sec
Forearm plank	148	30 sec
Downward dog	160	1 min
Come to seated and into rock and roll	130	1 min
Twisted root abdominals	131	2-3 min each side
Standing forward bend	54	30 sec
Rock and roll	130	30 sec
Lying spinal twist with block between knees, and drop knees left to right	126	2 min
Inverted table	139	1 min
Lying spinal twist with block between knees, and drop knees left to right	126	2 min
Bridge	136	1 min
Come up to seated and into inverted plank	138	1 min
Rock and roll	130	30 sec
Lying spinal twist with block between knees, and drop knees left to right	126	2 min
Rock and roll	130	30 sec
Boat pose	111	1 min
Boat (progression 3)	112	1-2 min
Roll legs over onto belly and into sphinx	171	3 min

POSE	PAGE	TIME/REPS
Downward dog	160	1 min
Plow	132	2 min
Hip flexor opener	189	5 min

ABDOMINALS SEQUENCE 3

POSE	PAGE	TIME/REPS
Perform typical warm-up before you begin		
Rock and roll, and after last roll, go into standing forward bend	130, 54	1 min
*Plank	147	1 min
Plank with wrist openers	147, 156	1 min each wrist position
Remain in plank and bring right knee to right elbow, then bring left knee to left elbow	147	30 sec each; 4 times
Low push-up to upward dog to downward dog	150, 163, 160	10 times
Standing forward bend	54	1 min
Remain in standing forward bend, interlace fingers at low back, and stretch arms up	54	1 min
Release arms and roll up to standing into standing backbend	53	30 sec
Standing crescent	53	30 sec each side; 2 times
Standing backbend	53	30 sec
Standing forward bend	54	30 sec
Lower to plank to low push-up to upward dog to downward dog	147, 150, 163, 160	3 times
Step right foot forward, then turn to left into half side squat (right knee bent, left leg straight)	96	30 sec
Come back to front with one hand on each side of right foot and into standing split (left leg up)	88	1 min
Come to standing forward bend, drop hips down into rock and roll	54, 130	1 min
Bridge	136	30 sec; 3 times
Twisted root abdominals	131	2 min each side
Roll over into plank	147	1 min
Repeat from * and then repeat from beginning for 3-5 times		
Leg raises in corpse	188	3 min
Leg flutters	188	3 min
Hip flexor opener	189	5 min
Supported fish	185	5 min

ABDOMINALS SEQUENCE 4

POSE	PAGE	TIME/REPS
Perform typical warm-up before you begin		
Rock and roll	130	30 sec
Standing forward bend to plank to low push-up to upward dog to downward dog, and back to standing forward bend	54, 147, 150, 163, 160, 54	2 min
*Downward dog	160	30 sec
Step right foot forward into crescent lunge	69	30 sec
Crescent lunge twist	71	30 sec
Lower to plank and onto belly into cobra push-ups	147, 164	2 min
Return to downward dog and repeat on other side from * for total of 3 times each side		
Forearm plank	148	1 min
Remain in forearm plank and alternate knees to upper arm	148	1 min
Puppy pose	158	30 sec
Plank	147	1 min
Downward dog	160	1 min
Come to seated and into boat pose	111	1 min
Cobbler's pose	104	1 min
Seated mountain pose with arms up	106	1 min
Repeat from boat pose for total of 3 times		
Bridge	136	30 sec; 3 times
Lying spinal twist	126	3 min each side
Lying banana pose	188	3 min each side

ABDOMINALS SEQUENCE 5

POSE	PAGE	TIME/REPS
Perform typical warm-up before you begin		
Rock and roll	130	5 times
Standing forward bend	54	3 breaths
Downward dog	160	1 min
*Bring right leg up into three-legged dog	94	1 min
Step right leg forward into warrior 2	84	1 min
Reverse warrior	85	30 sec
Right angle	67	30 sec
Reverse warrior	85	30 sec

POSE	PAGE	TIME/REPS
Right angle	67	30 sec
Half moon	68	1 min
Standing split (left leg up)	88	1 min
Standing forward bend	54	1 min
Remain on toes, then stand up and back down to standing forward bend	54	1 min
Camel	117	30 sec
Boat pose	111	30 sec
Boat (progression 3)	112	30 sec
Downward dog	160	30 sec
Repeat on other side from *		
Rock and roll	130	30 sec
Bridge	136	5 breaths; 3 times
Lower to floor, lie on back, and bring knees into chest, then roll up to seated and back down		2 min
Lying spinal twist	126	3 min each side
Twisted root abdominals	131	3 min each way
Bridge lifts	137	3 min
Twisted root abdominals	131	3 min each way

GLUTE AND BACK YOGA SEQUENCES

Strong glutes and a stable back are the cornerstone of speed, power, and protection of the spine. Consider these routines for athletes who need to focus on running, twisting, and powerful jumping.

GLUTES AND BACK SEQUENCE 1

POSE	PAGE	TIME/REPS
Perform typical warm-up before you begin		
Rock and roll; after last roll, go into standing forward bend	130	1 min
Plank	147	3 breaths
Low push-up to upward dog to downward dog	150, 163, 160	1 time
*Step right foot forward into warrior 2	84	1 min
Straighten right leg into triangle	61	1 min
Right angle	67	1 min
Step forward into half moon	68	1 min

(continued)

Glutes and Back Sequence 1 *(continued)*

POSE	PAGE	TIME/REPS
Release to standing split (left leg up)	88	3 breaths
Split kicks (left leg)	89	1 min
Bend left knee behind right and crouch, then shoot left leg back to standing split	88	5 times
Standing forward bend	54	30 sec
Squat	79	1 min
Lift halfway up to flat back, bring right arm under right thigh for binding twist in squat	79	1 min
Come to standing while holding bind		10 breaths
Release, bring arms up, and then fold into standing forward bend	54	3 breaths
Low push-up to upward dog to downward dog	150, 163, 160	4 times
Repeat on other side from * and for 2-4 times each side		
Pigeon	178	4 min each side
Double pigeon	179	3 min each side
Cow face pose	119	3 min each side

GLUTES AND BACK SEQUENCE 2

POSE	PAGE	TIME/REPS
Perform typical warm-up before you begin		
Standing mountain pose	52	1 min
*Standing forward bend	54	1 min
Lower into plank	147	30 sec
Side plank (right)	152	30 sec
Plank	147	30 sec
Side plank (left)	152	30 sec
Plank	147	30 sec
Low push-up to upward dog to downward dog	150, 163, 160	1 min
Step right foot forward into crescent lunge	69	1 min
Warrior 2	84	1 min
Warrior 1	82	1 min
Remain in warrior 1 and twist right	82	30 sec
Lower into plank to low push-up to upward dog to downward dog	147, 150, 163, 160	1 min
Drop knees into hero's pose with toes tucked	115	30 sec
Camel	117	30 sec

POSE	PAGE	TIME/REPS
Downward dog	160	30 sec
Jump forward into squat	147	30 sec
Squat to standing	147	10 times
From standing, interlace fingers behind head and into standing backbend	53	30 sec
Repeat on other side from * and for 2-4 times each side		
Rock and roll	130	30 sec
Reclining cobbler pose with block	145	3 min
Lying spinal twist	126	3 min each side
Happy baby	143	30 sec
Supported fish	185	4 min

GLUTES AND BACK SEQUENCE 3

POSE	PAGE	TIME/REPS
Perform typical warm-up before you begin		
Rock and roll; after last roll, go into standing forward bend	130, 54	1 min
Plank to low push-up to upward dog to downward dog	147, 150, 163, 160	4 times
*Step right foot forward between hands and turn left into half side squat; alternate sides	96	4 times each side
Face front of mat and fold into pyramid with right leg forward	64	1 min
Bring left leg up into standing split	88	1 min
Standing split kicks	89	1 min
Bring left leg down into standing forward bend	54	5 breaths
Bring right thigh over left thigh into eagle	76	1 min
Pulse in eagle	76	30 sec
Bring right leg around into crescent lunge with right knee down, keeping arms in eagle	69, 76	30 sec
Remain in crescent lunge, lifting chest and arms to sky	69	30 sec
Remain in crescent lunge, bring hands to heart center, and twist left	69	30 sec
Remain in crescent lunge, lift knee off floor, and twist left	69	30 sec
Come back to center and lower into plank	147	30 sec
Low push-up to upward dog to downward dog	150, 163, 160	3 times
Hold downward dog	160	1 min
Repeat on other side from * 2-5 times each side		
Squat	79	1 min

(continued)

Glutes and Back Sequence 3 *(continued)*

POSE	PAGE	TIME/REPS
Squat to standing	79	1 min
Lower onto back into rock and roll	130	1 min
Bow pose	165	30 sec; 3 times
Child's pose	176	30 sec
Frog	183	5 min

GLUTES AND BACK SEQUENCE 4

POSE	PAGE	TIME/REPS
Perform typical warm-up before you begin		
Rock and roll	130	30 sec
Plank to low push-up to upward dog to downward dog	147, 150, 163, 160	3 times
*Step right foot forward into warrior 2	84	30 sec
Reverse warrior	85	30 sec
Right angle with left arm up and right arm down	67	30 sec
Circle left arm around face		5 times
Triangle	61	30 sec
Circle left arm while it is in air		5 times
Turn to left into standing straddle, fold over into straddle forward bend, back up quickly	75	1 min
From standing, windmill arms forward and come to front of mat into standing split (left leg up)	88	1 min
Standing split kicks with left leg	89	30 sec
Standing forward bend	54	5 breaths
Chair	58	30 sec
Remain in chair and make backstrokes with both arms	58	5 times
Stand up and into standing backbend with cow face arms	53, 119	5 breaths
Keep arms in cow face, fold into standing forward bend, then release and shake out arms	119, 54	5 breaths
Repeat on other side from * for total of 3 times each side		
**Step right foot forward into crescent lunge	69	5 breaths
Remain in crescent lunge and bring chest and belly to right thigh	69	5 breaths; 3 times
Lunge push-offs forward and back off back foot	71	10 times
Remain in crescent lunge, lower knee to floor, and twist right	69	30 sec
Come back to center and into warrior 3	86	30 sec

POSE	PAGE	TIME/REPS
Crescent lunge to warrior 3	69, 86	3 times
Standing split (left leg up)	88	30 sec
Standing forward bend	54	30 sec
Squat	79	1 min
Repeat on other side from ** 1-2 times each side		
Supported fish	185	5 min

What if I have to teach a mixed class—athletes from different sports in the same class?

Dividing your classes by sport and by position is best, but there are times when this is not possible. I suggest you poll your group about the area most want to work on that day. When in doubt, the best fallback is to work on the hips and back.

LEG AND HIP YOGA SEQUENCES

These challenging sequences constantly test the power of the mind through intense leg-building poses. Hips that are strong yet flexible help protect the knees, and legs that are strong and supple help propel athletes across the field of play. Every athlete can benefit from stronger legs and hips, but these routines are especially good for running sports, jumping plays, and power moves.

LEGS AND HIPS SEQUENCE 1

POSE	PAGE	TIME/REPS
Perform typical warm-up before you begin		
Reclining cobbler's pose	145	2 min
Rock and roll	130	1 min
Standing forward bend	54	1 min
*Bring right leg up into standing split	88	30 sec
Step right foot forward between hands and into half side squat to left	96	2 times each side
Straddle forward bend	75	1 min
Lift halfway up to flat back		30 sec
Fold back down into straddle forward bend	75	1 min
Stand up, turn to front of mat, and windmill arms down into plank	147	1 min
Low push-up to upward dog	150, 163	1 min

(continued)

Legs and Hips Sequence 1 *(continued)*

POSE	PAGE	TIME/REPS
Downward dog	160	1 min
Lower into plank	147	5 breaths
Plank with opposite-arm opposite-leg reach	147, 122	1 min each way
From plank, bend left leg and reach around with right arm, grab hold and switch	147	30 sec each way
Come to downward dog and jump to standing forward bend	160, 54	1 min
Tree (right leg up)	90	1 min
In tree, extend right leg out in front	90	1 min
Tree (left leg up)	90	1 min
In tree, extend left leg out in front	90	1 min
Jump back into plank to low push-up to upward dog to downward dog	147, 150, 163, 160	1 min
Repeat on other side from *		
**Stand up and lower into figure-four chair with right leg crossed over	60	1 min
Remain in figure-four chair and fold chest over	60	1 min
Remain in figure-four chair and lift chest back up	60	1 min
Toe balance	60	30 sec
Repeat on other side from ** 1-4 times		
Pigeon	178	5 min each leg
Squat	79	2 min
Rock and roll	130	1 min
Hip flexor opener	189	3 min
Supported fish	185	5 min

LEGS AND HIPS SEQUENCE 2

POSE	PAGE	TIME/REPS
Perform typical warm-up before you begin		
Downward dog	160	1 min
Squat	79	1 min
Downward dog to squat	160, 79	3 times
*Step right foot forward into crescent lunge with left knee down	69	1 min
Remain in crescent lunge and twist right	69	1 min
Return to center in crescent lunge	69	30 sec
Remain in crescent lunge and place hands on floor inside of right leg into lizard	69, 71	2 min
Keeping left hand on floor, lizard twist to right	71	1 min

POSE	PAGE	TIME/REPS
Sit back into half hero's (right leg extended)	114	1 min
Return to lizard	71	1 min
Half hero's pose with toes tucked		1 min
Press legs and stand up into squat	79	1 min
Lower to table and into plank to low push-up to upward dog	147, 150, 163	1 time
Downward dog	160	1 min
Repeat on other side from * 2-3 times each side		
Half side squat	96	20 sec each side; 2 times
*Lie on back and bring right knee into chest		1 min
Half happy baby (right leg)	190	1 min
Keeping hold of toe, bring right leg straight up to sky		1 min
Keeping hold of toe, bring right leg straight out to right		1 min
Switch hands on toe and bring right leg across		1 min
Bring leg back to center and bring knee into chest		5 breaths
Repeat from * on other side		
Bring both knees into chest		5 breaths
Bring both legs straight up		1 min
Bring both legs out wide into straddle		1 min
Bring legs into reclining cobbler's pose	145	1 min
Happy baby	143	30 sec
Repeat from * 1-3 times		
Cobbler's pose and bring knees up and down	104	2 min
**Bring knees into chest then drop knees to left into lying spinal twist with arms to sides	126	3 min
Bend right elbow and come into face-up shoulder stretch	134	3 min
Come back to center and repeat on other side from **		
Hip flexor opener	189	5 min
Supported fish	185	5 min

LEGS AND HIPS SEQUENCE 3

POSE	PAGE	TIME/REPS
Perform typical warm-up before you begin		
Rock and roll	130	1 min
Plank to side plank	147, 152	30 sec each side; 2 times

(continued)

Legs and Hips Sequence 3 *(continued)*

POSE	PAGE	TIME/REPS
Plank to low push-up to cobra push-up	147, 150, 164	1 min
Downward dog	160	30 sec
Low push-up to upward dog to downward dog	150, 163, 160	30 sec
*Step right foot forward into crescent lunge with left knee down	69	30 sec
Remain in crescent lunge with knee down and twist	71	30 sec
Sit back with control onto left heel into half hero's pose	114	30 sec
Come back up to crescent lunge and into warrior 3	69, 86	30 sec
Go back to crescent lunge and down into half hero's and back up to crescent lunge for total of 3 times		
From crescent lunge, lower to knees into camel leans	118	1 min
Lower butt to heels into seated hero's pose with arms up to sky, then come up	113	10 times
Plank to low push-up and then down onto belly into bow pose	147, 150, 165	30 sec
Upward dog to downward dog	163, 160	30 sec
Repeat on other side from * 2 times		
Standing forward bend to squat	54, 79	30 sec
Plank to side plank	147, 152	30 sec each; 3 times each side
Come to plank and lower onto belly into cobra push-ups	147, 164	1 min
Camel	117	30 sec
Downward dog	160	1 min
**Step right foot forward outside of right hand into lizard	71	1 min
Keep left hand down and twist right into lizard twist	71	1 min
Lower to plank and repeat on other side from *		
Squat	79	1 min
Squat twist	81	30 sec each way
Squat to standing	79	1 min
Lower into reclining hero's	114	5 min
Come to table and into cat and cow	173	1 min
Thread the needle	174	30 sec each side; 2 times
Child's pose	176	1 min
Frog	183	5 min
Supported fish	185	5 min

LEGS AND HIPS SEQUENCE 4

POSE	PAGE	TIME/REPS
Perform typical warm-up before you begin		
Rock and roll	130	10 times
Plank to low push-up to upward dog to downward dog	147, 150, 163, 160	10 breaths
*Step right foot forward into crescent lunge with left knee down	69	30 sec
Remain in crescent lunge and twist right	69	30 sec
Come back to center, bend and straighten left knee		30 sec
Release and come into warrior 3 to crescent lunge	86, 69	4 times
Standing split (right leg up)	88	1 min
Bring left knee behind right knee and lower into seated spinal twist	128	2 min each way
Lower onto back into rock and roll	130	30 sec
Standing forward bend	54	30 sec
Plank to low push-up to upward dog to downward dog	147, 150, 163, 160	30 sec
Repeat on other side from *		
**Step right foot forward into crescent lunge	69	30 sec
Remain in crescent lunge, bring hands to heart center, and twist right	69	30 sec
Return to center and bring chest and belly to right thigh and back up into warrior 3	86	5 times
Standing split (left leg up)	88	30 sec
King dancer	92	30 sec
Release left leg, bring it across right thigh into figure-four chair with hands in prayer	60	1 min
Standing forward bend	54	30 sec
Jump back to plank to low push-up to upward dog to downward dog	147, 150, 163, 160	30 sec
Repeat on other side from ** 2-4 times each side		
Seated forward bend with legs crossed	108	1 min each way
Twisted root abdominals	131	3 min each way
Lying spinal twist	126	3 min each way
Reclining cobbler pose	145	3 min
Heavy legs	140	2 min

LEGS AND HIPS SEQUENCE 5

POSE	PAGE	TIME/REPS
Perform typical warm-up before you begin		
Rock and roll	130	10 times
Standing forward bend	54	30 sec
Lower to plank	147	30 sec
Low push-up to upward dog to downward dog	150, 163, 160	1 time
Standing forward bend	54	30 sec
*Stand up, grab right leg into king dancer	92	30 sec
From king dancer, touch floor with left hand	92	5 times
Release into standing forward bend	54	30 sec
Lower to plank to low push-up to upward dog to downward dog	147, 150, 163, 160	1 time
Standing forward bend	54	30 sec
Stand up, grab left leg into king dancer	92	30 sec
Lower to plank to low push-up to belly into cobra push-ups	147, 150, 164	1 min
Bow pose	165	30 sec
Upward dog to downward dog	163, 160	1 min
Standing forward bend	108	30 sec
Repeat from * for total of 3 times		
**Seated forward bend	108	2 min
Hero's pose	113	3 min
Half hero's with left leg bent	114	1 min
Remain in half hero's and bring right knee to chest while holding shin	114	5 breaths
Remain in half hero's and extend right leg to sky then lower leg	114	1 min
Repeat other side from **		
***Half hero's with left leg bent	114	1 min
One-leg seated forward bend (right leg straight)	109	1 min
Bring right leg into chest and then to sky		5 breaths each
Lower leg and into one-leg seated forward bend	109	10 breaths
Repeat on other side from * for total of 2 times each side**		
Pigeon	178	5 min each side
Cobbler's pose	104	3 min
Diamond pose	146	3 min
Supported fish	185	5 min

TWISTING YOGA SEQUENCES

Twists are great poses for detoxification of the organs while also encouraging rotation of the spine. When the spine can deeply rotate, it can offset some of the blows a player might take in a play. If you can twist deeply, you can absorb some shock and lessen a blow to the shoulder and even the knee. Tennis players and golfers in particular can benefit from these sequences, as well those who need to change direction quickly and efficiently.

TWISTS SEQUENCE 1

POSE	PAGE	TIME/REPS
Perform typical warm-up before you begin		
Rock and roll	130	10 times
Downward dog	160	1 min
*Three-legged dog (right leg up)	94	10 breaths
Step right foot forward outside of right hand and lizard twist right, keeping left hand down	71	1 min
Right angle	67	1 min
Twist right and back into right angle	71, 67	3 times
Bring both hands down and into three-legged dog (right leg up)	94	
Remain in three-legged dog, bend knee and twist to open, then flip the dog	94, 95	30 sec
Flip back by bringing right leg forward between hands and into triangle with left arm up	61	1 min
Revolving triangle	63	1 min
Triangle	61	30 sec
Half moon	68	2 min
Standing forward bend	54	1 min
Repeat on other side from * 2-4 times each side		
Rock and roll	130	10 times
Happy baby	143	30 sec
Face-down shoulder stretch	169	3 min each side
Child's pose	176	1 min
Frog	183	5-10 min

TWISTS SEQUENCE 2

POSE	PAGE	TIME/REPS
Perform typical warm-up before you begin		
Rock and roll	130	10 times
Plank	147	30 sec

(continued)

Twists Sequence 2 *(continued)*

POSE	PAGE	TIME/REPS
Lower to low push-up to upward dog to downward dog	150, 163, 160	5 times
Hold downward dog	160	1 min
*Three-legged dog with right leg up and lower into plank	94, 147	5 breaths
Remain in plank and bring right knee to right elbow	147	5 breaths
Circle right knee		3 times
Three-legged dog, then bend knee and twist to open	94	30 sec
Flip the dog	95	30 sec
Flip back to three-legged dog	94	5 breaths
Circle right knee		3 times
Three-legged dog (right leg up)	94	30 sec
Remain in three-legged dog, then bend knee and twist to open	94	30 sec
Flip the dog	95	30 sec
Flip back to three-legged dog, and then lower into plank, bringing right knee to forehead	94, 147	3 times
Circle right knee		3 times
Three-legged dog (right leg up)	94	30 sec
Remain in three-legged dog, then bend knee and twist to open	94	30 sec
Flip the dog	95	30 sec
Flip back to three-legged dog, then lower into plank	94, 147	5 breaths
Drop heels to right into side plank with left arm to sky	152	30 sec
Remain in side plank, bring left leg up, stomp left foot in front as you lift hips high	152	30 sec
Return to side plank	152	30 sec
Plank to forearm plank	147, 148	30 sec each; 4 times
Forearm side plank (right)	154	5 breaths
Remain in side plank and lower right hip so it kisses floor	152	10 times
Forearm plank	148	30 sec
Child's pose	176	1 min
Downward dog	160	1 min
Repeat on other side from * 2-4 times each side		
Puppy pose	158	2 min
Hip flexor opener	189	5 min
Heavy legs	140	2 min
Straddle heavy legs	141	2 min
Supported fish	185	5 min

TWISTS SEQUENCE 3

POSE	PAGE	TIME/REPS
Perform typical warm-up before you begin		
Rock and roll	130	10 times
Lower to plank to low push-up to upward dog to downward dog	147, 150, 163, 160	5 breaths
*Step right foot forward outside of right hand and lizard twist right, then circle arm around into extended side angle and return to twist	71	1 min each; 4 times
Lower into plank	147	30 sec
Low push-up to upward dog to downward dog	150, 163, 160	1 time
Repeat on other side from * for total of 4 times each side		
**Step right foot forward and turn to left into half side squat	96	30 sec each side; 3 times each side
Pyramid	64	30 sec
Triangle to revolving triangle	61, 63	30 sec each; 4 times
Standing split (left leg up)	88	30 sec
Warrior 3	86	30 sec
Half moon	68	30 sec
Grab left big toe with left hand and extend leg as you stand up		30 sec
Warrior 3	86	30 sec
Half moon	68	30 sec
Standing split (left leg up)	88	30 sec
King dancer	92	30 sec
Warrior 3	86	30 sec
Standing split (left leg up)	88	30 sec
Warrior 3	86	30 sec
Tree (left leg up)	90	1 min
Step out into squat	79	1 min
Squat to standing mountain pose	79, 52	10 times
Standing forward bend	54	1 min
Lower into plank to low push-up to upward dog to downward dog	147, 150, 163, 160	1 time
Repeat on other side from ** 1-2 times each side		
Pigeon	178	5 min
Wheel of life	181	5 min
Face-down shoulder stretch	169	3 min
Repeat on other side from pigeon		

TWISTS SEQUENCE 4

POSE	PAGE	TIME/REPS
Perform typical warm-up before you begin		
Plank	147	5 breaths
Chaturanga (low plank) to upward dog to downward dog	150, 163, 160	5 breaths
Remain in downward dog, bring right arm underneath, grab left ankle, and twist	160	1 min each side
Lower to plank	147	5 breaths
Side plank (right)	152	1 min
Remain in side plank and circle arm around face	152	5 times
Plank to low push-up to upward dog to downward dog	147, 150, 163, 160	5 breaths
Plank to side plank (left)	147, 152	1 min
Remain in side plank and circle arm around face	152	5 times
Plank to low push-up to upward dog to downward dog	147, 150, 163, 160	5 breaths
Drop knees and sit back into hero's pose	113	1 min
Remain in hero's pose and twist	113	1 min each way
From hero's pose, cross and roll over ankles into boat pose	111	30 sec
Remain in boat pose and bring knees in and out	111	1 min
*Lie down with left leg straight and bend right knee into chest		30 sec
Grab outside of right ankle with left hand and straighten leg, then twist		1 min each way
Boat pose	111	30 sec
Open wider in boat	111	30 sec
Lift up into inverted plank	138	30 sec
Repeat on other side from *		
Lower butt to floor and roll over legs into plank to low push-up to upward dog to downward dog	147, 150, 163, 160	5 breaths
Standing forward bend	54	1 min
**Standing split (alternating kicks)	88	2 min
Warrior 3 (right) to standing split	86, 88	3 times
Standing forward bend	54	1 min
Repeat on other side from **		
***Roll up into chair	58	5 breaths
Chair twist (right)	60	30 sec
Chair	58	5 breaths
Chair twist (left)	60	30 sec

POSE	PAGE	TIME/REPS
Repeat from *** 1-4 times		
Seated forward bend	108	3 min
Seated straddle forward bend	109	3 min
Seated straddle side bend	109	2 min each side
Seated forward bend	108	1 min
Cobbler's pose	104	2 min
Supported fish	185	5 min

TWISTS SEQUENCE 5

POSE	PAGE	TIME/REPS
Perform typical warm-up before you begin		
Rock and roll	130	30 sec
*Three-legged dog (left leg up) and pulse up and down on toes of right foot	94	10 times
From three-legged dog, bring left knee forward to nose	94	10 times
From three-legged dog, twist and open, then flip the dog	94, 95	30 sec
Return to three-legged dog, then step left foot forward into warrior 2	94, 84	1 min
Windmill arms around, bringing right hand to floor, come off back heel into lizard twist to left	71	1 min
Repeat warrior 2 to lizard twist to left	84, 71	3 times, 30 sec each
Plank to side plank right with left hand up, and then lift leg	147, 152	1 min
Release and lower into plank	147	30 sec
Side plank (alternate sides)	152	30 sec each side; 4 times
Plank to low push-up to upward dog	147, 150, 163	1 time
Downward dog	160	1 min
Jump to standing forward bend	54	30 sec
Eagle with left leg over right and left arm under	76	1 min
Remain in eagle and lower as much as you can	76	3 breaths
Return to eagle	76	30 sec
Remain in eagle and lower as much as you can	76	3 breaths
Stand up and lower to standing forward bend to plank to low push-up to upward dog	54, 147, 150, 163	1 time
Downward dog	160	1 min
Repeat on other side from * 1-4 times each side		

(continued)

Twists Sequence 5 *(continued)*

POSE	PAGE	TIME/REPS
Rock and roll	130	30 sec
Happy baby	143	30 sec
Lying spinal twist	126	3 min each side
Plow	132	2 min
Shoulder stand	192	2 min
Heavy legs	140	2 min
Supported fish	185	5 min

FULL-BODY YOGA SEQUENCES

Any athlete can use these routines for complete opening, strengthening, and stretching of the entire body. On days when the body feels great and the athlete does not have any tight spots to focus on, then you turn to the full-body routines. While performing these routines, remain focused on the symmetry of the body and on deep breaths.

FULL-BODY SEQUENCE 1

POSE	PAGE	TIME/REPS
Perform typical warm-up before you begin		
Rock and roll	130	1 min
Easy cross-legged twist	103	30 sec each side
Easy cross-legged pose with arm-ups	103	30 sec; 2 times
Remain in easy cross-legged pose and bring arms straight out with flexed wrists	102	30 sec
*Lie on back with block between knees into lying spinal twist	126	1 min
Reclining cobbler pose and bring knees up and down	145	1 min
Rock and roll	130	10 times
Standing forward bend	54	30 sec
Chair and fold forward	58	30 sec each; 5 times
Remain in chair and twist	60	30 sec each; 5 times each side
Lower into plank	147	1 min
Plank push-offs	148	30 sec
Plank with opposite arm and leg reach	147, 122	30 sec
Repeat from * 2 times		
Low push-up to upward dog to downward dog	150, 163, 160	30 sec

POSE	PAGE	TIME/REPS
**Step right foot forward outside of right hand and easy twist right, keeping left hand on floor		30 sec
Reach right arm to front of room		30 sec
Bring right hand to floor inside right foot and open into right angle	67	1 min
Twist chest open into triangle	61	30 sec
Revolving triangle	63	30 sec
Lower to plank to low push-up to upward dog to downward dog	147, 150, 163, 160	1 time
Lower to belly into face-down snow angel	168	30 sec
Bow pose	165	30 sec
Roll to side bow	165, 166	2 times each side
Face-down snow angel	168	30 sec
Child's pose	176	1 min
Downward dog	160	1 min
**Repeat on other side from **		
Lying spinal twist with block	126	1 min each side
Face-down shoulder stretch	169	4 min each side
Wheel of life	181	4 min each side
Frog	183	5 min
Half happy baby	190	2 min each side

FULL-BODY SEQUENCE 2

POSE	PAGE	TIME/REPS
Perform typical warm-up before you begin		
Rock and roll	130	30 sec
Downward dog	160	30 sec
*Step right foot forward into warrior 1	82	1 min
Warrior 2	84	1 min
Reverse warrior	85	1 min
Windmill arms down into plank	147	3 breaths
Low push-up to upward dog to downward dog	150, 163, 160	30 sec
Repeat on other side from * for total of 3 times each side		
From downward dog, jump to squat	79	1 min
Drop back to seated straddle forward bend	109	2 min

(continued)

Full-Body Sequence 2 *(continued)*

POSE	PAGE	TIME/REPS
Bring legs together into rock and roll	130	10 times
Standing forward bend	54	30 sec
Jump back to plank	147	5 breaths
Low push-up to upward dog to downward dog	150, 163, 160	5 breaths
Repeat from * for total of 3 times each side; after last downward dog, lower into plank		
**In plank, bend right knee and pulse foot to sky	147	30 sec
Side plank (left) and bring right knee to right elbow	152	10 times
Plank to low push-up to upward dog to downward dog	147, 150, 163, 160	1 time
Repeat on other side from **		
Jump into squat and squat turn to right	79, 80	1 time
Lower to seated straddle forward bend	109	3 min
Bring legs together and into rock and roll	130	30 sec
Repeat from * for total of 3 times each side		
Plank to low push-up to upward dog to downward dog	147, 150, 163, 160	1 time
Step forward to standing forward bend and into standing split with alternating kicks	54, 88	1 min
Return to standing forward bend to plank to low push-up to upward dog to downward dog	54, 147, 150, 163, 160	1 time
Step forward into squat, grab ankles, and jump	79	10 times
Lower into seated straddle forward bend	109	3 min
Repeat from * for total of 2 times each side		
**Standing split (right leg up)	88	30 sec
Warrior 3 to king dancer (stay or touch floor with left hand)	86, 92	5 times
Repeat on other side from **		
Squat	79	30 sec
Plank to low push-up to upward dog to downward dog	147, 150, 163, 160	1 time
Rock and roll	130	30 sec
Pigeon (right)	178	4 min
Double pigeon	179	2 min
Pigeon (left)	178	4 min
Double pigeon	179	2 min
Face-down shoulder stretch	169	3 min each side
Supported fish	185	5 min

FULL-BODY SEQUENCE 3

POSE	PAGE	TIME/REPS
Perform typical warm-up before you begin		
Rock and roll	130	10 times
Downward dog	160	30 sec
*Step right foot forward on outside of right hand into lizard	71	30 sec each side; 3 times each side
Step right forward on outside of right hand and open into triangle	61	1 min
Revolving triangle	63	1 min
Triangle to revolving triangle	61, 63	30 sec each pose, 3 times
Come up to warrior 3 on right leg	86	30 sec
Bring left leg over right into eagle	76	30 sec
Warrior 3 to eagle	86, 76	3 times
Standing split (left leg up)	88	30 sec
Tuck left leg behind right and into seated spinal twist	128	30 sec
Rock and roll	130	10 times
Jump back to plank to low push-up to upward dog to downward dog	147, 150, 163, 160	1 min
Repeat on other side from * 3-5 times each side		
**Forward into plank, then bring right leg forward into pigeon	147, 178	5 breaths; 2 times each side
Pigeon (right)	178	4 min
Remain in pigeon, interlace fingers behind low back, and raise arms up and down	178	3 times
**Repeat on other side from **		
Hero's pose with toes tucked	115	2 min
Hero's pose	113	4 min
Plow	132	2 min
Shoulder stand	192	2 min
Happy baby	143	1 min
Lying spinal twist	126	3 min each side

FULL-BODY SEQUENCE 4

POSE	PAGE	TIME/REPS
Perform typical warm-up before you begin		
Rock and roll	130	1 min
Happy baby	143	5 breaths
Remain in happy baby and open legs in and out	143	2 min
Bring knees into chest and into rock and roll	130	1 min
***Roll up into standing forward bend	54	1 min
Chair	58	30 sec
Remain in chair and twist right	60	30 sec
Chair	58	30 sec
Remain in chair and twist left	60	30 sec
Remain in chair and breast stroke arms	58	1 min
Remain in chair, interlace fingers behind back, and open chest	58	5 breaths
Remain in chair and fold into standing forward bend, keeping fingers interlaced behind back	58, 54	1 min
Come back up to chair, keeping fingers interlaced behind back	58	1 min
Remain in chair, bring hands to heart center and twist left	60	30 sec
Come back to center in chair and backstroke arms	58	1 min
Interlace fingers opposite way from normal habit and into standing forward bend	54	1 min
Release to standing mountain pose and back down into standing forward bend	52, 54	5 min
Lower into plank with wrist openers	147, 156	30 sec each wrist position; 2 times each
Plank push-offs	148	1 min
Low push-up to upward dog to downward dog	150, 163, 160	5 breaths
*Step right foot forward into warrior 2	84	30 sec
Right angle with left arm up to sky	67	30 sec
Remain in right angle, circle left arm up and around to front of room, and make big circles	67	10 times
In right angle, tuck left arm behind back and open shoulder and chest	67	30 sec
Warrior 2	84	30 sec
Crescent lunge to front of mat	69	30 sec
Crescent lunge twist to right	71	30 sec
Return to warrior 2	84	30 sec
Repeat on other side from * for total of 3 times each side		
**Straighten right leg into triangle	61	30 sec
Remain in triangle and bring left arm behind back	61	30 sec

POSE	PAGE	TIME/REPS
Come up to standing and into reverse triangle	63	30 sec
Remain in reverse triangle and bring right arm up and over as left hand comes up to meet it	63	5 breaths
Triangle	61	30 sec
Repeat from ** 2-3 times each side		
Come up to standing and square feet into standing with feet wide and face left		2 min
Bring legs wider and turn feet out into goddess pose, then twist torso back and forth	72	2 min
Straighten legs and turn to front of room into warrior 1	82	5 breaths
Remain in warrior 1 and bring arms into cow face arms	82, 119	30 sec
Pyramid with cow face arms	64, 119	30 sec
Lift halfway up to flat back and fold back down		3 times
Warrior 3 with cow face arms	86, 119	30 sec
Without touching left leg to floor, come to standing, bring left knee to chest, and then press left leg straight out		30 sec
Bend left knee back to chest and press back into warrior 3	86	30 sec
Come to standing with knee to chest and press back to warrior 3	86	30 sec each pose, 3 times
Squat with cow face arms	79, 119	1 min
Squat to standing	79	10 times
Squat turn	80	1 time each way
Standing forward bend	54	1 min
Repeat on other side from * 1-3 times each side**		
Plow	132	2 min
Shoulder stand	192	2 min
Happy baby	143	1 min
Wall walks	196	1-4 sets of 4
Pigeon	178	3 min each side
Face-down shoulder stretch	169	3 min each side

FULL-BODY SEQUENCE 5

POSE	PAGE	TIME/REPS
Perform typical warm-up before you begin		
Mountain pose to standing forward bend	52, 54	30 sec
Lower into plank	147	30 sec
Low push-up to upward dog to downward dog	150, 163, 160	30 sec
*Step with right foot into warrior 1	82	30 sec
Lower into plank	147	30 sec

(continued)

Full-Body Sequence 5 *(continued)*

POSE	PAGE	TIME/REPS
Low push-up to upward dog to downward dog	150, 163, 160	30 sec
Step with left foot into warrior 1	82	30 sec
Lower into plank	147	30 sec
Low push-up to upward dog to downward dog	150, 163, 160	30 sec
Child's pose	176	1 min
Slither into upward dog and back to child's pose	163, 176	1 min
Downward dog	160	30 sec
Jump to standing forward bend	54	30 sec
Standing backbend	53	30 sec
Standing forward bend	54	30 sec
Jump back to plank to low push-up to upward dog to downward dog	147, 150, 163, 160	30 sec
Step with right foot into warrior 1	82	30 sec
Warrior 2	84	30 sec
Lower to plank to low push-up to upward dog to downward dog	147, 150, 163, 160	30 sec
Step right foot forward into warrior 1	82	30 sec
Warrior 2	84	30 sec
Lower to plank to low push-up to upward dog to downward dog	147, 150, 163, 160	30 sec
Lower to belly into cobra push-ups	164	1 min
Downward dog	160	30 sec
Standing forward bend	54	30 sec
Standing backbend	53	30 sec
Standing forward bend	54	30 sec
Lower to plank to low push-up to upward dog to downward dog	147, 150, 163, 160	30 sec
Repeat on other side from * 2-5 times each side		
Downward dog to upward dog	160, 163	2 min
Come to seated, then into inverted table and move hips up and down	139	2 min
Leg raises in corpse	188	2 min
Roll over legs into plank to low push-up to upward dog to downward dog	147, 150, 163, 160	1 time
Standing forward bend	54	30 sec
Standing backbend	53	30 sec

Full-Body Sequence 5 *(continued)*

POSE	PAGE	TIME/REPS
Standing forward bend	54	30 sec
Lower to plank to low push-up to upward dog to downward dog	147, 150, 163, 160	1 time
Step right foot forward into warrior 1 to warrior 2 to reverse warrior to right angle to warrior 2 to plank to low push-up to upward dog to downward dog	82, 84, 85, 67, 84, 147, 150, 163, 160	One breath each pose, 3-5 times each side
Jump to squat	79	1 min
Squat to standing mountain pose	79, 52	3 min
Standing forward bend	54	1 min
Rock and roll	130	1 min
Pigeon (right)	178	3 min
Double pigeon	179	3 min
Pigeon (left)	178	3 min
Double pigeon	179	3 min
Supported fish	185	5 min

How soon will I notice a difference in performance?

With consistent practice two to four times a week, within three months your athletes with feel more open, stronger, more pliable, and better able to recover on regeneration days. Encourage them to make this commitment for their success.

Restorative Sequences

10

Restorative sessions are your go-to activities for before or after a game to prepare or rejuvenate the body but not overburden it. The poses used in restorative sessions should be meticulous in form and should be held for lengthy periods to allow the body to sink in and open to its greatest extent. Breath is a cornerstone of restoration; ease into each pose with depth of breath. These routines can also begin with the typical warm-up to best prepare the body. Be creative, and be attentive to what your athletes need.

The best poses to hold for a long period of time include the following:

Plow to open the posterior spine, reduce neck strain and injury, and encourage lymph drainage

Supported fish to counteract poor posture, open the thoracic spine, improve breathing, and stretch the chest and shoulders

Forward bend against a wall to open the hamstrings and posterior spine

Pigeon to increase deep hip flexibility, reduce knee strain, and increase power in the lower body

Frog for the inner thigh to also reduce knee strains and increase hip range of motion

Hero's pose toes untucked to stretch ankles, quads, and protect knee health

Hero's pose toes tucked to open the plantar fascia; decrease foot cramping; and stretch the Achilles tendon, calves, and feet for better power to push off and better elusiveness on the field of play

Lying spinal twist to increase spinal rotation and attain better field of vision and spinal health

Face-down shoulder stretch to increase flexibility in the chest and anterior shoulder and therefore to protect the shoulder from overworking

Heavy legs for lymph drainage to lighten the legs and quicken the step

Reclining cobbler's pose to open the groin, relax the back, and protect the knees

What are long, deep holds?

These are the types of holds that characterize yin-style yoga. They are typically performed for 1 to 10 minutes. You should mostly use them on regeneration days and on days when your athletes have a lot of soreness to work through. These holds are good for increasing flexibility.

Your Power Yoga for Sports Warm-Up

Each yoga sequence in this chapter starts with a typical warm-up and takes athletes through the poses needed to help them thrive in their sport and to avoid injury. The typical warm-up is as follows:

POSE	PAGE	TIME
Easy cross-legged twist	103	2 min
Easy cross-legged pose with arm-ups	103	2 min
Seated cat and cow	173	2 min
Opposite-arm opposite-leg	122	2 min
Lying spinal twist (with block between thighs)	126	2 min
Reclining cobbler's pose	145	2 min
Diamond pose	146	2 min
Rock and roll	130	30 sec
Standing forward bend	54	30 sec

What are three of the most restorative poses?

Definitely do heavy legs on the wall for lymph drainage, supported fish for back health and neck safety, and long pigeon pose holds for deep hips and legs.

RESTORATIVE SEQUENCE 1

POSE	PAGE	TIME
Perform typical warm-up before you begin		
Standing forward bend	54	1 min
Squat	79	1 min
Standing forward bend	54	1 min
Downward dog	160	2 min

Pose	Page	Time
Hands and knees		
Wrist turns	148	30 sec each 2 times
Hero's pose with toes tucked	115	2 min
Lying spinal twist	126	4 min each side
Hip flexor opener	189	5 min
Reclining cobbler's pose (feet on block)	145	2 min
Reclining cobbler's pose	145	2 min
Rock and roll	130	1 min
*Pigeon right leg	178	4 min
Wheel of life	181	4 min
Straddle forward bend twist	74	3 min
Seated forward bend	108	3 min
Repeat on other side from *		

RESTORATIVE SEQUENCE 2

POSE	PAGE	TIME
Perform typical warm-up before you begin		
Standing forward bend	54	1 min
Squat	79	1 min
Standing forward bend	54	1 min
Squat	79	1 min
Downward dog	160	2 min
Downward dog, upward dog	160, 163	2 min
Cobra push-up	164	2 min
Face-down snow angels	168	2 min
Puppy pose	158	2 min
Thread the needle	174	2 min each side
*Crescent lunge right	69	2 min
Pigeon	178	3 min
Wheel of life	181	4 min
Repeat on other side from *		
Frog	183	5 min
Lying spinal twist	126	5 min each side

RESTORATIVE SEQUENCE 3

POSE	PAGE	TIME
Perform typical warm-up before you begin		
Rock and roll	130	1 min

(continued)

Restorative Sequence 3 *(continued)*

POSE	PAGE	TIME
Standing forward bend	54	1 min
Squat	79	1 min
Standing forward bend	54	1 min
Squat	79	1 min
Downward dog	160	1 min
Puppy pose	158	1 min
Sphinx	171	2 min
Face-down shoulder stretch	169	4 min each side
Child's pose	176	2 min
Hero's toes tucked	115	2 min
Hero's	113	4 min
Frog	183	5 min

RESTORATIVE SEQUENCE 4

POSE	PAGE	TIME/REPS
Perform typical warm-up before you begin		
Stand up, grab left wrist with right hand for standing crescent	53	1 min each side
Standing forward bend	54	1 min
Downward dog	160	2 min
*Crescent lunge (right knee down)	69	1 min
Press back and lower into low push-up to upward dog to downward dog	150, 163, 160	1 time
Repeat on other side from *		
Standing forward bend	54	1 min
Rock and roll	130	10 times
Standing forward bend	54	1 min
Squat (add twists)	79	2 min
Rock and roll	130	10 times
Reclining cobbler's	145	3 min
Seated forward bend	108	5 min
Reclining cobbler's	145	3 min
Hip flexor opener with two blocks	189	5 min
Lower to one block for heavy legs	140	2 min
Straddle heavy legs	140	2 min
Heavy legs	140	1 min
**Remain on block and bring right knee into chest with left leg long on floor		1 min
Half happy baby (right leg)	190	1 min

POSE	PAGE	TIME/REPS
Repeat on other side from ** for 2 times each side		
Bring legs down with feet flat		
Place one block under very low back for hip flexor opener	189	5 min
Place block between thighs and bring knees to chest (left to right)		2 min
Plow	132	3 min
Happy baby	143	1 min

RESTORATIVE SEQUENCE 5

POSE	PAGE	TIME
Perform typical warm-up before you begin		
Bridge	136	1 min
Wheel of life	181	1 min
Happy baby	143	1 min
Face-up shoulder stretch	134	4 min each side
Place a block between thighs and into lying spinal twist	126	2 min
Pigeon	178	4 min each side
Hero's pose with toes tucked	115	2 min
Hero's pose	113	4 min
Hip flexor opener on blocks	189	5 min
Heavy legs	140	2 min
Heavy legs straddle	140	2 min
Supported fish	185	5 min

What if my athletes cannot hold the long-hold poses for the recommended amount of time?

That is OK, and it is common when starting out. Make sure your athletes are working to their ability and are not just bowing out because it is uncomfortable. Succeeding in sports involves knowing how to get comfortable in an uncomfortable situation. This is a great time to encourage your athletes to work on their mental toughness and focus. If they must leave a pose, it is OK. Athletes will sometimes quit too soon because they are not good at the pose, and it is humbling. Encourage them to stay and feel.

POWER YOGA FOR SPORTS MANIFESTO

Don't look for the exit door

Find comfort in an uncomfortable situation

Pain is temporary

Everything you are is a result of everything you think

Breathe

Check your ego at the door

Don't go to Florida when you only need to go to New Jersey

Talk it out, out loud

Ask why!

There is no *can't, should*, or *try*

I am temporarily unable to comply

You'll achieve it in two weeks

Strength + flexibility = power

Be inspired and humbled every day

Trying is an excuse for future failure

Fearlessness

Change your habit and you automatically become conscious

Visualize change

Look, feel, and realize

Be positive

NOW!

The greatest form of suffering is in attachment

Be less reactive

ABOUT THE AUTHOR

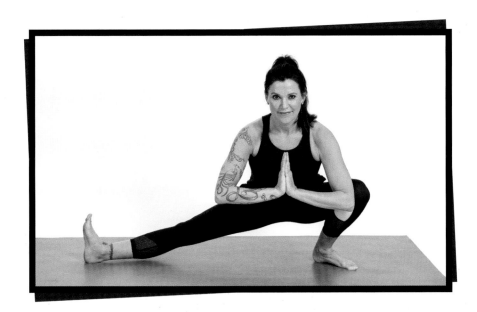

Gwen Lawrence, LMT, has been the team yoga coach for a number of professional sport teams, including the New York Giants, New York Knicks, New York Yankees, NYCFC, New York Redbulls, and New York Rangers. She is also an adjunct professor at Manhattanville College. She has been in the fitness industry for over 20 years and is an entrepreneur, business owner, massage therapist, yoga school owner, curriculum writer, speaker, yoga coach, author, and video producer. She earned her bachelor of science degree in art and dance, and she is a licensed massage therapist, registered yoga teacher, and registered yoga therapist. She is a member of the Yoga Teachers Association and Yoga Alliance.

Lawrence has been influential in gaining acceptance of yoga as an integral part of athlete training in the world of professional sports. She developed the Power Yoga for Sports™ program over a decade ago, and it was named Best Sports Medicine Innovation by *ESPN Magazine*. She created and teaches mindfulness programming (The Way of the Mindful Athlete); clients of the course include the coaches and players from the New York Giants and New York Knicks, New York state teachers, NCAA college athletes, and elite high school athletes. Another project close to her heart is her commitment to working with military veterans and helping them cope with PTSD and ease reentry into civilian life.

Lawrence has presented training workshops in more than 18 countries and 28 states. She is an official spokesperson for Gaia TV, a two-time ambassador for Lululemon, and ambassador for Kulae, Prismsport, and Torq-King. Her writing has appeared in *Men's Health, Women's Health, Fitness Magazine, Shape Magazine, Yoga Journal,* and *Details* magazine, as well as on Shape.com, ESPN.com, and ESPNW.com, where she also serves a monthly contributor. She makes regular appearances on NBC's *Today* show, *The Dr. Oz Show, Good Day New York,* and many TV news and national radio shows, and she is cohost of her own show, *The Better Man Show.*

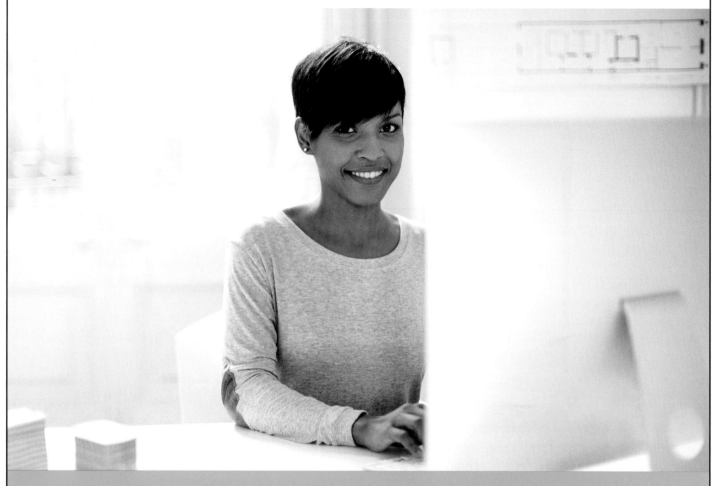
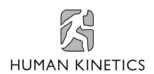